Official Congress Report

Celiac Disease and Other Small Bowel Disorders

Falk Symposium 193

Amsterdam, September 5–6, 2014

Editors
C.J.J. Mulder, Amsterdam
D. Schuppan, Mainz

27 figures and 19 tables, 2015

KARGER

Basel · Freiburg · Paris · London · New York · Chennai · New Delhi · Bangkok · Beijing · Shanghai · Tokyo · Kuala Lumpur · Singapore · Sydney

Reprint of **Digestive Diseases** (ISSN 0257–2753)
Vol. 33, No. 2, 2015

S. Karger
Medical and Scientific Publishers
Basel · Freiburg · Paris · London ·
New York · Chennai · New Delhi ·
Bangkok · Beijing · Shanghai · Tokyo ·
Kuala Lumpur · Singapore · Sydney

P.O. Box, CH–4009 Basel (Switzerland)
Printed on acid-free and non-aging paper (ISO 9706)
ISBN 978–3–318–03014–3

KARGER

E-Mail karger@karger.com
www.karger.com/ddi

Contents

KARGER

E-Mail karger@karger.com
www.karger.com/ddi

Dig Dis 2015;33:113–114
DOI: 10.1159/000371650

Small Bowel: From Sideline to Center Stage in Gastroenterology

The small bowel is not considered a central field in gastroenterology. However, celiac disease is the most frequent small intestinal disease in most populations of the world. It is characterized by intolerance to gluten, which causes damage to the resorptive mucosa, ranging from mild enteropathy, with only an increase in intraepithelial lymphocytes and crypt hyperplasia, to severe lesions, characterized by subtotal to total villous atrophy. Although being recognizable macroscopically by the experienced endoscopist, significant villous atrophy requires histological confirmation. However, other causes of villous atrophy, such as giardiasis, autoimmune enteropathy, combined variable immunodeficiency, some drugs, untreated HIV infection, or tropical sprue should be excluded. Notably, endoscopists cannot recognize an early MARSH 1 or MARSH 2 lesion.

Thus, celiac disease of the proximal small bowel, but also inflammatory diseases of the distal small bowel are key to important differential diagnoses of superficially unrelated (extraintestinal) diseases. Small bowel exploration has been facilitated since the early 2000 thanks to the availability of video capsule endoscopy, double-balloon enteroscopy, confocal endomicroscopy and magnetic resonance contrast imaging. Reports about small bowel diseases on many fronts continue to move so fast that a FALK symposium on this topic seemed mandatory to provide an update and evidence-based authoritative guidelines for an improved clinical practice and translational research. In this issue of *Digestive Diseases*, a community of internationally renowned experts in gastroenterology, celiac disease and small bowel research have summarized and highlighted advances in the understanding of intestinal immunology, the role of gut microbiota, the pathogenesis and treatment of celiac disease and its extraintestinal manifestations, nonceliac gluten sensitivity and important differential diagnoses.

It is only a short while ago that with the advent of the gluten-free diet (Willem Karel Dicke, Utrecht) in the late 1930s, the duodenal/jejunal biopsies in the 1950s and sensitive and specific serological tests in the 1980s and 1990s, it was realized that most cases of idiopathic steatorrhea were in fact celiac disease in adults and that gut symptoms were not always present in patients who were affected by this disorder. Thus, clinicians are now increasingly recognizing that the majority of patients lack the so-called typical picture of celiac disease, i.e. diarrheal illness with frequent bulky stools, anemia and weight loss. Instead, patients often present with atypical extraintestinal symptoms and coexisting autoimmunity like thyroiditis or type 1 diabetes.

KARGER 125

0257–2753/15/0332–0113$39.50/0

E-Mail karger@karger.com
www.karger.com/ddi

Celiac disease has also been recognized as a condition that requires (adjunctive) nondietary, i.e. pharmacological, therapy since it is very difficult to maintain a gluten-free diet in daily life because refined food may contain traces of gluten, and many patients do not reach remission even on a perceived strict gluten-free diet.

Refractory celiac disease, especially type 2, and the advanced stage of intestinal T cell lymphoma remain rare but difficult to treat and often deadly complications of celiac disease. But progress towards a potentially curative therapy including bone marrow transplantation or biologicals is being made.

Nonceliac gluten sensitivity, a diagnosis made after exclusion of celiac disease or wheat allergy, mainly manifests with worsening of extraintestinal diseases and is being recognized as a separate disease entity apparently due to innate immunity to wheat components.

Next to these topics, the clinical translational knowledge in this issue covers the basic small intestinal immunology, the role of the intestinal microbiome, relevant differential diagnoses, such as food allergies, eosinophilic enteritis, nonceliac gluten sensitivity, FODMAP intolerance, drug-induced inflammation like olmesartan enteropathy, Whipple's disease and motility disorders. We focus in this issue also on symptoms related to celiac disease, the epidemiology not only in the West but also in the African, South American and Asian subcontinents, preventive measures, nutrition and comorbidities of celiac disease such as microscopic colitis, extraintestinal autoimmunity, gluten ataxia and other neurological manifestations. Finally, we cover new diagnostic tools in serology, genetics and endoscopy, and we cover imaging techniques such as double balloon, capsule endoscopy and MRI endoscopy.

We hope that the proceedings of the FALK symposium of 4–5 September 2014 on Celiac Disease and Other Small Bowel Disorders will help to expand your knowledge and provide you with the best diagnostic and therapeutic tools currently available to manage small bowel disease in general and celiac disease in particular, and will further stimulate your interest in this growing research and clinical field.

This issue is also intended to enhance awareness amongst hepatogastroenterologists of celiac disease and other small intestinal disorders, which are more common than inflammatory bowel diseases and at least as common as Barrett's esophagus. If their experience does not accord with this, they should do biopsy diagnosis and imaging. We feel that a higher awareness and a lower threshold to suspect and clearly diagnose small bowel disease are extremely important to improve diagnostics compared to what we did in the 1990s and 2000s. We hope that this issue of *Digestive Diseases* will also serve as a handbook for clinicians and researchers dealing with these diseases. The assembly of this issue would not have been possible without the invaluable input of the experts, the unrestrained support of the Falk Foundation and the editing staff of S. Karger AG.

Chris J. Mulder, Amsterdam
Detlef Schuppan, Mainz

Dig Dis 2015;33:115–121
DOI: 10.1159/000369512

Small Bowel, Celiac Disease and Adaptive Immunity

Ludvig M. Sollid[a] Rasmus Iversen[a] Øyvind Steinsbø[a] Shuo-Wang Qiao[a] Elin Bergseng[a] Siri Dørum[a] M. Fleur du Pré[a] Jorunn Stamnaes[a] Asbjørn Christophersen[a] Inês Cardoso[a] Kathrin Hnida[a] Xi Chen[a] Omri Snir[a] Knut E.A. Lundin[a, b]

[a]Centre for Immune Regulation and Department of Immunology, University of Oslo and Oslo University Hospital – Rikshospitalet, and [b]Department of Gastroenterology, Oslo University Hospital – Rikshospitalet, Oslo, Norway

Key Words
Adaptive immunity · B cells · Celiac disease · Gluten · MHC genes · T cells

Abstract
Background: Celiac disease is a multifactorial and polygenic disease with autoimmune features. The disease is caused by an inappropriate immune response to gluten. Elimination of gluten from the diet leads to disease remission, which is the basis for today's treatment of the disease. There is an unmet need for new alternative treatments. ***Key Messages:*** Genetic findings point to adaptive immunity playing a key role in the pathogenesis of celiac disease. MHC is by far the single most important genetic factor in the disease. In addition, a number of non-MHC genes, the majority of which have functions related to T cells and B cells, also contribute to the genetic predisposition, but each of them has modest effect. The primary MHC association is with HLA-DQ2 and HLA-DQ8. These HLA molecules present gluten epitopes to CD4+ T cells which can be considered to be the master regulators of the immune reactions that lead to the disease. The epitopes which the T cells recognize are usually deamidated, and this deamidation is mediated by the enzyme transglutaminase 2 (TG2). Celiac disease patients have disease-specific antibodies. In addition to antibodies to gluten, these include autoantibodies to TG2. Antibodies to deamidated gluten are nearly as specific for celiac disease as the anti-TG2 antibodies. Both types of antibodies appear only to be produced in subjects who are HLA-DQ2 or HLA-DQ8 when they are consuming gluten. ***Conclusion:*** It is hardly coincidental that TG2 is implicated in T-cell epitope formation and at the same time a target for autoantibodies. Understanding this connection is one of the major challenges for obtaining a complete understanding of how gluten causes tissue destruction and remodeling of the mucosa in the small bowel.

The Gut and Its Immune System

The small bowel is essential for digestion and breakdown of food and absorption of nutrients. Only a single layer of epithelium is lining and protecting the gut. Along with nutrients, pathogenic bacteria and viruses are constantly hitting this epithelial surface layer. Bacteria and viruses that do not cause disease and which are in a symbiotic relationship with the host moreover colonize the

KARGER 125
© 2015 S. Karger AG, Basel
0257–2753/15/0332–0115$39.50/0

E-Mail karger@karger.com
www.karger.com/ddi

Ludvig M. Sollid
Centre for Immune Regulation and Department of Immunology
University of Oslo and Oslo University Hospital – Rikshospitalet
NO–0372 Oslo (Norway)
E-Mail l.m.sollid@medisin.uio.no

gut surface. To be well functioning, the body should thus respond to and expel harmful bacteria and viruses, but at the same time not respond to foodstuff or to symbiotic bacteria and viruses. This is a formidable challenge to the immune system, and it is no wonder that the gut immune system is large and intricate.

The immune system can broadly be separated into innate and adaptive immunity. Whereas innate immunity is based on nonspecific and generic recognition, adaptive immunity is based on specific recognition by antigen receptors of B and T lymphocytes. Another hallmark of adaptive immunity is clonal expansion of specific cells, and usually there is also establishment of memory. The same division of innate and adaptive immunity also applies to the immune system of the gut. The involvement of the adaptive immune system in the pathogenesis is more obvious for some gut diseases than others.

Celiac Disease and Involvement of the Adaptive Immune System

Celiac disease is an acquired disorder caused by an inappropriate immune response to cereal gluten proteins of wheat, barley and rye with clear signs of involvement of the adaptive immune system. It is a multifactorial disorder with influence of genes and environment. Gluten is obviously an important environmental factor as the disease goes in remission when gluten is eliminated from the diet. MHC is the single most important genetic factor which may account for as much as half of the genetic risk. The non-MHC genes have been extensively mapped by genome-wide association studies [1, 2], and most recently by the so-called ImmunoChip analysis [3]. Altogether 40 loci (including the MHC locus) have been identified with evidence of 54 independent signal genes. Many of these contain genes coding for molecules thought to be implicated in adaptive immunity, in particular the function of T cells and B cells.

The culprit MHC genes implicated in celiac disease encode for HLA-DQ2.5 (*DQA1**05, *DQB1**02), HLA-DQ8 (*DQA1**03, *DQB1**03:02) and HLA-DQ2.2 (*DQA1**02:01, *DQB1**02:02). One or more of these MHC allotypes are carried by all celiac disease patients. However, many healthy individuals also carry one of these MHC allotypes, so MHC is a necessary but not sufficient factor in celiac disease development. The risks for celiac disease associated with the various MHC allotypes are widely different. DQ2.5 confers the highest risk, whereas DQ2.2 and DQ8 confer much lower risks [4]. HLA-DQ molecules predispose to celiac disease by presenting gluten peptides to CD4 T cells [5]. Celiac disease patients have expansions of CD4 T-cell clones reactive to gluten peptides. Once these clonal expansions have taken place, a strong immune response to gluten will follow after an exposure to gluten, likely explaining why celiac disease patients have a lifelong intolerance to gluten. T cells recognize gluten peptides that are posttranslationally modified [6, 7]. The modification, the conversion of glutamine to glutamate, is called deamidation, and is mediated by the enzyme transglutaminase 2 (TG2). The TG2 enzyme targets in a sequence-specific manner certain glutamine residues [8, 9], and either crosslinks the glutamine with a primary amine which could be a lysine residue of another polypeptide, or converts the glutamine to glutamate by a reaction with water.

In addition to T cells reactive to gluten, celiac disease patients have antibodies reactive to gluten as well as antibodies reactive to TG2 [10]. The anti-gluten antibodies react particularly well with gluten peptides that are deamidated [11]. Both anti-TG2 and anti-gluten antibodies disappear in subjects with celiac disease upon commencement of a gluten-free diet and reappear upon gluten challenge. Serologic examination plays an increasingly important role in the diagnostic workup of celiac disease [12]. The anti-TG2 antibodies and probably also the anti-deamidated gluten antibodies are HLA dependent in the sense that they are only formed in individuals who are HLA-DQ2 or HLA-DQ8 [13].

Immune Responses Initiated by Gluten Exposure: Priming and Effector Sites

Antibodies are produced by plasma cells, which differentiate from B cells after recognition of antigen by surface immunoglobulin which serves as the B-cell receptor (BCR). The intestinal mucosa of celiac disease patients is characterized by massive plasmacytosis. There is an increase in density of jejunal plasma cells producing IgA, IgM and IgG by 2.4, 4.6 and 6.5 times, respectively, when compared to healthy controls [14]. As IgA-producing plasma cells are dominating and IgG-producing plasma cells are few in the intestine, the increase in absolute numbers of plasma cells is by far the biggest for IgA, while there are still few IgG-producing plasma cells in the celiac lesion.

The gluten-reactive CD4 T cells and plasma cells in the lamina propria are effector cells in the immune response (fig. 1). The mucosa can hence be considered an effector

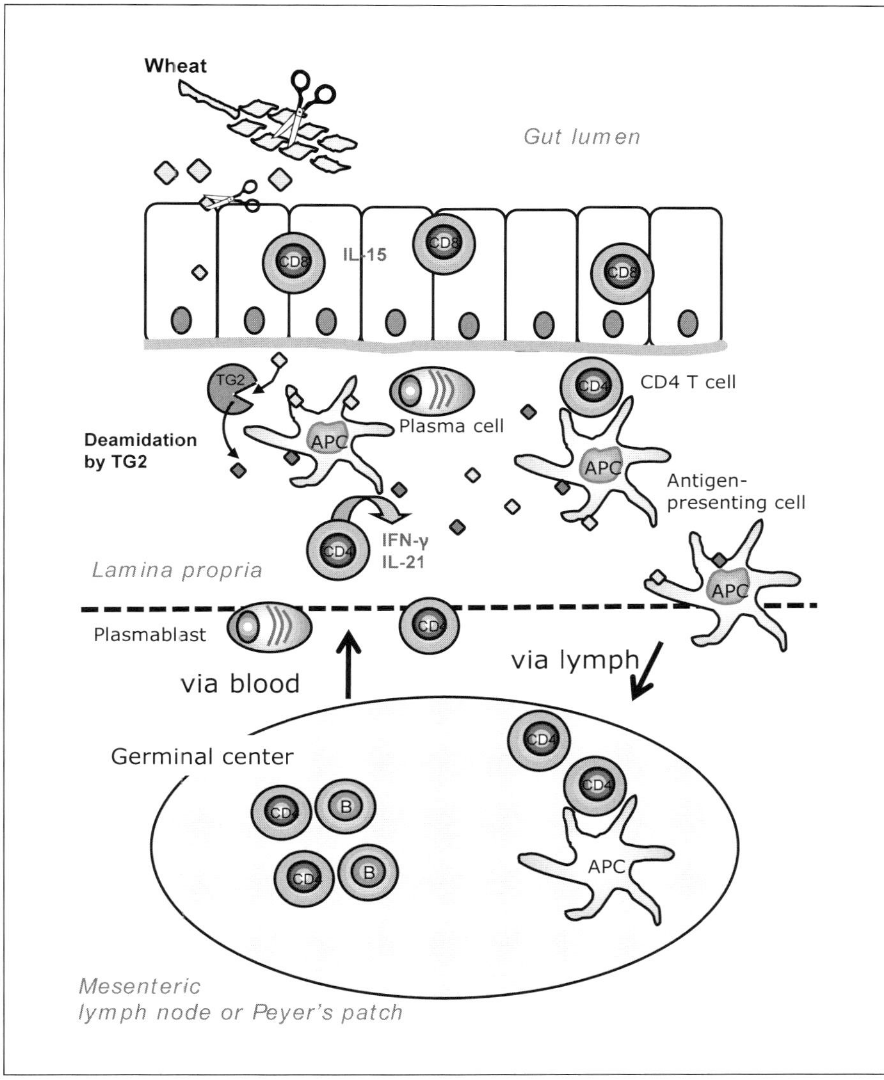

Fig. 1. Important events involving the adaptive immune system in the pathogenesis of celiac disease. Two key players in the disease are CD4+ T cells specific for deamidated gluten peptides and plasma cells specific for TG2 or gluten. The CD4+ T cells recognize gluten peptides in the context of the disease-associated HLA-DQ2.5 or HLA-DQ8 molecules. The immune reaction is initiated in organized lymphoid tissue (mesenteric lymph nodes or Peyer's patches), which serves as a priming site for the immune responses. Primed cells (T cells and plasma blasts) migrate via blood to seed into the lamina propria to become effector cells. The enzyme TG2 is the target of autoantibodies, and it is also responsible for creating deamidated gluten peptides.

Color version available online

site for the anti-gluten immune response. The induction of the immune response, however, likely takes place in organized lymphoid tissue, be that mesenteric lymph nodes or Peyer's patches. In these structures, naïve T cells will be primed to become effector T cells that circulate via blood to seed into the mucosa. Likewise, B cells will be primed to become plasma blasts that circulate via blood and seed into the mucosa to end-differentiate into plasma cells. In this priming of B cells, CD4 T cells are usually instrumental in providing cognate help. This happens either in germinal centers or extrafollicularly. Binding of antigen by the surface immunoglobulin BCR will lead to increased uptake of this antigen into the endosomes for antigenic processing. As a consequence, by mass action, there is high likelihood that MHC class II molecules of the B cell will display peptide fragments for which the BCR is specific. It is currently not known how gluten peptides access these organized lymphoid structures, nor is it known how TG2, which seems to be mainly catalytically inactive in situ [15], is active at these sites.

A particularly interesting question in relation to anti-TG2 antibodies is what dictates the formation of autoantibodies in response to exposure to a foreign antigen. As a first step to analyze this, we have established a panel of recombinant monoclonal antibodies from single TG2-specific plasma cells of the celiac lesion, and compared these with monoclonal antibodies established from gluten-specific plasma cells.

TG2 and Gluten-Specific IgA Antibodies Produced by Plasma Cells of the Celiac Lesion

IgA and IgM plasma cells have surface expression of immunoglobulins. This allows selection of antigen-specific cells by use of labeled antigen. We used biotinylated TG2 multimerized on fluorophore-conjugated streptavidin to stain and flow sort TG2-specific plasma cells [16]. We further found that on average 10% of plasma cells in the celiac lesion are specific for TG2, and that the percentage of anti-TG2-positive cells goes down in patients who are on a gluten-free diet. We PCR amplified and sequenced the VH and VL genes of single plasma cells and inserted them into expression vectors for expression as human IgG1 in HEK cells. We found that there is a restricted repertoire of immunoglobulin heavy and light chains among TG2-specific antibodies with overusage of the heavy-chain gene segments *IGVH5-51*, *IGVH3* and *IGVH4*. Many of the cells also use *IGVK1* light-chain gene segments. The antibodies display limited somatic hypermutation, yet the mutations introduced do affect binding affinity indicative of affinity maturation and that T-cell help is important for the formation of the antibodies. The epitopes recognized by the antibodies are conformational. Competitive ELISA experiments indicate that the antibodies recognize at least four different epitopes which are spatially related [17]. The epitopes correspond broadly to the *IGVH* gene segments used by the antibodies. The localization of the epitopes has been mapped by hydrogen-deuterium exchange, by analysis of interference with TG2 binding to fibronectin and by single amino acid mutation analysis [35]. The so-called epitope 1 used by *IGVH5-51* antibodies involves residues Glu8 and Lys30; epitope 2 used by *IGVH3* antibodies involves Arg19, and epitope 3 used by *IGVH4* antibodies involves Glu94. Epitope 1 and epitope 4 overlap with the fibronectin-binding site of TG2.

In parallel with anti-TG2 antibodies, the celiac disease patients make antibodies to gluten. We established gluten-specific monoclonal antibodies by two distinct approaches [18]. In one approach, VH and VL genes were established from cultures of intestinal biopsy single-cell suspensions which by ELISA were shown to contain antibodies reactive with deamidated complex gluten antigen. In the second approach, VH and VL genes were established from single plasma cells of biopsies sorted by flow cytometry using synthetic gluten peptides known to harbor epitopes recognized by serum antibodies of celiac disease patients. A panel of 38 antibodies was established. Typically, the antibodies bind gluten peptides related to T-cell epitopes and many have higher reactivity to deamidated peptides. There is restricted VH and VL combination and usage among the antibodies, with many antibodies carrying the *IGVH3-23/IGVL4-69* and *IGVH3-15/IGVK4-1* combinations. These gluten-specific antibodies also have limited somatic hypermutations.

Mechanisms for Formation of Anti-TG2 Antibodies

It is striking that TG2 which is essential to create deamidated gluten epitopes recognized by CD4 T cells is also the target of highly celiac disease-specific TG2 autoantibodies. This is unlikely to be coincidental, and suggests a causal link between the two phenomena. T-cell help to TG2-specific B cells by gluten-specific T cells is a model that would explain a causal link [19]. It would also explain why the TG2 antibodies are only formed in HLA-DQ2- or HLA-DQ8-expressing subjects and only when the subjects consume gluten. Gluten peptides are good substrates for TG2. When incubating gluten peptides with TG2, covalent complexes of gluten and TG2 are formed. Such complexes can be bound by TG2-specific B cells, which upon internalization and processing can present gluten epitopes in the context of HLA-DQ2 or HLA-DQ8 to T cells. The T cells recognize deamidated peptides, and one can envisage three ways deamidated peptides are generated from such complexes. These are: (a) The covalent bond is the thioester bond between TG2-active site cysteine and peptide glutamine in the enzyme substrate intermediate. Upon reaction of the enzyme substrate intermediate with water, the deamidated peptide is formed. (b) The covalent bond is the isopeptide bond between a lysine residue of TG2 and a glutamine residue of the peptide. Isopeptidase activity of TG2 could regenerate the enzyme substrate intermediate, which again could react with water for formation of a deamidated peptide. (c) The peptide could at least contain two glutamine residues targeted by TG2, one could be deamidated and one could be isopeptide bonded to TG2. Upon internalization in B cells, endoproteases in endosomes would cleave the peptide and release the deamidated epitope. If TG2-specific B cells would be able to present gluten peptides to T cells, the B cells would get their help, but at the same time the T cells would become activated, clonally expand and likely generate memory T cells. Interaction between TG2-specific B cells and gluten-specific T cells could thus be an important amplification loop for the anti-gluten T-cell response.

Mechanisms for Formation of Anti-Gluten Antibodies

B cells specific for gluten antigen could receive cognate help from gluten-specific T cells. The observation that anti-gluten antibodies bind peptides related to T-cell epitopes speaks in favor of this mechanism. B cells which bind and internalize deamidated gluten epitopes would load HLA-DQ2 or HLA-DQ8 molecules with deamidated epitopes and would hence be particularly well suited to receive help from T cells recognizing deamidated gluten antigen. This may explain why anti-deamidated gliadin antibodies and anti-TG2 antibodies both are excellent markers of disease with high clinical diagnostic performance as they both reflect the action of gluten-specific T cells recognizing deamidated peptides.

Selection of T-Cell Epitopes

Which parts of gluten proteins are recognized by T cells is the result of several processes. T-cell epitopes are localized to proline-rich regions of gluten proteins [20]. This is so partly because proline-rich sequences are resistant to proteolytic degradation by digestive enzymes [21]. It is also reflecting that proline is part of the recognition sequence of TG2. Typically, TG2 is targeting glutamine residues in the sequence QXP where Q is glutamine, X is any amino acid and P is proline [8, 9]. The central role of TG2 in selection of T-cell epitopes is signified by the finding that among the peptides being targeted by TG2 in a very complex gluten digest mixture, peptides harboring T-cell epitopes were heavily overrepresented [22]. Finally, binding of peptides to MHC is a selective force. The importance of this is reflected by the observation that T cells of celiac patients which recognize gluten peptides in the context of the disease predisposing HLA molecules DQ2.5, DQ2.2 and DQ8 by and large recognize different cohorts of gluten peptides.

T-Cell Epitopes Presented by DQ2.5, DQ2.2 and DQ8

Gluten peptides recognized by T cells in the context of DQ2.5 have deamidations at positions P4, P6 and occasionally P7, whereas gluten peptides recognized in the context of DQ8 have deamidations at position P1 or P4 [23]. This different distribution of glutamate residues reflects the different peptide-binding motifs of DQ2.5 and DQ8. Early experiments using DQ2.2-expressing cells for presentation of DQ2.5-restricted T-cell epitopes revealed presentation of most epitopes [24, 25]. These observations were in apparent contrast to the huge difference in risk to celiac disease conferred by the two HLA-DQ2 variants. Later, it was found that incubating the antigen-presenting cells after pulsing with the antigen epitopes before the addition of T cells to the culture revealed striking differences between DQ2.5 and DQ2.2 antigen-presenting cells [26]. The gluten epitopes were only being effectively presented by DQ2.5-expressing cells speaking to stable binding of gluten epitopes as prerequisite for establishing the in vivo T-cell response. This led to the prediction that DQ2.2 would present other gluten epitopes which bind stably to DQ2.2. Recent research has revealed that this indeed is the case [26]. Using HLA molecules as affinity matrix for isolation of DQ2.2-binding peptides of gluten digests, three DQ2.2 epitopes were identified [27], one of which was previously characterized as an immunodominant epitope [28]. Characteristically, these epitopes all have serine at position P3. This suggests that Ser at P3 is a unique characteristic of DQ2.2-restricted epitopes. Moreover, peptide binding experiments indicated that Ser and Thr are anchor residues for binding of peptides to DQ2.2 but not to DQ2.5 [28, 29]. This notion was further established by elution of endogenous peptides from B-lymphoblastoid cell lines [36]. This analysis revealed big differences in the repertoires of peptides eluted from DQ2.2 compared to DQ2.5, with a minority of peptides being presented by both HLA-DQ molecules. Characterization of the binding motifs by neural network analysis of the eluted peptides revealed a preference of serine, threonine and aspartate at P3 by DQ2.2, which was not found for DQ2.5. Thus, DQ2.5 and DQ2.2 appear to have similar peptide-binding motifs, with DQ2.2 having an additional anchor requirement at P3. Gluten peptides that shall bind stably to DQ2.2 will need to fulfill this extra requirement. Hence, fewer peptides in the gluten proteome will be able to bind stably to DQ2.2 than DQ2.5, and this likely explains the differential celiac disease risks of the two HLA-DQ2 variants.

Conserved Usage of Celiac Disease-Relevant BCRs and T-Cell Receptors

T-cell receptors (TCRs) and BCRs have enormous diversity due to receptor rearrangement with recombination of variable (V), diversity (D) and joining (J) gene segments during T-cell and B-cell development. Despite this diversity, similar and clonally dominant BCRs and TCRs are observed across celiac disease patients. This is the case for anti-TG2 antibodies predominantly using the *IGVH5-51*, *IGVH3* or *IGVH4* heavy-chain gene segments together with *IGVK1* light-chain gene segment [16]. It is the case for anti-gluten antibodies with many antibodies using the *IGVH3-23/IGVL4-69* and *IGVH3-15/IGVK4-1* combinations [18]. It is also the case for TCRs recognizing certain peptide-MHC complexes. It is particularly prominent for TCRs recognizing the DQ2.5-glia-α2 epitope with overusage and preferred pairing of the *TRAV26-1* and *TRBV7-2* gene segments [30–33]. In addition to the overusage of the *TRAV26-1/TRBV7-2* gene segments, these TCRs have a conserved arginine residue in their complementarity-determining region (CDR) 3β loop [30]. Recently resolved crystal structures of peptide-MHC-TCR complexes revealed this CDR3β arginine in the TCR serves as a lynchpin in the recognition of the DQ2.5-glia-α2 epitope, yet the arginine is not making any direct contact with the glutamate at the P4 in the epitope [33]. Similar preferred usage and pairing seem to be the case for TCRs recognizing the DQ8-glia-α1 epitope with overusage of the *TRAV26-2* and *TRBV9* gene segments [34] as well as for TCRs recognizing DQ2.5-glia-α1 with overusage of *TRBV20-1*, *TRBV29-1* and *TRAV4* gene segments [33]. Whether similar types of biased usage and chain pairing occur in TCRs recognizing other gluten T-cell epitopes remains to be established.

Further work should shed light on why there is this conserved antigen receptor usage among presumably disease-relevant BCRs and TCRs in celiac disease. It is possible that the basis lies in a competition for which antigen receptors are best at recognizing certain structures, and that this selection follows the same rules in different subjects. Another interesting avenue to pursue in future studies is whether the conserved receptor usage that seems to be a hallmark of the disease can be harnessed in DNA-based diagnostic approaches.

Conclusions

The adaptive immune system appears to be central in the pathogenesis of celiac disease. Current understanding advocates that gluten-specific CD4 T cells orchestrate an immune response to gluten which also involves an antibody response to the self-antigen TG2. Interactions between gluten-reactive CD4 cells and B cells appear to be key steps in the pathogenesis giving rise to antibodies to gluten (including deamidated gluten fragments) and to TG2. These antibodies serve as excellent surrogate markers for celiac disease. The interaction between T cells and B cells not only gives rise to antibodies, but also amplifies the anti-gluten T-cell response. Interference with the distinct steps in the immune reactions that lead to gluten hypersensitivity could control celiac disease and would represent strategies for novel therapies of this prevalent disorder.

Acknowledgements

The work in the authors' laboratory is supported by grants from the Research Council of Norway (partially through its Centres of Excellence funding scheme, grant No. 179573/V40), the European Commission (grant Nos. ERC-2010-Ad-268541, FP7-People-2011-ITN-289964), the University of Oslo, the South-East Norway Regional Health Authority as well as by a Research Prize of the United European Gastroenterology.

Disclosure Statement

The authors declare no conflicts of interest.

References

1 Hunt KA, Zhernakova A, Turner G, Heap GA, et al: Newly identified genetic risk variants for celiac disease related to the immune response. Nat Genet 2008;40:395–402.

2 Dubois PC, Trynka G, Franke L, Hunt KA, et al: Multiple common variants for celiac disease influencing immune gene expression. Nat Genet 2010;42:295–302.

3 Trynka G, Hunt KA, Bockett NA, Romanos J, et al: Dense genotyping identifies and localizes multiple common and rare variant association signals in celiac disease. Nat Genet 2011;43:1193–1201.

4 Sollid LM, Lie BA: Celiac disease genetics: current concepts and practical applications. Clin Gastroenterol Hepatol 2005;3:843–851.

5 Lundin KEA, Scott H, Hansen T, Paulsen G, Halstensen TS, Fausa O, Thorsby E, Sollid LM: Gliadin-specific, HLA-DQ(α1*0501, β1*0201) restricted T cells isolated from the small intestinal mucosa of celiac disease patients. J Exp Med 1993;178:187–196.

6 Molberg O, McAdam SN, Körner R, Quarsten H, Kristiansen C, Madsen L, Fugger L, Scott H, Roepstorff P, Lundin KEA, Sjöström H, Sollid LM: Tissue transglutaminase selectively modifies gliadin peptides that are recognized by gut-derived T cells. Nat Med 1998;4:713–717.

7 van de Wal Y, Kooy Y, van Veelen P, Pena S, Mearin L, Papadopoulos G, Koning F: Selective deamidation by tissue transglutaminase strongly enhances gliadin-specific T cell reactivity. J Immunol 1998;161:1585–1588.

8 Vader LW, de Ru A, van Der WY, Kooy YM, Benckhuijsen W, Mearin ML, Drijfhout JW, van Veelen P, Koning F: Specificity of tissue transglutaminase explains cereal toxicity in celiac disease. J Exp Med 2002;195:643–649.

9 Fleckenstein B, Molberg, Qiao SW, Schmid DG, Von Der MF, Elgstoen K, Jung G, Sollid LM: Gliadin T cell epitope selection by tissue transglutaminase in celiac disease. Role of enzyme specificity and pH influence on the transamidation versus deamidation process. J Biol Chem 2002;277:34109–34116.

10 Dieterich W, Ehnis T, Bauer M, Donner P, Volta U, Riecken EO, Schuppan D: Identification of tissue transglutaminase as the autoantigen of celiac disease. Nat Med 1997;3:797–801.

11 Osman AA, Gunnel T, Dietl A, Uhlig HH, Amin M, Fleckenstein B, Richter T, Mothes T: B cell epitopes of gliadin. Clin Exp Immunol 2000;121:248–254.

12 Husby S, Koletzko S, Korponay-Szabo IR, Mearin ML, Phillips A, Shamir R, Troncone R, Giersiepen K, Branski D, Catassi C, Lelgeman M, Maki M, Ribes-Koninckx C, Ventura A, Zimmer KP; ESPGHAN Working Group on Coeliac Disease Diagnosis; ESPGHAN Gastroenterology Committee; European Society for Pediatric Gastroenterology, Hepatology, and Nutrition: European Society for Pediatric Gastroenterology, Hepatology, and Nutrition guidelines for the diagnosis of coeliac disease. J Pediatr Gastroenterol Nutr 2012;54:136–160.

13 Bjorck S, Brundin C, Lorinc E, Lynch KF, Agardh D: Screening detects a high proportion of celiac disease in young HLA-genotyped children. J Pediatr Gastroenterol Nutr 2010;50:49–53.

14 Baklien K, Brandtzaeg P, Fausa O: Immunoglobulins in jejunal mucosa and serum from patients with adult coeliac disease. Scand J Gastroenterol 1977;12:149–159.

15 Siegel M, Strnad P, Watts RE, Choi K, Jabri B, Omary MB, Khosla C: Extracellular transglutaminase 2 is catalytically inactive, but is transiently activated upon tissue injury. PLoS One 2008;3:e1861.

16 Di Niro R, Mesin L, Zheng NY, Stamnaes J, Morrissey M, Lee JH, Huang M, Iversen R, du Pre MF, Qiao SW, Lundin KE, Wilson PC, Sollid LM: High abundance of plasma cells secreting transglutaminase 2-specific IgA autoantibodies with limited somatic hypermutation in celiac disease intestinal lesions. Nat Med 2012;18:441–445.

17 Iversen R, Di Niro R, Stamnaes J, Lundin KE, Wilson PC, Sollid LM: Transglutaminase 2-specific autoantibodies in celiac disease target clustered, N-terminal epitopes not displayed on the surface of cells. J Immunol 2013;190:5981–5991.

18 Steinsbo O, Henry Dunand CJ, Huang M, Mesin L, Salgado-Ferrer M, Lundin KE, Jahnsen J, Wilson PC, Sollid LM: Restricted VH/VL usage and limited mutations in gluten-specific IgA of coeliac disease lesion plasma cells. Nat Commun 2014;5:4041.

19 Sollid LM, Molberg, McAdam S, Lundin KE: Autoantibodies in coeliac disease: tissue transglutaminase – guilt by association? Gut 1997;41:851–852.

20 Arentz-Hansen H, McAdam SN, Molberg, Fleckenstein B, Lundin KE, Jorgensen TJ, Jung G, Roepstorff P, Sollid LM: Celiac lesion T cells recognize epitopes that cluster in regions of gliadins rich in proline residues. Gastroenterology 2002;123:803–809.

21 Shan L, Molberg, Parrot I, Hausch F, Filiz F, Gray GM, Sollid LM, Khosla C: Structural basis for gluten intolerance in celiac sprue. Science 2002;297:2275–2279.

22 Dørum S, Arntzen MO, Qiao SW, Holm A, Koehler CJ, Thiede B, Sollid LM, Fleckenstein B: The preferred substrates for transglutaminase 2 in a complex wheat gluten digest are peptide fragments harboring celiac disease T-cell epitopes. PLoS One 2010;5:e14056.

23 Tollefsen S, Arentz-Hansen H, Fleckenstein B, Molberg, Raki M, Kwok WW, Jung G, Lundin KE, Sollid LM: HLA-DQ2 and -DQ8 signatures of gluten T cell epitopes in celiac disease. J Clin Invest 2006;116:2226–2236.

24 Qiao SW, Bergseng E, Molberg O, Jung G, Fleckenstein B, Sollid LM: Refining the rules of gliadin T cell epitope binding to the disease-associated DQ2 molecule in celiac disease: importance of proline spacing and glutamine deamidation. J Immunol 2005;175: 254–261.

25 Vader W, Kooy Y, van Veelen P, de Ru A, Harris D, Benckhuijsen W, Pena S, Mearin L, Drijfhout JW, Koning F: The gluten response in children with celiac disease is directed toward multiple gliadin and glutenin peptides. Gastroenterology 2002;122:1729–1737.

26 Fallang LE, Bergseng E, Hotta K, Berg-Larsen A, Kim CY, Sollid LM: Differences in the risk of celiac disease associated with HLA-DQ2.5 or HLA-DQ2.2 are related to sustained gluten antigen presentation. Nat Immunol 2009;10: 1096–1101.

27 Dørum S, Bodd M, Fallang LE, Bergseng E, Christophersen A, Johannesen MK, Qiao SW, Stamnaes J, de Souza GA, Sollid LM: HLA-DQ molecules as affinity matrix for identification of gluten T-cell epitopes. J Immunol 2014;193:4497–4506.

28 Bodd M, Kim CY, Lundin KE, Sollid LM: T-cell response to gluten in patients with HLA-DQ2.2 reveals requirement of peptide-MHC stability in celiac disease. Gastroenterology 2012;142:552–561.

29 van de Wal Y, Kooy YC, Drijfhout JW, Amons R, Papadopoulos GK, Koning F: Unique peptide binding characteristics of the disease-associated DQ(α1*0501, β1*0201) vs the non-disease-associated DQ(α1*0201, β1*0202) molecule. Immunogenetics 1997;46:484–492.

30 Qiao SW, Raki M, Gunnarsen KS, Loset GA, Lundin KE, Sandlie I, Sollid LM: Posttranslational modification of gluten shapes TCR usage in celiac disease. J Immunol 2011;187: 3064–3071.

31 Qiao SW, Christophersen A, Lundin KE, Sollid LM: Biased usage and preferred pairing of α- and β-chains of TCRs specific for an immunodominant gluten epitope in coeliac disease. Int Immunol 2014;26:13–19.

32 Han A, Newell EW, Glanville J, Fernandez-Becker N, Khosla C, Chien YH, Davis MM: Dietary gluten triggers concomitant activation of CD4+ and CD8+ αβ T cells and γδ T cells in celiac disease. Proc Natl Acad Sci USA 2013;110:13073–13078.

33 Petersen J, Montserrat V, Mujico JR, Loh KL, Beringer DX, van Lummel M, Thompson A, Mearin ML, Schweizer J, Kooy-Winkelaar Y, van Bergen J, Drijfhout JW, Kan WT, La Gruta NL, Anderson RP, Reid HH, Koning F, Rossjohn J: T-cell receptor recognition of HLA-DQ2-gliadin complexes associated with celiac disease. Nat Struct Mol Biol 2014;21: 480–488.

34 Broughton SE, Petersen J, Theodossis A, Scally SW, Loh KL, Thompson A, van Bergen J, Kooy-Winkelaar Y, Henderson KN, Beddoe T, Tye-Din JA, Mannering SI, Purcell AW, McCluskey J, Anderson RP, Koning F, Reid HH, Rossjohn J: Biased T cell receptor usage directed against human leukocyte antigen DQ8-restricted gliadin peptides is associated with celiac disease. Immunity 2012;37:611–621.

35 Iversen R, Mysling S, Hnida K, Jørgensen TJ, Sollid LM: Activity-regulating structural changes and autoantibody epitopes in transglutaminase 2 assessed by hydrogen/deuterium exchange. Proc Natl Acad Sci USA 2014;111:17146–17151.

36 Bergseng E, Dørum S, Arntzen MØ, Nielsen M, Nygård S, Buus S, de Souza GA, Sollid LM: Different binding motifs of the celiac disease-associated HLA molecules DQ2.5, DQ2.2, and DQ7.5 revealed by relative quantitative proteomics of endogenous peptide repertoires. Immunogenetics 2015;67:73–84.

Dig Dis 2015;33:122–130
DOI: 10.1159/000369521

Interleukin-15, a Master Piece in the Immunological Jigsaw of Celiac Disease

Bertrand Meresse[a, b] Natalia Korneychuk[a, b] Georgia Malamut[a–c]
Nadine Cerf-Bensussan[a, b]

[a]INSERM UMR1163, Laboratory of Intestinal Immunity, [b]Université Paris Descartes-Sorbonne Paris-Cité and Institut Imagine, and [c]Gastroenterology Department, Hôpital Georges-Pompidou, APHP, Paris, France

Key Words
Interleukin-15 · Celiac disease · Refractory celiac disease · Intraepithelial lymphocytes

Abstract
Background: The immune response causing celiac disease (CD) depends on the activation of intestinal CD4+ T cells by gluten-derived peptides presented by HLA-DQ2 or HLA-DQ8 molecules, the main genetic risk factor. However, additional factors are necessary to impair immune tolerance to dietary gluten, to stimulate intraepithelial lymphocytes (IEL) and to induce intestinal damage. ***Key Messages:*** Current data point to a central role of interleukin-15 (IL-15). In situ and ex vivo studies indicate that IL-15 stimulates the accumulation and cytotoxic activation of CD8+ T IEL in active CD, and that of the malignant innate-like IEL in type II refractory CD (RCDII). Other studies show that IL-15 impairs the immunoregulatory control of effector T cells, notably CD8+. Recently, animal models have been designed to investigate the respective role of CD4+ T cells and IL-15 in CD. We discuss more particularly our results in such a model, which shows that IL-15 produced in excess in the intestine can cooperate with CD4+ T cells specific for a dietary antigen to trigger a celiac-like enteropathy. In this mouse model, CD4+ T cells activated by dietary ovalbumin secreted IL-2 which, along with IL-15, stimulated the expansion of noncognate intestinal cytotoxic CD8+ T cells containing large amounts of granzyme B. In the presence of IL-15, the latter cells did not respond to regulatory T cells, and accumulated in the intestine close to epithelial damage. ***Conclusion:*** On the basis of these data, we propose that, in CD, gluten-specific CD4+ T cells synthesize cytokines that synergize with IL-15 to license the expansion and activation of cytotoxic IEL, which drive tissue damage. We suggest that IL-15 is a meaningful therapeutic target, notably in patients with RCDII in which malignant IEL can respond to IL-15 independently of signals provided by CD4+ T cells.

Introduction

Celiac disease (CD) is a complex disease generally defined as an autoimmune-like enteropathy triggered by dietary gluten in genetically predisposed individuals. Typical epithelial lesions of villous flattening and crypt hyperplasia predominate in the proximal part of the small intestine in which gluten peptides incompletely digested by luminal and brush border enzymes can stimulate the

KARGER 125
E-Mail karger@karger.com
www.karger.com/ddi

0257–2753/15/0332–0122$39.50/0

Nadine Cerf-Bensussan
INSERM UMR1163, Laboratory of Intestinal Immunity
Institut Imagine
24, boulevard du Montparnasse, FR–75015 Paris (France)
E-Mail nadine.cerf-bensussan@inserm.fr

chronic activation of CD4+ T and IgA plasma cells and the expansion of intraepithelial CD8+ granzyme B+ lymphocytes [reviewed in 1, 2]. Since the discovery in the 1990s that the MHC class II haplotypes encoding HLA-DQ2.5 and HLA-DQ8 represent the main genetic risk factor for CD, a considerable amount of work has demonstrated how these two molecules expressed at the surface of antigen-presenting cells can orchestrate the activation of an adaptive immune response against gluten [1, 2]. Yet, it is increasingly clear that the recognition of dietary gluten by CD4+ T cells generally leads to local and systemic tolerance, and additional events are necessary to disrupt tolerance, to drive the activation of intraepithelial lymphocytes (IEL) and to induce tissue damage. Herein, we discuss how interleukin-15 (IL-15), a cytokine upregulated in the intestine of CD patients, can impair local immunoregulation and, in concert with gluten-specific CD4+ T cells, drive the activation of cytotoxic intestinal T cells, the onset of epithelial lesions and promote the onset of IEL-derived lymphomas, a rare but most severe complication of CD.

The HLA-DQ-Restricted Anti-Gluten Adaptive Immune Response Is Necessary but Not Sufficient to Develop CD

The molecular mechanisms by which HLA-DQ2.5 or HLA-DQ8 molecules orchestrate an adaptive immune response against gluten are now well established [reviewed in 1, 2]. Briefly, gluten peptides incompletely digested in the intestinal lumen can enter into the intestinal mucosa, where they can be deamidated by tissue transglutaminase TG2, an ubiquitous enzyme, which is also the target of CD-specific IgA autoantibodies. Gluten peptides modified by TG2 bind with high avidity to HLA-DQ2.5 or HLA-DQ8 molecules at the surface of antigen-presenting cells and activate naive CD4+ T cells in organized intestinal lymphoid tissue. Gluten-specific CD4+ T cells can then migrate into intestinal lamina propria and become tissue-resident memory T CD4+ cells and secrete large amounts of cytokines upon reencounter with gluten. In active CD, gluten-activated intestinal CD4+ T cells can produce conspicuous amounts of IFNγ and IL-21, two cytokines absent or very weakly expressed in the normal duodenal mucosa [reviewed in 2, 3]. Gluten-specific CD4+ T cells can also provide help to intestinal B cells, which differentiate into plasma cells producing IgA against gluten peptides and TG2 [4–6]. Paradoxically, in active CD, anti-gluten IgA are secreted in very large amounts in the intestinal lumen but fail to play their protective barrier function. Due to their interactions with the CD71 receptor abnormally expressed at the apical enterocyte surface, anti-gluten SIgA rather behave as a Trojan horse and facilitate transcellular permeability to gluten [7–9].

The HLA-DQ-restricted adaptive anti-gluten response is indispensable to develop CD. Yet, large evidence indicates that it is not sufficient. Only a small fraction of individuals carrying the HLA-DQ2.5 or HLA-DQ8 haplotypes develop CD even if the risk is increased in individuals homozygous for HLA-DQ2.5 [10]. Moreover, no celiac-like enteropathy could be induced in humanized mice in which endogenous MHC class II molecules have been replaced by HLA-DQ8 or -DQ2.5, even if mice were also engineered to express a human CD4 (hCD4) molecule to facilitate T-cell interaction with HLA-DQ8 [11] or a T-cell receptor specific for a gluten peptide in the context of HLA-DQ2.5 [12, 13]. One important pitfall was however the difficulty to activate the deamidation activity of TG2 in vivo in mice. This was notably the case in hDQ2 mice, which exclusively responded to deamidated gliadin [12, 13]. Interestingly, a gluten-sensitive blistering skin disease reminiscent of dermatitis herpetiformis was observed in hCD4-DQ8 mice backcrossed on the autoimmune NOD background after intraperitoneal immunization and 2–5 months of gluten-containing diet [14]. Yet, again, there was no evidence of enteropathy [14]. A mild enteropathy associated with increased epithelial conductance and a modest increase in IEL was however observed when NOD/hCD4-DQ8 mice were fed with gluten and cholera toxin, a strong mucosal adjuvant that impairs the intestinal barrier [15]. Overall, these data are in keeping with observations in adult wild-type mice, which respond to dietary gluten but develop active tolerance [16]. It suggests that the anti-gliadin CD4+ T cell response elicited by dietary gluten generally leads to active immune tolerance even when facilitated by HLA-DQ presentation and that additional mechanisms are necessary to break tolerance and trigger tissue damage. Work led by our group and others suggests the role of the cytokine IL-15.

IL-15 Is an Interesting Candidate in the Pathogenesis of CD

IL-15 is a member of the γc family of cytokines, which also includes IL-2, IL-4, IL-9 and IL-21. γc cytokines share a 4-α helix-bundled structure and are defined by their use of a receptor containing the common γc chain

(CD132) [17]. IL-15 and IL-2 receptors also share a β-chain (CD122), which combines with γc to form a common signaling module. This receptor can autonomously bind IL-2, albeit with a weak avidity and IL-15 with an intermediate avidity. As a consequence, the two cytokines display largely overlapping in vitro functions and both stimulate CD8+ T and NK cell survival, proliferation and cytotoxicity [18–20]. Their in vivo functions are however strikingly distinct, likely because the two cytokines differ markedly by their cellular source, by the distribution and functions of the private α-chains of their receptors and by their regulation [19–21]. IL-2 is mostly secreted by activated T cells, and the private IL-2Rα chain (CD25) of its receptor is restricted to activated T cells and to the subset of FOXP3 regulatory T cells (Tregs) [19, 21]. Inactivation of IL-2 or CD25 in mice and loss-of-function mutations of CD25 in humans result in a marked deficiency in Tregs and in the onset of severe autoimmune disorders, indicating that the main in vivo function of IL-2 is to maintain Tregs homeostasis and survival [19, 21]. The deficiency in Tregs is however less pronounced than in mice or individuals lacking FOXP3, the nuclear transcription factor indispensable for the differentiation and function of Tregs, suggesting compensatory mechanisms [22]. This role may be held by IL-15, which can expand Tregs in vitro as well in vivo [23, 24]. The overlapping signaling functions of IL-2 and IL-15 on lymphocytes sharing the βγc module might also explain why IL-2 or CD25 deficiencies have only a minor impact on other expected functions of IL-2 during T cell activation. IL-15 has however important in vivo functions that are nonredundant with those of IL-2. Indeed, IL-15 and the private IL-15Rα chain of its receptor are synthesized by many cell types of either hematopoietic or stromal origins [3, 18]. Also, in marked contrast with IL-2, IL-15 is generally not secreted but is rather exported at the cell surface together with IL-15Rα, and they form a membrane-bound complex [18]. This complex can however be shed from the cell surface and bind the βγc receptor with much higher affinity than soluble IL-15 [20]. Compelling evidence indicates that, in vivo, IL-15 signals are mainly delivered to βγc+ lymphocytes via transpresentation of IL-15/IL-15Rα complexes. IL-15 thus delivers signals instrumental to maintain the homeostasis of NK and NK/T cells, memory CD8+ T cells and intestinal CD8αα IEL [25–27]. These cell subsets are either absent or markedly decreased in mice lacking IL-15 or IL-15Rα [3, 18]. Conversely, they expand in transgenic mice overexpressing IL-15, and these mice can develop malignant lymphoproliferations of NK cells or of CD8 T cells displaying NK receptors [28, 29].

One hallmark of CD is a massive expansion of IEL combining a considerable increase in CD8+ TCRαβ+ IEL exclusively observed in active CD and an increase in TCRγδ+ IEL CD8+ or CD8– that persists for prolonged periods in patients on gluten-free diet (GFD) [reviewed in 2]. In active CD, a high frequency of IEL expresses activating NK receptors of the lectin-like family, notably CD94 and NKG2D, that can be upregulated by IL-15. A large fraction of IEL also upregulate granzyme B, a protein under the transcriptional control of IL-15, which is necessary for the cytotoxicity of NK and T cells [reviewed in 2]. Moreover, enteropathy-associated lymphoma, a rare but characteristic complication of CD, was shown to develop from a subset of IEL lacking surface T cell receptors but expressing NK receptors and strongly responsive to IL-15 [reviewed in 30]. Recent work further indicates that the malignant lymphocytes derived from a normal subset of innate-like IEL, which depend on IL-15 not only for their survival but also for their differentiation [31; Montcuquet et al., in preparation]. Overall, these observations led us and others to investigate whether IL-15 might be upregulated in the celiac mucosa and participate in CD pathogenesis.

IL-15 Is Chronically Upregulated in CD

IL-15 production is tightly controlled at multiple checkpoints [reviewed in 18]. Transcription is regulated by signals via Toll-like receptors or interferons [32]. It is also developmentally regulated in hematopoietic cells and shut down in mature T cells [33]. Yet, IL-15 expression is mainly regulated at the posttranscriptional level. IL-15 translation is notably strongly restrained by the presence of multiple AUG initiation codons in the 5′UTR and of a regulatory sequence in the 3′UTR [18]. Expression of active IL-15 might also be restrained via the production of alternatively spliced isoforms of IL-15 [34] or of IL-15Rα [35]. In agreement with these data, IL-15 transcripts are present in the normal human intestinal mucosa and are not significantly increased in active CD [36]. However, IL-15Rα transcription is upregulated in active CD, suggesting increased export of IL-15/IL-15Rα complexes to the cell surface [37]. Accordingly, IL-15 was detected at the cell surface of enterocytes isolated from biopsies of active or with type II refractory CD (RCDII) but not of controls [36]. Increased expression of IL-15 was also detected in intestinal biopsies of active CD patients by immunohistochemistry, Western blot or ELISA [36, 38–40]. IL-15 was present both in epithelial cells and lamina propria mononuclear cells, and its expression de-

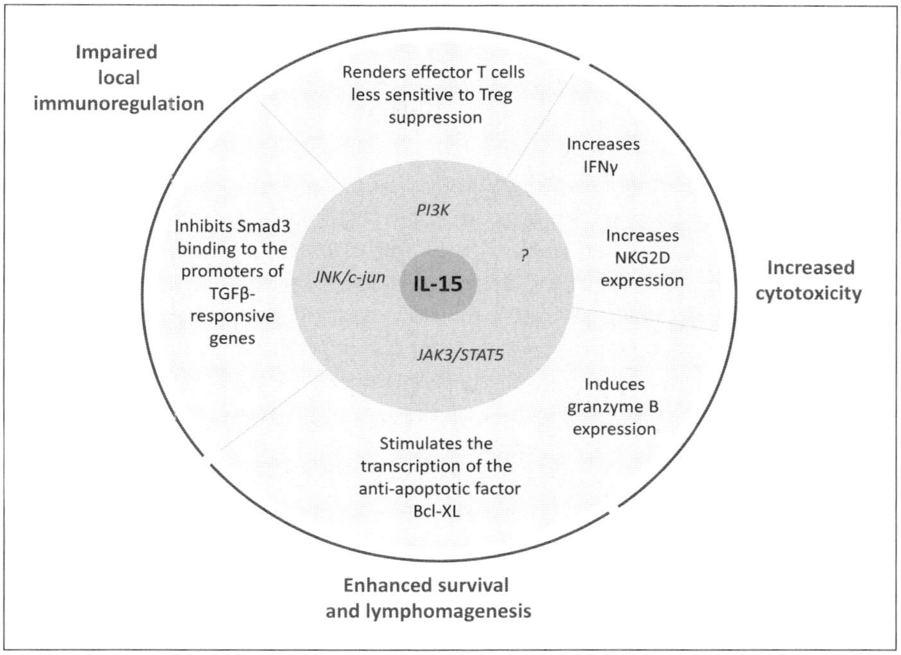

Fig. 1. Mechanisms of action of IL-15 in CD. IL-15 impairs the response of effector lymphocytes, notably CD8+ to immunoregulation by TGF-β and Tregs through activation of the JNK/c-jun and PI3K pathways, respectively. Via a cascade implicating the phosphorylation of JAK3 and STAT5 and the transcription of Bcl-xL, IL-15 exerts potent anti-apoptotic effects that promote IEL accumulation and lymphomagenesis. IL-15 also stimulates IEL cytotoxic functions through STAT5-dependent induction of granzyme B transcription and upregulation of NKG2D. IL-15 can also increase IFN-γ production by CD4+ T cells and IEL.

creased after GFD, albeit not always to the basal normal level [36, 39]. Quantitative and reproducible detection of IL-15 is however difficult, probably due to the small amounts of IL-15 that are produced, and to the inadequacy of most IL-15 antibodies, notably to detect IL-15 bound to IL-15Rα. Therefore, the analysis of IL-15 in CD tissue is not yet established in routine. The mechanisms that drive IL-15 overexpression in CD remain also poorly understood. The inducing effect of one gluten peptide in organ cultures [41] is likely indirect as no direct effect on enterocyte cell lines could be demonstrated [unpubl. results]. Functional interactions between CD susceptibility genes and IL-15 have been suggested but remain to be demonstrated [3].

IL-15 Can Participate in Multiple Steps of CD Pathogenesis

Upregulation of IL-15 in the Gut Epithelium Might Drive the Accumulation of IEL in Active CD and in RCDII

Upregulation of IL-15 in the gut epithelium might drive the accumulation of IEL in active CD and in RCDII as it does in mice overexpressing a human IL-15 transgene under the control of a gut epithelium-specific promoter (hIL-15 TgE mice) [29]. In the latter mice, as in CD and RCDII, IEL did not actively proliferate but rather accumulated due to the delivery of potent anti-apoptotic signals by IL-15. Accordingly, administration of a blocking anti-IL-15 antibody to hIL-15TgE mice induced massive apoptosis of IEL within 24–48 h and subsequent normalization of IEL numbers [42]. The signaling pathways by which IL-15 exerts its potent anti-apoptotic effects are debated. In human CD and RCDII, the IL-15 anti-apoptotic signal depended on phosphorylation of the kinase JAK3, recruitment of the nuclear factor Stat 5 and transcription of the anti-apoptotic factor BCL-xL [42] (fig. 1).

IL-15 Can Orchestrate a Cytolytic Attack of the Gut Epithelium

Thus, both normal T-IEL from active CD or innate-like IEL from RCDII patients could in vitro kill epithelial targets after incubation in IL-15 [41, 43–45]. IL-15 can promote IEL cytotoxicity by different mechanisms [2] (fig. 1). Via Stat5, IL-15 stimulates the transcription of granzyme B, indispensable for lymphocyte killing activity [46]. Innate-like IEL from RCDII patients do not express surface T cell receptors but can use activating NK receptors, notably NKG2D, to kill epithelial targets [41, 45]. IL-15 can also increase the surface expression of activating NK receptors such as NKG2D and CD94/NKG2C in CD8+ TCRαβ+ IEL and stimulate their cytotoxicity against targets expressing the nonclassical MHC class I

Dig Dis 2015;33:122–130
DOI: 10.1159/000369521

molecules MICA/B and HLA-E, the respective ligands of these two NK receptors [39, 43, 44, 47]. IL-15 can even endorse T-IEL from active CD patients with lymphokine-activated killer activity and allow their killing of MICA+ or HLA-E+ targets independently of any T cell recognition [43, 44]. Since both HLA-E and in MICA are strongly upregulated in the epithelium in active CD and/or RCDII [41, 44], IL-15-activated T-IEL might exert innate-like killer properties and thereby participate in epithelial damage. Signals provided by IL-15 or activating NK receptors can also facilitate T cell receptor-dependent cytotoxicity [41]. In vivo, this mechanism may facilitate the activation of CD8+ IEL with T cell receptors of low avidity for self-antigens and license an autoimmune attack of the gut epithelium. The key role of IL-15 in epithelial damage is illustrated in hIL-15TgE mice, which progressively develop severe epithelial lesions [29]. Despite the early development of IEL infiltration, epithelial damage develops only late in life (in our animal farm not before 8–9 months) and not in all animals [23], suggesting that additional events may be necessary to uncover the cytotoxic activity of IEL.

lL-15 Can Impair Local Immunoregulation

In humans, IL-15 impedes the Smad3 pathway of TFGβ, which plays an important role in intestinal homeostasis [48] (fig. 1). In humans and in mice, IL-15 can also impair immunoregulation by Tregs, a subset of cells indispensable for tolerance to the self but also to dietary antigens [22, 49, 50] (fig. 1). An inhibitory effect of IL-15 on the generation of induced Tregs by dendritic cells was reported in mice. Yet this effect was only observed in combination with retinoic acid [51]. It is unclear whether this mechanism can operate in vivo in CD when the absorption of dietary vitamin A, the only source of retinoic acid, is reduced. Our own data in hIL-15TgE mice suggest that IL-15 alone is not sufficient to impair the conversion of naïve CD4+ T cells into Tregs [23]. However, in agreement with previous work, we observed that IL-15 rendered human effector CD8+ T cells and, at a lesser degree, memory CD4+CD45RO+ T cells, insensitive to the immunosuppressive effects of Tregs [52]. This mechanism likely operates in CD, as intestinal and peripheral T cell from active CDs, notably CD8+, responded less well in vitro to suppression by autologous or heterologous Tregs [53, 54]. These data might explain why, despite increased numbers of Tregs in their intestinal mucosa [53–55], CD patients can develop adverse immune responses to dietary gluten. IL-15-induced resistance to Tregs might also promote the onset of extraintestinal autoimmunity, a complication affecting approximately 20% CD patients [56]. In keeping with this hypothesis, loss of systemic tolerance to gluten was observed in mice expressing HLA-DQ8 and a murine IL-15 transgene under the control of the H2-Dd promoter [51]. Similar to hIL-15TgE mice, the latter mice also developed low levels of anti-TG2 antibodies [51]. However, no enteropathy was observed in these mice, probably due to the lack of expression of the IL-15 transgene in the gut epithelium [51]. Data discussed below support this hypothesis.

Cooperation between CD4+ T Cells Specific for a Dietary Antigen and IL-15 Is Necessary and Sufficient to Induce a Celiac-Like Enteropathy

Data discussed above suggest that HLA-DQ2-restricted gluten-specific CD4+ T cells and IL-15 are two important players in CD pathogenesis. Yet, how they may cooperate to induce tissue damage remained unclear. We have recently designed an animal model to address this question [23]. To mimic the in vivo CD4+ T cell response to dietary gluten, we chose to use OTII mice that possess CD4+ T cells bearing a T cell receptor specific for an ovalbumin (OVA) peptide [57]. In contrast to gluten peptides, this OVA peptide does not require any posttranslational modification to be presented to T cells, precluding the need to activate TG2 for efficient antigen presentation. To recapitulate chronic intestinal IL-15 overexpression, we used the heterozygous C57BL/6 (B6) × hIL-15TgE mice generated by Ohta et al. [29] that express a human IL-15 transgene under the control of the T3b promoter. Due to the substitution of the IL-15 peptide sequence by that of IL-2, IL-15 is not only strongly expressed in the small intestinal epithelium but is also secreted and present in lamina propria and serum [29]. Mothers and offspring were either left on OVA-free diet or exposed to an OVA-containing diet initiated during the last 2 weeks of gestation [23]. The offspring was sacrificed at 3 months. This early and prolonged exposure was chosen as preliminary results suggested that no clinical signs of enteropathy developed in mice fed with OVA after weaning. The delay of 3 months was chosen to analyze mice largely before the spontaneous development of epithelial damage that is observed in hIL-15TgE mice after 4–5 months [29] (after 8–9 months in our colony [23]).

OTII$^{+/-}$ B6 control mice chronically exposed to OVA developed active tolerance to OVA [23]. Thus, the frequency of OVA-specific FoxP3+ T cells was increased in the intestinal lamina propria, while OVA-specific effector

Fig. 2. Cooperation between gluten-specific CD4+ T cells and IL-15 in CD. In healthy individuals (A), basal levels of IL-15 are sufficient to maintain IEL homeostasis but not to impair immunoregulation by TGF-β and Tregs. In active CD (B), gluten-activated CD4+ T cells secrete IL-2 and IL-21, while epithelium and dendritic cells produce more IL-15. IL-2 and IL-21 synergize with IL-15 and stimulate the activation of noncognate cytotoxic IEL, notably by inducing their expression of granzyme B and of NKG2D. IL-15 opposes the immunoregulatory effects of TGF-β and Tregs and, on the contrary, provides potent anti-apoptotic signals, overall leading to the accumulation of activated CD8+ T IEL that can induce epithelial lesions. In RCD (C), cooperation between gluten-specific CD4+ T cells and IL-15 might also promote the accumulation and cytotoxic activation of clonal innate-like IEL. Yet, the latter cells are highly sensitive to IL-15, and IL-15 remains upregulated in epithelial cells, so that RCDII IEL can continue to expand and to induce tissue damage after a strict GFD which switches off CD4 help.

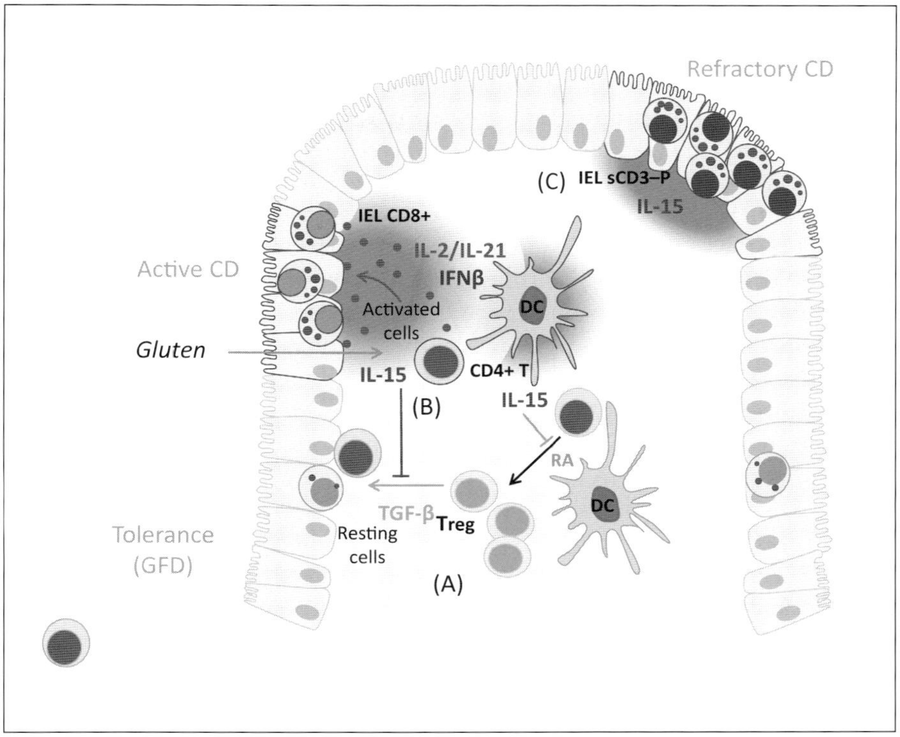

CD4+ T cells were depleted in and outside the gut [23]. Accordingly, mice showed normal growth and intestinal architecture. In contrast, a substantial fraction of OTII$^{+/-}$ hIL-15TgE^{+} mice exposed to OVA and notably almost all females, developed growth retardation, villous atrophy and a conspicuous expansion of granzyme B-expressing CD8+ T cells in the duodenal mucosa [23]. These changes occurred despite the expansion of lamina propria OVA-specific Foxp3+ Tregs. Yet, as discussed above, in the presence of IL-15, effector T cells, notably CD8+ T cells, failed to respond in vitro to Tregs and to restrain the production of IFNγ or of granzyme B induced by T cell receptor stimulation [23]. Consistent with impaired control of effector T cell responses by Tregs and previous observation in H2-Dd-IL-15Tg mice, hIL-15TgE$^{+/-}$ mice displayed increased frequency of IFNγ-secreting CD4+ or CD8+ cells in and outside the gut. Interestingly, this change was observed in all hIL-15TgE mice irrespective of the diet and of the presence of intestinal lesions [23]. In contrast and as observed in CD, intestinal damage correlated with an increase in granzyme B+ CD8+ T cells, and the two changes were observed exclusively in OTII$^{+/-}$ hIL-15TgE mice fed with OVA, indicating their dependence on the cooperation between IL-15- and OVA-activated CD4+ T cells [23].

As already alluded to above, T cell receptor specificity of CD8+ IEL in CD is unknown. MHC class I-restricted recognition of gluten peptides by CD8+ T cells has been suggested but remains debated [58, 59]. Results in our model plead against this hypothesis. Thus, intestinal CD8+ T cells of OTII$^{+/-}$ hIL-15TgE mice exposed to OVA showed no reactivity against the immunodominant H2-Kb-restricted OVA257–264 peptide [23]. In contrast, we observed that, in the presence of IL-15, activated OVA-specific CD4+ T cells induced the expansion of noncognate memory CD8+ T cells and their differentiation into cytotoxic cells expressing granzyme B and NKG2D [23]. CD4+ T cell help depended exclusively on a soluble factor and could be recapitulated in vitro as well as in vivo by IL-2 (fig. 1) [23]. Thus, injection of IL-2 into hIL-15TgE mice (but not into B6 mice) resulted in the expansion of granzyme B+ IEL and simultaneous reduction of the villous/crypt ratio [23]. Importantly, only effector/memory but not naïve CD8+ T cells responded to the complementary signals provided by IL-15- and OVA-specific CD4+ T cells [23]. Interestingly, our findings are reminiscent of very recent observations demonstrating that reactivation of a small number of resident memory T cells (TRM) by their cognate antigen induced the rapid mobilization of many more noncognate granzyme B+ CD8+ TRM able to confer protection against a distinct pathogen [60, 61]. Protection required IL-2Rβ-dependent cytokines [60]. In these reports, activation of noncognate CD8+ TRM was initiated through the stimulation of a few cognate CD8+ T cells [60, 61]. In CD, cognate help delivered by gluten-specific CD4+ T cells might, in the presence of epithelium-derived IL-15, also result in the cytotoxic activation of noncognate resident CD8+ T-IEL. Accumulation of cytotoxic IEL might then be sustained by anti-apoptotic signals delivered by IL-15 and granzyme B release triggered via NK receptors or T cell receptor recognition of self-antigens (fig. 2). After GFD, CD8+ T-IEL lose the CD4 help required for their activation, allowing clinical and histological remission. Noncognate help by gluten-specific T cells might also drive the expansion and cytotoxic activation of clonal innate-like IEL in RCDII patients. Yet in RCDII, clonal IEL are so exquisitely sensitive to IL-15 that their expansion becomes at least partially independent of CD4 help (fig. 2). Epithelial damage and expansion of clonal malignant IEL are however severely worsened by a gluten-containing diet.

Conclusion and Perspectives

Our experimental data support the hypothesis that co-operation between HLA-DQ-restricted gluten-specific CD4+ T cells and IL-15 plays a central role in the pathogenesis of CD. Yet, the mouse model used to substantiate this hypothesis differs in many aspects from CD, and several questions remain unanswered. In OVA-fed OTII$^{+/-}$ hIL-15TgE mice, CD4 help to IL-15-activated resident CD8+ TRM was recapitulated by IL-2 [23]. Why IL-2 and IL-15, which largely share their signaling pathways [20], are both necessary to drive the expansion of granzyme B+ CD8+ TRM? What is the role of IL-21? This cytokine was not detected in our model but is produced by gluten-specific CD4+ T cells of CD patients [62] and can potentiate IL-15 signals in CD8+ T cells and NK cells [63]. Which signal(s) present in CD but not in our mouse model stimulate(s) the production of IL-21 by CD4+ T cells? What are the respective roles of IL-2 and IL-21 in human CD? Strikingly, both cytokines are encoded in the same chromosomal region, which contains variants associated with CD and other autoimmune diseases [64]. Finally, many data converge to substantiate the role of IL-15 in CD and to indicate that IL-15 is a meaningful therapeutic target, notably in cases refractory to GFD. Yet the mechanisms which upregulate IL-15 in CD remain elusive. This question is challenging given the complex regulation of IL-15 but needs to be solved to fully delineate the role of IL-15 in CD pathogenesis.

Acknowledgments

The authors are supported by Institutional grants from Institut National pour la Santé et la Recherche and Université Paris Descartes, and by grants from La Ligue contre le Cancer and La Fondation Princesse Grace. Institut Imagine is recipient of Investissement d'Avenir ANR-10-IAHU-01. Natalia Korneychuk was supported by fellowships from the Ministère de l'Enseignement Supérieur et de la Recherche and La Fondation pour la Recherche Médicale (code FDT20130927989).

Disclosure Statement

The authors declare no conflict of interest.

References

1 Abadie V, Sollid LM, Barreiro LB, Jabri B: Integration of genetic and immunological insights into a model of celiac disease pathogenesis. Annu Rev Immunol 2011;29:493–525.

2 Meresse B, Malamut G, Cerf-Bensussan N: Celiac disease: an immunological jigsaw. Immunity 2012;36:907–919.

3 Abadie V, Jabri B: IL-15: a central regulator of celiac disease immunopathology. Immunol Rev 2014;260:221–234.

4 Di Niro R, Mesin L, Zheng NY, Stamnaes J, Morrissey M, Lee JH, Huang M, Iversen R, du Pre MF, Qiao SW, et al: High abundance of plasma cells secreting transglutaminase 2-specific IgA autoantibodies with limited somatic hypermutation in celiac disease intestinal lesions. Nat Med 2012;18:441–445.

5 Steinsbo O, Henry Dunand CJ, Huang M, Mesin L, Salgado-Ferrer M, Lundin KE, Jahnsen J, Wilson PC, Sollid LM: Restricted VH/VL usage and limited mutations in gluten-specific IgA of coeliac disease lesion plasma cells. Nat Commun 2014;5:4041.

6 Qiao SW, Iversen R, Raki M, Sollid LM: The adaptive immune response in celiac disease. Semin Immunopathol 2012;34:523–540.

7 Matysiak-Budnik T, Moura IC, Arcos-Fajardo M, Lebreton C, Menard S, Candalh C, Ben-Khalifa K, Dugave C, Tamouza H, van Niel G, et al: Secretory IgA mediates retrotranscytosis of intact gliadin peptides via the transferrin receptor in celiac disease. J Exp Med 2008;205:143–154.

8 Lebreton C, Menard S, Abed J, Moura IC, Coppo R, Dugave C, Monteiro RC, Fricot A, Traore MG, Griffin M, et al: Interactions among secretory immunoglobulin A, CD71, and transglutaminase-2 affect permeability of intestinal epithelial cells to gliadin peptides. Gastroenterology 2012;143:698–707, e691–e694.
9 Abed J, Lebreton C, Champier G, Cuvillier A, Cogne M, Meresse B, Dugave C, Garfa-Traore M, Corthesy B, Cerf-Bensussan N, et al: Abnormal apical-to-basal transport of dietary ovalbumin by secretory IgA stimulates a mucosal Th1 response. Mucosal Immunol 2014; 7:315–324.
10 Vader W, Stepniak D, Kooy Y, Mearin L, Thompson A, van Rood JJ, Spaenij L, Koning F: The HLA-DQ2 gene dose effect in celiac disease is directly related to the magnitude and breadth of gluten-specific T cell responses. Proc Natl Acad Sci USA 2003;100:12390–12395.
11 Black KE, Murray JA, David CS: HLA-DQ determines the response to exogenous wheat proteins: a model of gluten sensitivity in transgenic knockout mice. J Immunol 2002; 169:5595–5600.
12 de Kauwe AL, Chen Z, Anderson RP, Keech CL, Price JD, Wijburg O, Jackson DC, Ladhams J, Allison J, McCluskey J: Resistance to celiac disease in humanized HLA-DR3-DQ2-transgenic mice expressing specific anti-gliadin CD4+ T cells. J Immunol 2009;182:7440–7450.
13 Du Pre MF, Kozijn AE, van Berkel LA, ter Borg MN, Lindenbergh-Kortleve D, Jensen LT, Kooy-Winkelaar Y, Koning F, Boon L, Nieuwenhuis EE, et al: Tolerance to ingested deamidated gliadin in mice is maintained by splenic, type 1 regulatory T cells. Gastroenterology 2011;141:610–620, 620, e611–e612.
14 Marietta E, Black K, Camilleri M, Krause P, Rogers RS 3rd, David C, Pittelkow MR, Murray JA: A new model for dermatitis herpetiformis that uses HLA-DQ8 transgenic NOD mice. J Clin Invest 2004;114:1090–1097.
15 Galipeau HJ, Rulli NE, Jury J, Huang X, Araya R, Murray JA, David CS, Chirdo FG, McCoy KD, Verdu EF: Sensitization to gliadin induces moderate enteropathy and insulitis in nonobese diabetic-DQ8 mice. J Immunol 2011; 187:4338–4346.
16 Troncone R, Ferguson A: Gliadin presented via the gut induces oral tolerance in mice. Clin Exp Immunol 1988;72:284–287.
17 Rochman Y, Spolski R, Leonard WJ: New insights into the regulation of T cells by gamma(c) family cytokines. Nat Rev Immunol 2009;9:480–490.
18 Fehniger TA, Caligiuri MA: Interleukin 15: biology and relevance to human disease. Blood 2001;97:14–32.
19 Waldmann TA: The biology of interleukin-2 and interleukin-15: implications for cancer therapy and vaccine design. Nat Rev Immunol 2006;6:595–601.
20 Ring AM, Lin JX, Feng D, Mitra S, Rickert M, Bowman GR, Pande VS, Li P, Moraga I, Spolski R, et al: Mechanistic and structural insight into the functional dichotomy between IL-2 and IL-15. Nat Immunol 2012;13:1187–1195.
21 Liao W, Lin JX, Leonard WJ: Interleukin-2 at the crossroads of effector responses, tolerance, and immunotherapy. Immunity 2013; 38:13–25.
22 Josefowicz SZ, Lu LF, Rudensky AY: Regulatory T cells: mechanisms of differentiation and function. Annu Rev Immunol 2012;30: 531–564.
23 Korneychuk N, Ramiro-Puig E, Ettersperger J, Schulthess J, Montcuquet N, Kiyono H, Meresse B, Cerf-Bensussan N: Interleukin 15 and CD4(+) T cells cooperate to promote small intestinal enteropathy in response to dietary antigen. Gastroenterology 2014;146: 1017–1027.
24 Passerini L, Allan SE, Battaglia M, Di Nunzio S, Alstad AN, Levings MK, Roncarolo MG, Bacchetta R: STAT5-signaling cytokines regulate the expression of FOXP3 in CD4+CD25+ regulatory T cells and CD4+CD25- effector T cells. Int Immunol 2008;20:421–431.
25 Sandau MM, Schluns KS, Lefrancois L, Jameson SC: Cutting edge: transpresentation of IL-15 by bone marrow-derived cells necessitates expression of IL-15 and IL-15R alpha by the same cells. J Immunol 2004;173:6537–6541.
26 Schluns KS, Klonowski KD, Lefrancois L: Transregulation of memory CD8 T-cell proliferation by IL-15Ralpha+ bone marrow-derived cells. Blood 2004;103:988–994.
27 Schluns KS, Nowak EC, Cabrera-Hernandez A, Puddington L, Lefrancois L, Aguila HL: Distinct cell types control lymphoid subset development by means of IL-15 and IL-15 receptor alpha expression. Proc Natl Acad Sci USA 2004;101:5616–5621.
28 Fehniger TA, Suzuki K, Ponnappan A, VanDeusen JB, Cooper MA, Florea SM, Freud AG, Robinson ML, Durbin J, Caligiuri MA: Fatal leukemia in interleukin 15 transgenic mice follows early expansions in natural killer and memory phenotype CD8+ T cells. J Exp Med 2001;193:219–231.
29 Ohta N, Hiroi T, Kweon MN, Kinoshita N, Jang MH, Mashimo T, Miyazaki J, Kiyono H: IL-15-dependent activation-induced cell death-resistant Th1 type CD8 alpha beta+NK1.1+ T cells for the development of small intestinal inflammation. J Immunol 2002;169:460–468.
30 Malamut G, Meresse B, Cellier C, Cerf-Bensussan N: Refractory celiac disease: from bench to bedside. Semin Immunopathol 2012;34:601–613.
31 Schmitz F, Tjon JM, van Bergen J, Koning F: Dendritic cells promote expansion and survival of aberrant TCR-negative intraepithelial lymphocyte lines from refractory celiac disease type II patients. Mol Immunol 2014;58: 10–16.
32 Colpitts SL, Stoklasek TA, Plumlee CR, Obar JJ, Guo C, Lefrancois L: Cutting edge: the role of IFN-alpha receptor and MyD88 signaling in induction of IL-15 expression in vivo. J Immunol 2012;188:2483–2487.
33 Colpitts SL, Stonier SW, Stoklasek TA, Root SH, Aguila HL, Schluns KS, Lefrancois L: Transcriptional regulation of IL-15 expression during hematopoiesis. J Immunol 2013; 191:3017–3024.
34 Tan X, Lefrancois L: Novel IL-15 isoforms generated by alternative splicing are expressed in the intestinal epithelium. Genes Immun 2006;7:407–416.
35 Muller JR, Waldmann TA, Kruhlak MJ, Dubois S: Paracrine and transpresentation functions of IL-15 are mediated by diverse splice versions of IL-15Ralpha in human monocytes and dendritic cells. J Biol Chem 2012;287: 40328–40338.
36 Mention JJ, Ben Ahmed M, Begue B, Barbe U, Verkarre V, Asnafi V, Colombel JF, Cugnenc PH, Ruemmele FM, McIntyre E, et al: Interleukin 15: a key to disrupted intraepithelial lymphocyte homeostasis and lymphomagenesis in celiac disease. Gastroenterology 2003; 125:730–745.
37 Bernardo D, Garrote JA, Allegretti Y, Leon A, Gomez E, Bermejo-Martin JF, Calvo C, Riestra S, Fernandez-Salazar L, Blanco-Quiros A, et al: Higher constitutive IL15R alpha expression and lower IL-15 response threshold in coeliac disease patients. Clin Exp Immunol 2008;154:64–73.
38 Di Sabatino A, Ciccocioppo R, Cupelli F, Cinque B, Millimaggi D, Clarkson MM, Paulli M, Cifone MG, Corazza GR: Epithelium derived interleukin 15 regulates intraepithelial lymphocyte Th1 cytokine production, cytotoxicity, and survival in coeliac disease. Gut 2006;55:469–477.
39 Jabri B, de Serre NP, Cellier C, Evans K, Gache C, Carvalho C, Mougenot JF, Allez M, Jian R, Desreumaux P, et al: Selective expansion of intraepithelial lymphocytes expressing the HLA-E-specific natural killer receptor CD94 in celiac disease. Gastroenterology 2000;118: 867–879.
40 Maiuri L, Ciacci C, Auricchio S, Brown V, Quaratino S, Londei M: Interleukin 15 mediates epithelial changes in celiac disease. Gastroenterology 2000;119:996–1006.
41 Hue S, Mention JJ, Monteiro RC, Zhang S, Cellier C, Schmitz J, Verkarre V, Fodil N, Bahram S, Cerf-Bensussan N, et al: A direct role for NKG2D/MICA interaction in villous atrophy during celiac disease. Immunity 2004;21:367–377.
42 Malamut G, El Machhour R, Montcuquet N, Martin-Lanneree S, Dusanter-Fourt I, Verkarre V, Mention JJ, Rahmi G, Kiyono H, Butz EA, et al: IL-15 triggers an antiapoptotic pathway in human intraepithelial lymphocytes that is a potential new target in celiac disease-associated inflammation and lymphomagenesis. J Clin Invest 2010;120:2131–2143.

43 Meresse B, Chen Z, Ciszewski C, Tretiakova M, Bhagat G, Krausz TN, Raulet DH, Lanier LL, Groh V, Spies T, et al: Coordinated induction by IL15 of a TCR-independent NKG2D signaling pathway converts CTL into lymphokine-activated killer cells in celiac disease. Immunity 2004;21:357–366.
44 Meresse B, Curran SA, Ciszewski C, Orbelyan G, Setty M, Bhagat G, Lee L, Tretiakova M, Semrad C, Kistner E, et al: Reprogramming of CTLs into natural killer-like cells in celiac disease. J Exp Med 2006;203:1343–1355.
45 Tjon JM, Kooy-Winkelaar YM, Tack GJ, Mommaas AM, Schreurs MW, Schilham MW, Mulder CJ, van Bergen J, Koning F: DNAM-1 mediates epithelial cell-specific cytotoxicity of aberrant intraepithelial lymphocyte lines from refractory celiac disease type II patients. J Immunol 2011;186:6304–6312.
46 Ye W, Young JD, Liu CC: Interleukin-15 induces the expression of mRNAs of cytolytic mediators and augments cytotoxic activities in primary murine lymphocytes. Cell Immunol 1996;174:54–62.
47 Roberts AI, Lee L, Schwarz E, Groh V, Spies T, Ebert EC, Jabri B: NKG2D receptors induced by IL-15 costimulate CD28-negative effector CTL in the tissue microenvironment. J Immunol 2001;167:5527–5530.
48 Benahmed M, Meresse B, Arnulf B, Barbe U, Mention JJ, Verkarre V, Allez M, Cellier C, Hermine O, Cerf-Bensussan N: Inhibition of TGF-beta signaling by IL-15: a new role for IL-15 in the loss of immune homeostasis in celiac disease. Gastroenterology 2007;132:994–1008.
49 Hadis U, Wahl B, Schulz O, Hardtke-Wolenski M, Schippers A, Wagner N, Muller W, Sparwasser T, Forster R, Pabst O: Intestinal tolerance requires gut homing and expansion of FoxP3+ regulatory T cells in the lamina propria. Immunity 2011;34:237–246.
50 Torgerson TR, Linane A, Moes N, Anover S, Mateo V, Rieux-Laucat F, Hermine O, Vijay S, Gambineri E, Cerf-Bensussan N, et al: Severe food allergy as a variant of IPEX syndrome caused by a deletion in a noncoding region of the FOXP3 gene. Gastroenterology 2007;132:1705–1717.
51 DePaolo RW, Abadie V, Tang F, Fehlner-Peach H, Hall JA, Wang W, Marietta EV, Kasarda DD, Waldmann TA, Murray JA, et al: Co-adjuvant effects of retinoic acid and IL-15 induce inflammatory immunity to dietary antigens. Nature 2011;471:220–224.
52 Ben Ahmed M, Belhadj Hmida N, Moes N, Buyse S, Abdeladhim M, Louzir H, Cerf-Bensussan N: IL-15 renders conventional lymphocytes resistant to suppressive functions of regulatory T cells through activation of the phosphatidylinositol 3-kinase pathway. J Immunol 2009;182:6763–6770.
53 Hmida NB, Ben Ahmed M, Moussa A, Rejeb MB, Said Y, Kourda N, Meresse B, Abdeladhim M, Louzir H, Cerf-Bensussan N: Impaired control of effector T cells by regulatory T cells: a clue to loss of oral tolerance and autoimmunity in celiac disease? Am J Gastroenterol 2012;107:604–611.
54 Zanzi D, Stefanile R, Santagata S, Iaffaldano L, Iaquinto G, Giardullo N, Lania G, Vigliano I, Vera AR, Ferrara K, et al: IL-15 interferes with suppressive activity of intestinal regulatory T cells expanded in celiac disease. Am J Gastroenterol 2011;106:1308–1317.
55 van Leeuwen MA, du Pre MF, van Wanrooij RL, de Ruiter LF, Raatgeep HR, Lindenbergh-Kortleve DJ, Mulder CJ, de Ridder L, Escher JC, Samsom JN: Changes in natural Foxp3(+) Treg but not mucosally-imprinted CD62L(neg)CD38(+)Foxp3(+)Treg in the circulation of celiac disease patients. PLoS One 2013;8:e68432.
56 Cosnes J, Cellier C, Viola S, Colombel JF, Michaud L, Sarles J, Hugot JP, Ginies JL, Dabadie A, Mouterde O, et al: Incidence of autoimmune diseases in celiac disease: protective effect of the gluten-free diet. Clin Gastroenterol Hepatol 2008;6:753–758.
57 Barnden MJ, Allison J, Heath WR, Carbone FR: Defective TCR expression in transgenic mice constructed using cDNA-based alpha- and beta-chain genes under the control of heterologous regulatory elements. Immunol Cell Biol 1998;76:34–40.
58 Han A, Newell EW, Glanville J, Fernandez-Becker N, Khosla C, Chien YH, Davis MM: Dietary gluten triggers concomitant activation of CD4+ and CD8+ alphabeta T cells and gammadelta T cells in celiac disease. Proc Natl Acad Sci USA 2013;110:13073–13078.
59 Mazzarella G, Stefanile R, Camarca A, Giliw berti P, Cosentini E, Marano C, Iaquinto G, Giardullo, N, Auricchio, S, Sette, A, et al: Gliadin activates HLA class I-restricted CD8+ T cells in celiac disease intestinal mucosa and induces the enterocyte apoptosis. Gastroenterology 2008;134:1017–1027.
60 Ariotti S, Hogenbirk M, Dijkgraaf F, Visser L, Hoekstra M, Song J.-Y, Jacobs H, Haanen J, Schumacher T: Skin-resident memory CD8+ T cells trigger a state of tissue-wide pathogen alert. Science 2014;346:101–105.
61 Schenkel JM, Fraser KA, Beura LK, Pauken KE, Vezys V, Masopust D: Resident memory CD8 T cells trigger protective innate and adaptive immune responses. Science 2014; 346:98–101.
62 Bodd M, Raki M, Tollefsen S, Fallang LE, Bergseng E, Lundin KE, Sollid LM: HLA-DQ2-restricted gluten-reactive T cells produce IL-21 but not IL-17 or IL-22. Mucosal Immunol 2010;3:594–601.
63 Zeng R, Spolski R, Finkelstein SE, Oh S, Kovanen PE, Hinrichs CS, Pise-Masison CA, Radonovich MF, Brady JN, Restifo NP, et al: Synergy of IL-21 and IL-15 in regulating CD8+ T cell expansion and function. J Exp Med 2005;201:139–148.
64 van Heel DA, Franke L, Hunt KA, Gwilliam R, Zhernakova A, Inouye M, Wapenaar MC, Barnardo MC, Bethel G, Holmes GK, et al: A genome-wide association study for celiac disease identifies risk variants in the region harboring IL2 and IL21. Nat Genet 2007;39:827–829.

Dig Dis 2015;33:131–136
DOI: 10.1159/000369534

Host-Microbiota Interactions in the Intestine

Charles O. Elson Katie L. Alexander

Departments of Medicine and Microbiology, University of Alabama at Birmingham, Birmingham, Ala., USA

Key Words
Microbiota · T cell · B cell · Innate lymphoid cell · Epithelial cell

Abstract
The comprehensive collection of bacterial species, termed microbiota, within human and other mammalian hosts has profound effects on both innate and adaptive immunity. Multiple host innate mechanisms contribute to intestinal homeostasis, including epithelial production of protective mucin layers maintaining spatial segregation in the intestine as well as epithelial cell secretion of a broad range of antimicrobial peptides. Additionally, epithelial cells employ autophagy to contain and eliminate invading bacteria; interestingly, genetic variants in specific autophagy genes are linked to susceptibility to Crohn's disease. Innate lymphoid cells, which rapidly respond to cytokine and microbial signals, have emerged as important regulators of the intestinal immune response to the microbiota. With regard to adaptive immunity, specific microbial species stimulate induction of regulatory T cells while others induce effector T cells within the gut. Such stimulation is subject to dysregulation during inflammation and disease, contributing to 'dysbiosis' or an abnormal microbiota composition that has been associated with a variety of immune-mediated inflammatory disorders, including celiac disease. The microbiota communicates with the immune system and vice versa; thus, an abnormal microbiota composition likely translates into an altered host immune response, though the exact mechanisms of such are not yet clear. Immunoglobulin A plays a critical role in limiting bacterial access to the host and in maintaining mutualism with the microbiota. Perturbation of the mucosal barrier via infection or other means can induce effector T cells reactive to the intestinal microbiota, and these cells can persist as memory cells for extended periods of time and potentially serve as pathogenic effector cells upon re-encounter with antigen. Health is associated with a diverse microbiota that functions to maintain the balance between T effector and T regulatory cells in the intestine. Whether dysbiosis can be reversed in immune-mediated disease, thus restoring health, is a question of intense interest for this active area of research.

Introduction

Interactions between mammalian hosts and their bacterial constituents, or microbiota, shape both innate and adaptive immunity [1]. The members of these bacterial communities have been elucidated in the Human Microbiome Project, which was launched in 2007 [2]. This initiative, as well as other studies, have helped to identify the

KARGER 125

© 2015 S. Karger AG, Basel
0257–2753/15/0332–0131$39.50/0

E-Mail karger@karger.com
www.karger.com/ddi

Charles O. Elson, MD
SHEL 607, Division of Gastroenterology and Hepatology
University of Alabama at Birmingham, 1825 University Blvd
Birmingham, AL 35294-0007 (USA)
E-Mail coelson@uab.edu

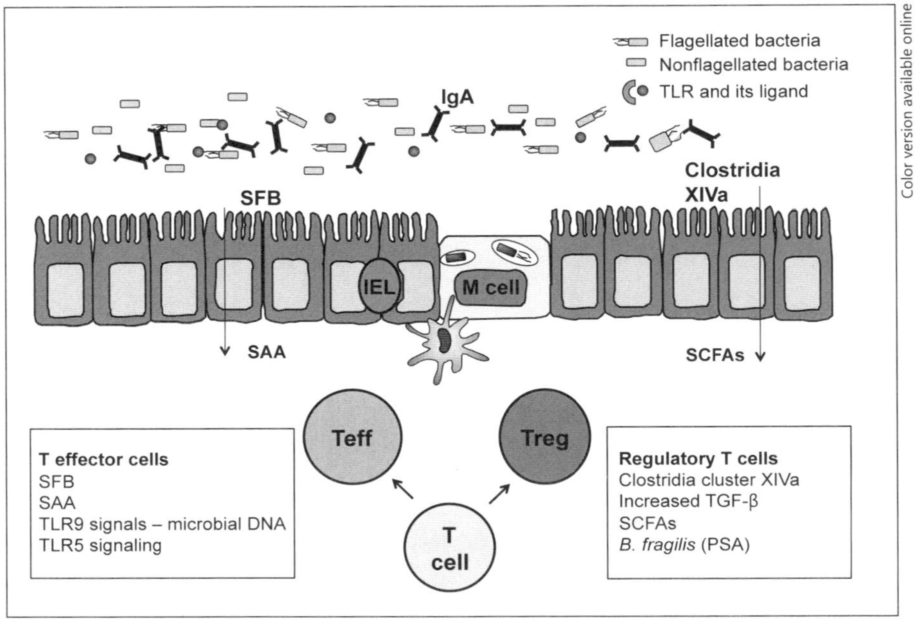

Fig. 1. Treg/Teff balance in the intestine. Differential expression of microbial species and components contributes to the balance of Teffs and Tregs in the lamina propria. SFB colonization is marked by increased SAA production and augmented T_H17 cells. Colonization of the colon with Clostridia XIVa and IV family members is associated with increased TGF-β from the epithelium and augmented Tregs. Numerous additional signals contribute to the balance of Teff/Treg including levels of short-chain fatty acids (SCFAs) and TLR ligand interactions. Figure used with permission [1]. PSA = Polysaccharide A; SAA = serum amyloid A.

microbiome, which refers to the collective genomes of the community of organisms that inhabit our bodies. Investigators have also begun to identify the metagenome, which usually denotes DNA sequencing of all the genes from a natural environment, such as the intestinal tract, and can be used to characterize the functions of the microbiome. Other 'omics' have been applied to understanding the microbiota, including metabolomics, which can identify sets of small-molecule metabolites that are produced by the microbiota, as well as transcriptomics, proteomics, among others.

The majority of studies of the microbiota involve sequencing the 16S rRNA gene, which contains highly conserved, invariant regions. Polymerase chain reaction is used to amplify across one or more of the variable regions, thus allowing identification of the organism by cross-referencing to a database of known bacterial sequences. The total cell number of the microbiota exceeds the aggregate of eukaryotic cells by about 10-fold, and its genes exceed the amount of human genes by approximately 100-fold. Despite the impressive sum of these bacteria, they come from a limited set of phyla, some 6 or 7. With regard to the intestine, the Firmicute and Bacteroidetes phyla comprise the vast majority of the microbiota, although there is a great deal of variation in the microbiota species composition from person to person. In an interesting study of the microbiota colonizing in the left hand versus the right hand, >150 species level phylotypes were identified, and the right and left hands from the same individuals shared only 17% of these phylotypes [3]. This illustrates the challenges inherent in defining what constitutes a healthy bacterial community. In the intestine, 99.9% of the bacteria are anaerobic. Collectively, they represent a biomass metabolically equivalent to the liver. In humans, these bacteria contribute approximately 10% of caloric intake, and immunologically they are the largest mass of microbial antigens and adjuvants encountered by the host during one's lifetime. The microbiota has profound effects on the host, including epithelial turnover, maturation and integrity, development of the mucosal and systemic immune systems, development of the enteric nervous system, development of the gut vasculature, and provision of energy, metabolites, and various vitamins to the host. When the immensely variable 16S sequence profiles are converted into functional categories, a remarkable homogenization of the functional profile of the microbiota results. In other words, different species combinations can lead to very similar functional profiles in the gut.

One acquires the gut microbiota at birth, and there are differences in the founder species depending on whether delivery is vaginal or via cesarean section. Microbial colonization at birth results in a dramatic development and maturation of the gut-associated lymphoid tissue in the intestine and also in the systemic immune system. Through early childhood up to approximately age 3, new strains colonize and can outcompete some of the existing ones, resulting in a rapid increase in diversity. As adults, the microbiota can continue to evolve and change, but at a much slower rate than is seen in childhood. The microbiota can clearly shift in response to diet, illness, and antibiotics. A favorable balance of regulatory T cells (Tregs) and effector T cells (Teffs) is critical for homeostasis in the intestine, and this balance is greatly affected by microbiota components (fig. 1) [1]. A highly diverse microbiota has been associated with health and a less diverse one with various illnesses.

Segregation of the Microbiota from the Epithelium

The expansive microbiota is separated from the host immune system by the single layer of columnar intestinal epithelium. On the host side of that epithelium, the number of T and B cells present in the intestine collectively represents the majority of the lymphoid cells in the body. In addition, there are abundant macrophages, dendritic cells, eosinophils and mast cells. Despite the array of potential antigenic stimulation below the membrane, in most individuals there is limited to no active inflammation. Part of this détente with the microbiota is mediated by the epithelial layer itself, which produces a variety of antimicrobial peptides, as well as mucus, thus providing a spatial separation of bacteria from the cell surface. In mice, it has been shown that there is a 50-μm zone devoid of bacteria between the surface of the epithelium and the lumen [4]. The formation of this protective zone is dependent on signaling through the signaling adaptor protein MyD88, and this zone is vital in limiting adaptive immune responses to the microbiota [4]. One of the antimicrobial peptides that mediates this spatial separation is RegIIIγ; mice deficient in RegIIIγ have increased quantities of Gram-positive mucosa-associated bacteria, increased intestinal immunoglobulin A (IgA) levels, and augmented numbers of CD4+ IFNγ-producing T cells in the intestine [4, 5]. A more recently described mechanism by which epithelial cells maintain homeostasis is the demonstration that autophagy is capable of coping with opportunistic commensals and pathogenic bacteria at the epithelial surface [6]. Again, this epithelial cell activity is dependent on MyD88 signaling and limits the spread of bacteria to sites beyond the epithelial layer [6]. Interestingly, defects in autophagy have been linked to susceptibility for Crohn's disease in genome-wide association studies [7–11]. In the colon, a thick mucus layer devoid of bacteria plays an important role in preventing direct contact between the microbiota and the epithelium [12].

Innate Lymphoid Cells

Innate lymphoid cells (ILCs) are a recently discovered entity. They are unusual in that they lack the typical lymphoid markers as well as receptors for antigen. ILCs play an important role in maintaining mucosal function and integrity and have been categorized into three functional groups (ILC1, ILC2, ILC3) according to their expression and dependence on specific transcription factors, namely T-bet, GATA3, and RORγ, respectively [13, 14]. ILCs participate in the immune response to pathogens in the intestine and do so more rapidly compared to adaptive immune cells. ILCs are stimulated by various cytokines to produce additional cytokines that function in host defense. For example, in *Citrobacter rodentium* infection, innate immune cells produce IL-23, which acts on group 3 ILCs, which, in turn, produce large quantities of IL-22 that act on the epithelium to induce the production of antimicrobial peptides [13]. Group 2 ILCs, which correspond roughly to the T_H2-type adaptive immune cells, seem to play a similar role in helminth infection [15]. In mice, IL-23-responsive/IL-22-producing ILC3 cells are required to contain the lymph node-resident commensal species *Alcaligenes xylosoxidans*, which, once disseminated, can cause systemic inflammation [16]. ILCs also contribute to the spatial segregation of the microbiota. ILCs expressing the aryl hydrocarbon receptor, which detects xenobiotics and polycyclic aromatic hydrocarbons, produce IL-22 that stimulates epithelial antimicrobial peptide production and contributes to the bacteria-free zone above villi [2]. The aryl hydrocarbon receptor has been recently shown to bind certain virulence factors of pathogens, which, in turn, causes this transcription factor to move into the nucleus and activate a variety of genes that contribute to pathogen clearance [17]. A subset of group 3 ILCs expresses major histocompatibility complex class II and can bind and present antigen. This MHC-positive ILC3 subset lacks co-stimulatory molecules and functions to limit CD4+ mucosal T cell responses in vivo [18]. ILCs are not limited to the intestine, but rather are expressed widely in the host and play various roles depending on the context of the microenvironment where they exist.

Despite this spatial segregation of whole bacteria from the epithelial surface, the microbiota is capable of signaling to the epithelium and can alter epithelial gene expression. For example, monocolonization of adult germ-free mice with *Bacteroides thetaiotaomicron* results in the induction of genes involved in nutrient absorption, mucosal barrier function, xenobiotic metabolism, as well as in intestinal maturation [19] via stimulation of Toll-like receptor (TLR) ligands. Signaling by TLR ligands also results in the maturation of the intestinal epithelium and the localization of the proliferative zone in the crypt.

Adaptive Immune Response to the Microbiota

The microbiota stimulates a vigorous adaptive immune response. This is demonstrated in germ-free mice following colonization with gut bacteria. The germ-free intestine has very few adaptive immune B or T cells, but these cells rapidly accumulate to form functional Peyer's patches and infiltrate through the intestinal lamina propria effector sites shortly after colonization. With regard to the B-cell response, it is well known that IgA is the predominant antibody at mucosal surfaces. IgA plays a multifaceted role in the body, and although it is often described as defending against pathogens, the primary function of IgA is to maintain a mutualistic relationship with the microbiota. In support of this idea, it has been found that Foxp3+ Tregs are the major helper cells for IgA [20]. In fact, Tregs in the intestine provide crucial survival signals for mucosal IgA+ B cells. Consistent with this role, adoptive transfer of CD4+CD25+ or CD4+Foxp3+ Tregs into immune-compromised mice induces greater levels of intestinal IgA than transfer of CD25– or Foxp3– T cells [20]. IgA also reduces uptake of microbial antigens into systemic immune sites, thus preventing systemic immunity to commensal bacteria [21]. Overall, these findings support a model in which Tregs aid and stimulate mucosal IgA+ B cells to both inhibit inflammatory responses and maintain the gut microbiota, which, in turn, protects the host against intestinal pathogens via a phenomenon known as colonization resistance. Interestingly, a subset of IgA-producing B cells in the lamina propria produces inducible nitric oxide synthase (iNOS), an antimicrobial factor, as well as tumor necrosis factor (TNF)α. Mice deficient in the iNOS+TNFα+IgA+ plasma cell population have decreased IgA production and are unable to clear infection with *C. rodentium*, a pathogenic *E. coli* equivalent in mice [22]. Because communication between the microbiota and the adaptive immune system is bidirectional, adaptive immunity is paramount in maintaining a healthy microbiota. This is manifest in mice deficient in T and B cells that also have a deletion of the T-bet transcription factor, $Tbet^{-/-}Rag2^{-/-}$ (TRUC mice). Such mice develop spontaneous colitis and abnormal barrier function [23]. TRUC colitis was demonstrated to be transmissible to normal mice by transfer of bacteria from colitic TRUC mice. This colitis was also vertically transmitted to both wild-type and $Rag2^{-/-}$ pups that were cross-fostered with TRUC mothers. Transfer of CD4+CD25+ Tregs was sufficient to prevent colitis [23]. Thus, the absence of a functional adaptive immune system can result in a pathogenic microbiota [24].

With regard to the T-cell compartment of the adaptive response, various subsets of bacteria have been found to induce Teffs, while others seem to preferentially induce Tregs. The most well-studied example of selective induction of Teffs is that of segmented filamentous bacteria (SFB). SFB is a member of the Clostridia cluster of the Firmicute phylum. It grows in the distal ileum and cecum of mice and is widely distributed in nature, including insects [25]. It grows in long strands with one end attaching to the intestinal epithelium, including Peyer's patch epithelium [26]. SFB-colonized mice have increased levels of Th17 cells in the small intestinal lamina propria [27, 28]. Interestingly, colonization by SFB has been shown to be necessary for induction of experimental models of autoimmunity that are mediated by Th17 cells [29].

A number of different bacteria have been found to induce Tregs selectively. This includes clusters IV and XIVa from Clostridia, which have been demonstrated to stimulate increased levels of transforming growth factor-β (TGF-β) from intestinal epithelial cells and encourage the induction of Tregs in the colon [30, 31]. Another bacterium, *Bacteroides fragilis*, produces polysaccharide A, which is able to induce IL-10 production in Tregs [32–34]. Such Tregs can suppress both systemic, as well as intestinal, inflammation. Between effector and regulatory activities, the balance appears to be shifted in favor of Tregs in the normal gut. This may be due to a TGF-β-rich environment, and TGF-β is a vital cytokine for the induction and maintenance of Tregs.

Thus, the microbiota has potent effects on the type of adaptive immune response that results in the intestine. The composition of the microbiota changes during various illnesses, including inflammatory bowel disease. In most cases, this involves a decrease in the richness or variety of stains present. Such abnormal composition of the microbiota has been termed 'dysbiosis'. The concept of 'dysbiosis' proposes that an abnormal composition of the multiple members of the microbiota can result in aberrant immune responses, which, in turn, fosters the development of disease, including autoimmune and metabolic. This is in distinction to the typical pathogen model where a single bacterial species is capable of inducing a given disease. Whether dysbiosis can be reversed in adults with immune-mediated or metabolic disease, thus restoring health, is an unanswered question of intense interest.

Infection of the gut itself by pathogens can induce immune responses to the microbiota. Thus, any inflammation of the mucosa on the surface of the intestine may be accompanied by the induction of effector cells to the microbiota that could then contribute to pathology upon re-encounter with microbiota antigens. For example, infection with *Toxoplasma gondii* induces CD4+ T cells reactive to CBir1 flagellin, an immunodominant microbiota antigen [35]. CBir1-specific memory CD4+ T cells persist in the host for long periods and can be reactivated upon subsequent antigen encounter; thus, it would not be surprising that a significant adaptive response to the microbiota could contribute to inflammation of the small intestine, such as that seen in celiac disease. Because gluten-free diet resolves the mucosal lesions, an adaptive immune response would not prevent remission of inflammation, but it might affect the tempo of recovery or contribute to the lack of response in some individuals despite a gluten-free diet.

Diet is known to affect microbiota composition; thus, it is likely that the small intestinal microbiota will be affected by gluten in the diet, as well as by its absence. The microbiota has been shown in rodents to alter neurotrophic factors in the brain [36] and affect behaviors such as anxiety. Assuming similar effects occur in humans, it is not a huge leap to postulate that the microbiota might affect food choices that humans make, and may do so in order to benefit themselves. This notion was a recent topic of an article in the *New York Times*. Might a microbiota favored by gluten ingestion induce a craving for breads and other gluten-containing foods and contribute to noncompliance with a gluten-free diet? This is a question that we would have never thought to ask before the 'microbiome era'. Our understanding of how the microbiota interacts with us in health and disease is meager, but this interaction surely will continue to surprise us as investigations progress.

Disclosure Statement

The authors have no conflicts of interest to declare.

References

1 Alexander KL, Targan SR, Elson CO 3rd: Microbiota activation and regulation of innate and adaptive immunity. Immunol Rev 2014;260:206–220.

2 Turnbaugh PJ, Ley RE, Hamady M, Fraser-Liggett CM, Knight R, Gordon JI: The human microbiome project. Nature 2007;449:804–810.

3 Fierer N, Hamady M, Lauber CL, Knight R: The influence of sex, handedness, and washing on the diversity of hand surface bacteria. Proc Natl Acad Sci USA 2008;105:17994–17999.

4 Vaishnava S, et al: The antibacterial lectin RegIIIgamma promotes the spatial segregation of microbiota and host in the intestine. Science 2011;334:255–258.

5 Cash H, Whitham C, Behrendt C, Hooper L: Symbiotic bacteria direct expression of an intestinal bactericidal lectin. Science 2006;313:1126–1130.

6 Benjamin JL, Sumpter R Jr, Levine B, Hooper LV: Intestinal epithelial autophagy is essential for host defense against invasive bacteria. Cell Host Microbe 2013;13:723–734.

7 Cho JH: The genetics and immunopathogenesis of inflammatory bowel disease. Nat Rev Immunol 2008;8:458–466.

8 Cooney R, et al: NOD2 stimulation induces autophagy in dendritic cells influencing bacterial handling and antigen presentation. Nat Med 2010;16:90–97.

9 Travassos LH, Carneiro LA, Girardin S, Philpott DJ: Nod proteins link bacterial sensing and autophagy. Autophagy 2010;6:409–411.

10 Travassos LH, et al: Nod1 and Nod2 direct autophagy by recruiting ATG16L1 to the plasma membrane at the site of bacterial entry. Nat Immunol 2010;11:55–62.

11 Homer CR, Richmond AL, Rebert NA, Achkar JP, McDonald C: ATG16L1 and NOD2 interact in an autophagy-dependent antibacterial pathway implicated in Crohn's disease pathogenesis. Gastroenterology 2010;139:1630–1641, 1641.e1–2.

12 Johansson M, Phillipson M, Petersson J, Velcich A, Holm L, Hansson G: The inner of the two Muc2 mucin-dependent mucus layers in colon is devoid of bacteria. Proc Natl Acad Sci USA 2008;105:15064–15069.

13 Sonnenberg G, Monticelli L, Elloso M, Fouser L, Artis D: CD4+lymphoid tissue-inducer cells promote innate immunity in the gut. Immunity 2011;34:122–134.

14 Sonnenberg G, Artis D: Innate lymphoid cell interactions with microbiota: implications for intestinal health and disease. Immunity 2012;37:601–610.

15 Tait Wojno ED, Artis D: Innate lymphoid cells: balancing immunity, inflammation, and tissue repair in the intestine. Cell Host Microbe 2012;12:445–457.

16 Sonnenberg GF, et al: Innate lymphoid cells promote anatomical containment of lymphoid-resident commensal bacteria. Science 2012;336:1321–1325.

17 Moura-Alves P, et al: AhR sensing of bacterial pigments regulates antibacterial defence. Nature 2014;512:387–392.

18 Hepworth M, et al: Innate lymphoid cells regulate CD4+ T-cell responses to intestinal commensal bacteria. Nature 2013;498:113–117.

19 Hooper LV, Wong MH, Thelin A, Hansson L, Falk PG, Gordon JI: Molecular analysis of commensal host-microbial relationships in the intestine. Science 2001;291:881–884.

20 Cong Y, Feng T, Fujihashi K, Schoeb T, Elson C: A dominant, coordinated T regulatory cell-IgA response to the intestinal microbiota. Proc Natl Acad Sci USA 2009;106:19256–19261.

21 Konrad A, Cong Y, Duck W, Borlaza R, Elson C: Tight mucosal compartmentation of the murine immune response to antigens of the enteric microbiota. Gastroenterology 2006;130:2050–2059.

22 Fritz JH, et al: Acquisition of a multifunctional IgA+ plasma cell phenotype in the gut. Nature 2012;481:199–203.
23 Garrett WS, et al: Communicable ulcerative colitis induced by T-bet deficiency in the innate immune system. Cell 2007;131:33–45.
24 Garrett WS, et al: Enterobacteriaceae act in concert with the gut microbiota to induce spontaneous and maternally transmitted colitis. Cell Host Microbe 2010;8:292–300.
25 Talham GL, Jiang HQ, Bos NA, Cebra JJ: Segmented filamentous bacteria are potent stimuli of a physiologically normal state of the murine gut mucosal immune system. Infect Immun 1999;67:1992–2000.
26 Klaasen HL, Koopman JP, Poelma FG, Beynen AC: Intestinal, segmented, filamentous bacteria. FEMS Microbiol Rev 1992;8:165–180.
27 Ivanov II, et al: Induction of intestinal Th17 cells by segmented filamentous bacteria. Cell 2009;139:485–498.
28 Gaboriau-Routhiau V, et al: The key role of segmented filamentous bacteria in the coordinated maturation of gut helper T cell responses. Immunity 2009;31:677–689.
29 Wu H-J, et al: Gut-residing segmented filamentous bacteria drive autoimmune arthritis via T helper 17 cells. Immunity 2010;32:815–827.
30 Atarashi K, et al: Induction of colonic regulatory T cells by indigenous *Clostridium* species. Science 2011;331:337–341.
31 Atarashi K, et al: Treg induction by a rationally selected mixture of Clostridia strains from the human microbiota. Nature 2013;500:232–236.
32 Round JL, et al: The Toll-like receptor 2 pathway establishes colonization by a commensal of the human microbiota. Science 2011;332:974–977.
33 Mazmanian SK, Round JL, Kasper DL: A microbial symbiosis factor prevents intestinal inflammatory disease. Nature 2008;453:620–625.
34 Round JL, Mazmanian SK: Inducible Foxp3+ regulatory T-cell development by a commensal bacterium of the intestinal microbiota. Proc Natl Acad Sci USA 2010;107:12204–12209.
35 Hand T, et al: Acute gastrointestinal infection induces long-lived microbiota-specific T cell responses. Science 2012;337:1553–1556.
36 Bercik P, et al: The intestinal microbiota affect central levels of brain-derived neurotropic factor and behavior in mice. Gastroenterology 2011;141:599–609, 609.e1–3.

Celiac Disease: Clinical Perspective

Dig Dis 2015;33:137–140
DOI: 10.1159/000370204

Clinical Manifestations of Celiac Disease

Peter H.R. Green Suneeta Krishnareddy Benjamin Lebwohl

The Celiac Disease Center at Columbia University, New York, N.Y., USA

Key Words
Clinical presentation · Diarrhea · Anemia · Screening

Abstract
Celiac disease (CD) is an immune-based condition affecting multiple organ systems. Clinical manifestations are manifold in form and number due to the multisystem nature of CD. There has been a progressive change in the clinical manifestations over the recent decades with fewer patients, both adults and children, presenting with a diarrheal, classical form. This, in children, is seen in only the youngest, while growth issues, screening at-risk groups and recurrent abdominal pain are the most common modes of presentation among children. Among adults, diarrhea is the most common presentation followed by anemia. Screening at-risk groups, metabolic bone disease and incidental recognition at endoscopy performed for reflux are the other main modes of presentation. The bulk of those with CD remain undiagnosed. The symptoms are often common, and increased medical education should lead to greater awareness in the medical community and an increased rate of diagnosis.

Introduction

The clinical manifestations of celiac disease (CD) are many [1]. Although CD was first characterized as a pediatric diarrheal illness with a prominent malabsorption syndrome, it is now considered a disease of any age with adults predominating. There is a vast array of symptoms originating in any organ system (table 1). As well as shifting to adults, there has been a shift in the mode of clinical presentation.

Recently, there have been attempts to define the nomenclature of the types or clinical presentations of CD [2]. The major classifications are classical and nonclassical CD. Regarding classical CD, these patients present with diarrhea, malabsorption, or a malnutrition syndrome. As for nonclassical CD, these patients do not have signs or symptoms of malabsorption or diarrhea. This group includes: asymptomatic CD – this category refers to patients who have no symptoms on presentation; subclinical CD – patients in this category have symptoms that fall below the threshold of clinical detection that would warrant testing for CD in routine clinical practice; potential CD – this category refers to patients with positive CD-related serologies but normal small intestinal biopsy; a subset of these patients may develop CD in the future. Some of these patients may have a temporary celiac or gluten autoimmunity, which is seen in both adults and children, though this is most well documented in the latter [3, 4].

We are not aware why some patients present with diarrhea and others do not. The classical presentation does not correlate with the degree of villous atrophy [5], or length of bowel involvement as assessed by video capsule imaging [6]. Neurohormonal mechanisms may be an important cause of symptoms as abnormalities in serotonin metabolism have been described in some patients [7].

While in the United States analysis of the NHANES data revealed that the prevalence of CD was 0.71% (95% CI 0.58–0.86%), the majority, 83%, were not diagnosed [8]. Among those diagnosed, women predominate (2:1), and the peak age at diagnosis is between 30 and 60 years of age [9].

KARGER 125

© 2015 S. Karger AG, Basel
0257–2753/15/0332–0137$39.50/0

E-Mail karger@karger.com
www.karger.com/ddi

Peter H.R. Green, MD
The Celiac Disease Center at Columbia University
180 Fort Washington Avenue, Suite 936
New York, NY 10032 (USA)
E-Mail Pg11@columbia.edu

Table 1. Clinical manifestations of CD

System	Symptoms directly related to CD	Symptoms due to conditions associated with CD
Constitutional	Fatigue Weight loss	
Cardiovascular		Dyspnea/edema (cardiomyopathy) Angina (ischemic heart disease) Palpitations (atrial fibrillation)
Gastrointestinal	Diarrhea Abdominal pain Bloating Dyspepsia Reflux	Dysphagia/reflux (eosinophilic esophagitis) Bloating (small intestinal bacterial overgrowth) Diarrhea (pancreatic insufficiency)
Hematologic	Iron deficiency Folate deficiency Copper deficiency	Thrombocytopenia (idiopathic thrombocytopenia purpura)
Respiratory	Dyspnea due to anemia	Pneumonia, influenza, tuberculosis Pulmonary hemosiderosis
Endocrine	Osteoporosis Infertility	Fatigue, cold intolerance (hypothyroidism)
Musculoskeletal	Myalgias, arthralgias	Arthritis (rheumatoid arthritis)
Neurologic	'Brain fog'	Gluten ataxia Migraine Peripheral neuropathy
Cutaneous	Dermatitis herpetiformis	Psoriasis Urticaria Acne

There has been a progressive decrease in the percentage of patients presenting with a diarrheal syndrome. This trend is attributed to a changing nature of CD, greater knowledge of the nonclassical manifestations among physicians and the advent of serological testing [10, 11].

Among adults seen in our Celiac Disease Center at Columbia University in New York, the major mode of presentation was diarrhea; however, it occurred in only 36% of patients. Other presentations included: anemia (13%); screening high-risk groups (8%), namely those with a family history, associated autoimmune diseases or Down syndrome; metabolic bone disease (5%), or incidental at endoscopy performed typically for esophageal reflux disease (4%). Twenty percent were classified as 'other' modes of presentation. This group included those with dermatitis herpetiformis (DH), abnormal liver function tests, low ferritin without anemia, abdominal pain, low cholesterol as well as a variety of mineral or vitamin deficiencies (fig. 1). Patients with DH have a similar degree of deficiencies irrespective of whether they present predominantly with DH or predominantly CD and coexistent DH as a minor concern [12].

Among the pediatric population seen at our Center, recurrent abdominal pain, growth issues (short stature and failure to thrive) and screening were the most common modes of presentation, each accounting for about 25%. Diarrheal presentations only accounted for <10% of cases [13]. However, most of those who presented with diarrhea were in the very young age group, ≤2 years of age [14]. Other age-specific presentations included screening that was mainly seen among older children, 2–12 and >12 years of age, and growth issues occurred in all age groups [14].

Overweight and obese adults and children may present with CD [13, 15]. Among adults seen in our center, 17.3% were underweight, 60.7% normal, 15.2% overweight, and 6.8% obese. Factors associated with low BMI were female sex, Marsh IIIb/c histology, and presentation with diarrhea. On a gluten-free diet, those who were underweight gained weight, whereas 54% of overweight and 47% of obese patients lost weight; this was associated with being followed by our dietitian [15]. Similarly, overweight children lost weight on the diet [13].

Anemia was the second most frequent presentation in our series and the most common hematologic manifestation of CD [16]. The anemia in CD is multifactorial in

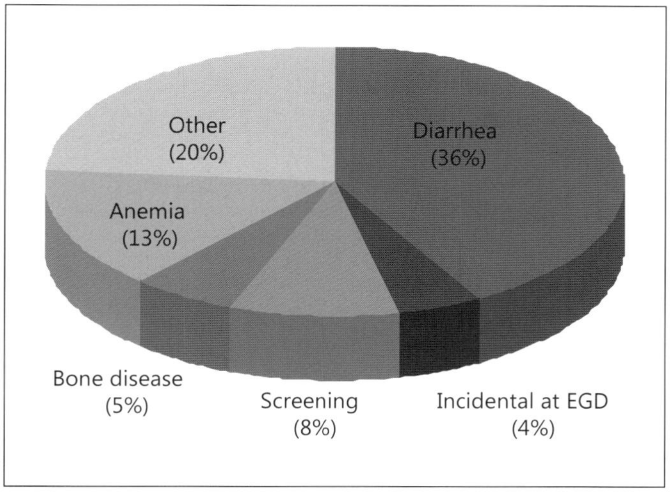

Fig. 1. Presentation of CD in adults (n = 1,499), Columbia University Medical Center. EGD = Esophagogastroduodenoscopy.

etiology with both iron deficiency and anemia of chronic disease predominating [17]. While patients may have folate or vitamin B_{12} deficiency, macrocytic anemia is uncommon.

There is no scoring system or disease activity index for CD like there is for Crohn's disease. However, our recent study of patients who presented with diarrhea compared to those who presented with anemia suggested that those with anemia had more severe disease. The anemia group had higher ESR, serum tissue transglutaminase levels, more severe degrees of villous atrophy and worse bone disease [18].

At presentation, patients with CD typically have low total cholesterol and HDL levels that improve after treatment with a gluten-free diet [19]. We have utilized the patients' HDL levels to predict the presence of CD among those with iron deficiency anemia. We found that screening for CD should at least be done for iron deficiency anemia patients who present with HDL levels <40 mg/dl with an expectation that those with levels <30 mg/dl would have a greatly increased likelihood of CD positivity [20].

Endocrine manifestations in CD may be manifold, but the most prominent is reduced bone mineral density. This was the mode of presentation of about 10% of patients seen by us in the Celiac Disease Center at Columbia University [11]. Fracture risk is a major concern; patients with CD are at increased risk of fractures of any type, and are at particularly increased risk of hip fracture, with one population-based study finding a hazard ratio of 2.1 (95% CI 1.8–2.4) compared to age- and sex-matched controls without CD [21]. While this risk was present in both diagnosed and undiagnosed CD, a study comparing outcomes among those with mucosal healing with those with persistent villous atrophy in patients with CD undergoing follow-up biopsy found that those with persistent villous atrophy had an increased risk of hip fracture [22]. These results, together with data showing improvement of bone density after diagnosis of CD and institution of the gluten-free diet [23], suggest that the risk of osteoporotic fracture is due to the sequelae of dietary gluten and is, at least in some cases, reversible.

Screening of high-risk groups accounts for a considerable number of new diagnoses of CD, with those who have a family history of CD predominating. Among those diagnosed through screening, many patients have symptoms even if only in retrospect.

Abdominal pain is a mode of presentation of CD in both adults and children. One case-control study from the UK involving 300 consecutive adult patients presenting to the emergency room with acute abdominal pain revealed among those with nonsurgical abdominal pain a prevalence of CD of 10.5% [24]. The etiology of the abdominal pain is not clear; however, patients with CD have a high rate of small intestinal intussusceptions when imaged [25, 26]. Recurrent intussusceptions may be a presentation of CD in both children and adults [27, 28].

Many neurologic manifestations of CD have been reported, and the pathophysiology of most such manifestations is unknown. CD has been associated with common neurologic disorders such as migraine headaches [29], peripheral neuropathy which is characteristically due to a small fiber neuropathy [30, 31] and epilepsy [32], as well as uncommon forms of ataxia that are responsive to the gluten-free diet [33]. In some cases, neuropathy can be due to identifiable vitamin deficiencies due to malabsorption, such as thiamine (B_1), pyridoxine (B_6), cobalamin (B_{12}), and niacin, though in most cases a specific vitamin or mineral deficiency is not identified.

In conclusion, CD can present with a myriad of clinical signs and symptoms, but the majority of patients with CD remain undiagnosed. Greater awareness of the diverse clinical manifestations of CD among medical practitioners will be needed to increase the low rate of diagnosis that is currently found in many countries around the world.

Disclosure Statement

The authors declare that no financial or other conflict of interest exists in relation to the content of the article.

References

1 Green PH, Cellier C: Celiac disease. N Engl J Med 2007;357:1731–1743.
2 Ludvigsson JF, Leffler DA, Bai JC, et al: The Oslo definitions for coeliac disease and related terms. Gut 2013;62:43–52.
3 Liu E, Bao F, Barriga K, et al: Fluctuating transglutaminase autoantibodies are related to histologic features of celiac disease. Clin Gastroenterol Hepatol 2003;1:356–362.
4 Mahadev S, Bhagat G, Green PH: Transient celiac autoimmunity in an adult. J Clin Gastroenterol 2011;45:912–913.
5 Brar P, Kwon GY, Egbuna I, et al: Lack of correlation of degree of villous atrophy with severity of clinical presentation of coeliac disease. Dig Liver Dis 2007;39:26–29.
6 Murray JA, Rubio-Tapia A, Van Dyke CT, et al: Mucosal atrophy in celiac disease: extent of involvement, correlation with clinical presentation, and response to treatment. Clin Gastroenterol Hepatol 2008;6:186–193; quiz 25.
7 Coleman NS, Foley S, Dunlop SP, et al: Abnormalities of serotonin metabolism and their relation to symptoms in untreated celiac disease. Clin Gastroenterol Hepatol 2006;4: 874–881.
8 Rubio-Tapia A, Ludvigsson JF, Brantner TL, Murray JA, Everhart JE: The prevalence of celiac disease in the United States. Am J Gastroenterol 2012;107:1538–1544; quiz 1537, 1545.
9 Green PHR, Stavropoulos SN, Panagi SG, et al: Characteristics of adult celiac disease in the USA: results of a national survey. Am J Gastroenterol 2001;96:126–131.
10 Lo W, Sano K, Lebwohl B, Diamond B, Green PH: Changing presentation of adult celiac disease. Dig Dis Sci 2003;48:395–398.
11 Rampertab SD, Pooran N, Brar P, Singh P, Green PH: Trends in the presentation of celiac disease. Am J Med 2006;119:355.e9–e14.
12 Krishnareddy S, Lewis SK, Green PH: Dermatitis herpetiformis: clinical presentations are independent of manifestations of celiac disease. Am J Clin Dermatol 2014;15:51–56.
13 Reilly NR, Aguilar K, Hassid BG, et al: Celiac disease in normal-weight and overweight children: clinical features and growth outcomes following a gluten-free diet. J Pediatr Gastroenterol Nutr 2011;53:528–531.
14 Rizkalla Reilly N, Dixit R, Simpson S, Green PH: Celiac disease in children: an old disease with new features. Minerva Pediatr 2012;64: 71–81.
15 Cheng J, Brar PS, Lee AR, Green PH: Body mass index in celiac disease: beneficial effect of a gluten-free diet. J Clin Gastroenterol 2010;44:267–271.
16 Baydoun A, Maakaron JE, Halawi H, Abou Rahal J, Taher AT: Hematological manifestations of celiac disease. Scand J Gastroenterol 2012;47:1401–1411.
17 Harper JW, Holleran SF, Ramakrishnan R, Bhagat G, Green PH: Anemia in celiac disease is multifactorial in etiology. Am J Hematol 2007;82:996–1000.
18 Abu Daya H, Lebwohl B, Lewis SK, Green PH: Celiac disease patients presenting with anemia have more severe disease than those presenting with diarrhea. Clin Gastroenterol Hepatol 2013;11:1472–1477.
19 Brar P, Kwon GY, Holleran S, et al: Change in lipid profile in celiac disease: beneficial effect of gluten-free diet. Am J Med 2006;119:786–790.
20 Abu Daya H, Lebwohl B, Smukalla S, Lewis SK, Green PH: Utilizing HDL levels to improve detection of celiac disease in patients with iron deficiency anemia. Am J Gastroenterol 2014;109:769–770.
21 Ludvigsson JF, Michaelsson K, Ekbom A, Montgomery SM: Coeliac disease and the risk of fractures – a general population-based cohort study. Aliment Pharmacol Ther 2007;25: 273–285.
22 Lebwohl B, Michaelsson K, Green PH, Ludvigsson JF: Persistent mucosal damage and risk of fracture in celiac disease. J Clin Endocrinol Metab 2014;99:609–616.
23 Meyer D, Stavropolous S, Diamond B, Shane E, Green PH: Osteoporosis in a North American adult population with celiac disease. Am J Gastroenterol 2001;96:112–119.
24 Sanders DS, Hopper AD, Azmy IA, et al: Association of adult celiac disease with surgical abdominal pain: a case-control study in patients referred to secondary care. Ann Surg 2005;242:201–207.
25 Willingham FF, Opekun AR, Graham DY: Endoscopic demonstration of transient small bowel intussusception in a patient with adult celiac disease. Gastrointest Endosc 2003;57: 626–627.
26 Sanders DS, Azmy IA, Kong SC, Lee FK: Symptomatic small bowel intussusception: a surgical opportunity to diagnose adult celiac disease? Gastrointest Endosc 2004;59:161–162.
27 Gonda TA, Khan SU, Cheng J, Lewis SK, Rubin M, Green PH: Association of intussusception and celiac disease in adults. Dig Dis Sci 2010;55:2899–2903.
28 Reilly NR, Aguilar KM, Green PH: Should intussusception in children prompt screening for celiac disease? J Pediatr Gastroenterol Nutr 2013;56:56–59.
29 Dimitrova AK, Ungaro RC, Lebwohl B, et al: Prevalence of migraine in patients with celiac disease and inflammatory bowel disease. Headache 2013;53:344–55.
30 Chin RL, Latov N: Peripheral neuropathy and celiac disease. Curr Treat Options Neurol 2005;7:43–48.
31 Brannagan TH 3rd, Hays AP, Chin SS, et al: Small-fiber neuropathy/neuronopathy associated with celiac disease: skin biopsy findings. Arch Neurol 2005;62:1574–1578.
32 Ludvigsson JF, Zingone F, Tomson T, Ekbom A, Ciacci C: Increased risk of epilepsy in biopsy-verified celiac disease: a population-based cohort study. Neurology 2012;78:1401–1407.
33 Hadjivassiliou M, Grunewald RA, Chattopadhyay AK, et al: Clinical, radiological, neurophysiological, and neuropathological characteristics of gluten ataxia. Lancet 1998;352: 1582–1585.

Dig Dis 2015;33:141–146
DOI: 10.1159/000369518

World Perspective and Celiac Disease Epidemiology

Carlo Catassi[a] Simona Gatti[a] Elena Lionetti[b]

[a]Department of Pediatrics, Università Politecnica delle Marche, Ancona, and [b]Department of Pediatrics, University of Catania, Catania, Italy

Key Words
Celiac disease · Genetic predisposition · Geoepidemiology · Celiac disease screening

Abstract
In Europe and the USA, the mean frequency of celiac disease (CD) in the general population is approximately 1%, with some regional differences, the reasons for which remain elusive. A similar disease prevalence has been found in other countries mostly populated by individuals of European origin, e.g. Australia and Argentina. In Western countries, a true rise in overall CD prevalence of CD has been documented. CD is a common disorder in North Africa, the Middle East and India; however, the diagnostic rate is low in these countries due to low availability of diagnostic facilities and poor disease awareness. The highest CD prevalence in the world (5.6%) has been described in an African population originally living in Western Sahara, the Saharawi, of Arab-Berber origin. The reasons for this high CD frequency are unclear but could be primarily related to recent dietary changes and genetic factors, given the high level of consanguinity of this population. Further studies are needed to quantify the incidence of the celiac condition in apparently 'celiac-free' areas such as Sub-Saharan Africa and the Far East. In many developing countries, the frequency of CD is likely to increase in the near future given the diffuse tendency to adopt Western, gluten-rich dietary patterns. As most cases currently escape diagnosis all over the world, an effort should be made to increase the awareness of CD polymorphism. A cost-effective case-finding policy and new strategies of mass CD screening could significantly reduce the morbidity and mortality associated with untreated disease. The current high prevalence of CD is just the last link in a chain of events started about 10,000 years ago after wheat domestication and diffusion from the Middle East. We hypothesize different mechanisms to explain the so-called evolutionary celiac paradox of colocalization of gluten consumption and HLA CD-predisposing genotypes.

Introduction

In the past, celiac disease (CD) was considered a rare disorder, mostly affecting individuals of European origin, usually characterized by onset during the first years of life. At that time, diagnosis was entirely based on the detection of typical gastrointestinal symptoms and confirmation by the small-intestinal biopsy. The emergence of highly sensitive and specific serological tools, first the antigliadin and later the antiendomysium and the anti-transglutaminase antibodies, showed an unsuspected frequency of clinically atypical or even silent forms of CD. Using these sensitive serological tools, a huge number of studies have shown that CD is one of the commonest, lifelong disorders affecting mankind all over the world [1]. This widespread diffusion is not surprising at all, given that causal factors, i.e. HLA CD-predisposing genotypes (DQ2 and DQ8) and consumption of gluten-containing cereals,

0257–2753/15/0332–0141$39.50/0

E-Mail karger@karger.com
www.karger.com/ddi

Prof. Carlo Catassi
Department of Pediatrics, Università Politecnica delle Marche
Via F. Corridoni 11
IT–60123 Ancona (Italy)
E-Mail c.catassi@univpm.it

Table 1. Percent prevalence of selected CD-predisposing haplotypes in the world

Population	DQ2 (cis)	DQ8
Saharawi	23.0	2.7
Sardinia	22.4	5.0
Iran	20.0	12.0
Turkey	18.0	22.0
USA	13.1	4.2
Algeria	11.2	2.2
Scandinavia	11.0	15.0
North India	9.0	15.6
Italy	9.0	2.0
Cameroon	9.0	0.6
South African Blacks	6.2	2.8
Inuit	6.1	0
Gipsy	6.0	0
Mongolia	5.2	4.4
North American Indians	4.5	25.3
Japan	0.6	7.6
Mexico	0	28.3
Cayapa	0	41
Bushman	0	30.2
Highlanders (PNG)	0	0

PNG = Papua New Guinea.

show a worldwide distribution (table 1). CD is not only frequent in developed countries, but is increasingly reported in areas of the developing world, especially North Africa, the Middle East and India. CD can contribute substantially to childhood morbidity and mortality in many developing countries [2].

The knowledge of CD geographical distribution can help to clarify the complex interaction between genetic and environmental factors underlying this complex disorder. The aims of this review are (a) to present an updated picture of CD epidemiology, and (b) to briefly discuss the theoretical and practical issues arising from the knowledge of the geoepidemiology of this frequent disorder.

CD Frequency and Trends in Countries Populated by People of European Origin

In Western countries, several recent studies evaluated the overall prevalence of CD in the general population, usually by counting the number of clinically diagnosed CD patients plus those detected by serological screening of a population sample. In Europe and the USA, the mean frequency of CD in the general population is approximately 1%, with some regional differences, the reasons for which remain elusive. The prevalence of CD is as high as 2–3% in Finland and Sweden, whereas it is only 0.2% in Germany, although these areas share a similar distribution of causal factors (level of gluten intake and frequency of HLA-DQ2 and -DQ8). Although the incidence of clinically diagnosed CD cases is increasing, the larger part of the 'celiac iceberg' remains undetected, with a ratio of 1:3–1:5 between diagnosed and undiagnosed cases [3–5]. A 6.4-fold increase in incidence has been recently described in Scotland from 1990 to 2009 and particularly classical cases of CD are increasing, indicating a true rise in the incidence of pediatric CD [6]. This finding is mostly related to increased awareness of CD clinical polymorphism, as well as wider use of serological CD screening tests.

In Western countries, a true rise in overall CD prevalence of CD has also been documented [7]. A recent US study showed that CD prevalence was only 0.2% in the year 1975, and increased 5-fold during the following 35 years [8]. The reasons for these changes are unclear, but have to do with the environmental components of CD (changes in the quantity and quality of ingested gluten, infant feeding patterns, the spectrum of intestinal infections, gut microbiota colonization, etc.).

Apart from Europe and North America, the epidemiology of CD has been investigated in many other countries mostly populated by individuals of European origin. The disease epidemiology reported from these areas (e.g. Australia, New Zealand and Argentina) largely overlaps with European and American data [9]. A serologic CD screening was recently performed in a representative sample of a young adult general population in Israel. The prevalence of overt CD diagnosed before recruitment was 0.12% (0.1% in men and 0.14% in women). The overall prevalence based on positive serology was 1.1%. Six of 9 subjects with positive serology underwent endoscopy showing histological changes compatible with CD. The ratio of overt to silent CD was 1:8. These findings suggested that CD is highly prevalent in the young adult population in Israel [10].

CD Epidemiology in Other Areas of the World

CD is a common disorder in North Africa and Middle East countries as well; however, the diagnostic rate is mostly low in these countries due to low availability of diagnostic facilities and poor disease awareness. In the classical Anderson's textbook of *Pediatric Gastroenterology*, first published in 1975, the following was reported: 'The typical child with celiac disease, usually fair-haired, blue-eyed…'. The subsequent developments of CD epidemiology proved that this statement was incorrect. The highest CD prevalence in the world has indeed been described in a black-eyed, black-haired African population originally living in Western Sahara, the Saharawi, of Arab-Berber origin. In a sample of 990 Saharawi children screened by antiendomysium testing and intestinal biopsy, we found a CD prevalence of 5.6%, which is almost 5-fold higher than in most European countries [11]. The reasons for this spiking CD frequency are unclear but could be primarily related to genetic factors given the high level of consanguinity of this population. The main susceptibility genotypes, HLA-DQ2 and -DQ8, exhibit one of the highest frequencies in the world in the general background Saharawi population [12]. Gluten consumption is very high as well since wheat flour is the staple food of the Saharawi refugees. CD in the Saharawi children can be a severe disease characterized by chronic diarrhea, stunting, anemia, and increased mortality. There are only anecdotal reports of CD in Sub-Saharan African countries.

The knowledge of the epidemiology of CD in the Asia Pacific region is still limited and mostly confined to India, where CD is being more frequently recognized, both in children and adults. However, as efficiently described by an Indian task force, CD in India is 'submerged in an ocean of malnutrition' [13]. The frequency of CD in India seems to be higher in the northern part of the country, the so-called celiac belt, a finding that is at least partially explained by the wheat-rice shift from the north to the south. The prevalence of CD amongst apparently healthy blood donors (n = 1,610) was 1:179 (0.56%) [14], a finding that overlaps with data from Western countries. In a large population sample (n = 2,879), Makharia et al. [15] found CD prevalence to be 1.04% (1 in 96) and the prevalence of positive serological test (anti-transglutaminase antibodies) to be 1.44% (1 in 69). Based on these data, it is estimated that 5–8 million people are expected to have CD in India. Of such a large pool of patients, only a few thousand patients have been diagnosed so far. If there is a real difference in the prevalence of CD in northern and southern parts of India, India may prove to be a model to understand the interplay between genetics and environmental causes of CD. With >1.3 billion people, China is the most populous nation and the second largest by land area in the world. Both CD-causing factors – gluten consumption (particularly in the northern part of the country) and the HLA CD-predisposing genotypes DQ2 and DQ8 (even though with a lower prevalence than in Western countries) – are largely diffused in China [16]. Nevertheless, the evidence of the existence of CD in this huge population has been poor so far. In a recent series of 118 children with chronic diarrhea admitted to pediatric hospitals from 4 major Chinese cities (Shanghai, Wuhan, Jinan, and Chengdu), serology and duodenal biopsy results were consistent with CD diagnosis in 14 patients [17]. CD is on the map in China, too. However, epidemiological studies are needed to quantify the impact of this condition in this country. Finally, CD is likely to be rare in Japan, Indonesia, Korea, the Philippines and many smaller Pacific islands because of low wheat consumption and a low frequency of HLA-DQ2.

The Celiac Iceberg

The epidemiology of CD is efficiently conceptualized by the iceberg model, which retains its validity across different populations in the world [1]. The prevalence of CD can be conceived as the overall size of the iceberg, which is not only influenced by the frequency of the predisposing genotypes in the population, but also by the pattern of gluten consumption. In many countries, the prevalence of CD is roughly in the range of 0.5–1% of the general population. A sizable portion of these cases is properly diagnosed because of suggestive complaints (e.g. chronic diarrhea, unexplained iron deficiency) or other reasons (e.g. family history of CD). These cases make up the visible part of the celiac iceberg, in quantitative terms expressed by the incidence of the disease. In developed countries, for each diagnosed case of CD, an average of 5–10 cases remain undiagnosed (the submerged part of the iceberg), usually because of atypical, minimal or even absent complaints. These undiagnosed cases remain untreated and are therefore exposed to the risk of long-term complications. The 'water line', namely the ratio of diagnosed to undiagnosed cases, mostly depends on the physician's tendency to request serological CD markers in situations of low clinical suspicion, i.e. awareness of CD clinical polymorphism.

Concerning policies of disease detection, the debate on mass screening versus case finding is still open given that both policies present pros and cons (fig. 1). So far, case-finding has been the common approach to the iceberg of undiagnosed CD. Case-finding in at-risk groups minimizes costs and is ethically appropriate. Increased awareness of the clinical polymorphism of CD coupled with a low threshold for serological testing can theoretically uncover a large portion of the submerged CD iceberg,

	Pros	Cons
Scr	• Highly sensitive • Higher impact on CD-associated morbidity and mortality	• Treatment is different in silent cases • Expensive
CF	• Effective • Cheap • Ethically sound	• At least 50% of cases escape diagnosis

Color version available online

Fig. 1. Pros and cons of CD mass screening (Scr) and case-finding (CF).

primary care being the natural setting of this selective screening. However, the case-finding process has proven to be a poorly effective strategy [18]. The proportion of clinically detected CD remains lower than 30% even in countries with high disease awareness, such as Norway [19], and may be critically low in developing countries. On the other hand, there are new arguments in favor of mass screening that deserve consideration. The recently increased prevalence of gluten-related disorders (not only CD but also nonceliac gluten sensitivity) is contributing to break down barriers against the gluten-free diet (GFD), with the consequence that gluten-free food is more easily and diffusely available at lower prices [20]. The public attitude toward the GFD is also favorably changing. Interestingly, a recent Swedish survey among patients with screening-detected CD and their families showed that the most common opinion among both adolescents and parents was that future CD mass screening should be 'a right for everyone' and should be offered as early as possible [21]. At what age could a general CD screening be performed? New data on the natural history of gluten sensitization shed light on this previously unanswered question. In a cohort of newborns at family risk of CD prospectively followed from birth, it was found that the large majority of subjects developed CD autoimmunity within the first 5 years of life and 80% during the first 3 years [22]. These results suggest that efficient screening for CD may be carried out by testing school-age children. There is indeed a single country in the world where mass CD screening during childhood is the rule since the year 1993. In the small San Marino Republic (32,538 inhabitants in the year 2011), general CD screening is performed regularly in children at entry in primary school (age 6 years), at low cost and with a positive acceptance by the population. The screening program led to increased disease awareness among doctors and to the general education of people about CD. The screening program self-amplified because often nonsymptomatic relatives of affected children were investigated and diagnosed with CD [23].

We are aware that there are still several arguments, particularly economic considerations, against CD screening. Nevertheless, it is time to reconsider a more active policy of serological CD testing in our view, e.g. performing the anti-transglutaminase determination at least once in children undergoing blood testing for any reason [24].

The Geoepidemiology of Gluten Consumption and HLA CD-Predisposing Genotypes: A Clue to the History of CD

A recent geoepidemiological analysis [25] highlighted the paradoxical distribution of CD and its causative factors in the world, which are best exemplified by findings in Europe and the Middle East.

Domestication of gluten-containing cereals (particularly ancient varieties of wheat and barley) began approximately 10,000 years ago in Neolithic settlements in the northeastern (Turkey, Iran, and Iraq) and in the southwestern (Palestine, Syria, and Lebanon) regions of the so-called Fertile Crescent area. Cultivation of wheat and barley slowly spread northwestward across Europe to reach Western countries, as Britain, 'only' 4,000 years ago [26]. The agriculture revolution paved the way to new diseases, such as CD. Since treatment with the GFD was not available in the ancient time, the CD geno-/phenotype could have exerted a negative impact on human reproductive fitness and survival over 1,000 years. As a consequence of a prolonged negative selective pressure, CD and the genotypes predisposing to it should be less common in the Middle East than in European countries (as originally theorized by Simoons [27]). On the contrary, nowadays CD is equally common in the UK and Turkey, and the frequency of HLA-DQ2 (the major CD-predisposing haplotype) is even higher in Turkey and Iran, i.e. countries consuming more wheat and for a longer duration of time than Finland and Ireland, i.e. countries consuming less gluten and for a shorter duration of time. This evolutionary celiac paradox is strengthened by the co-localization of gluten consumption and HLA-DQ2 observed in other areas of the world, e.g. Africa and India. To explain these counterintuitive findings, we suggested that the high diffusion of the HLA CD-predisposing genotypes and the diffusion of the high prevalence of CD are unrelated phenomena that occurred at different times. The currently high prevalence of CD is most likely a recent event explained by recent changes in environmental conditions that occurred in the last centuries/decades, e.g. related to the quantity and quality of ingested gluten, dough fermentation, human intestinal microbioma and pattern of infant nutrition [8, 28].

On the other hand, the parallel geographical distribution of gluten intake and HLA-DQ2 and DQ8 genotypes could be explained by different mechanisms which are not mutually exclusive:

(a) A founder effect reflecting the higher prevalence of DQ2/DQ8 in the early farmers that 10,000 years ago spread from the Middle East and gradually colonized Europe determining a South/East-North/West genetic gradient (so-called demic diffusion model of Cavalli-Sforza and Ammerman) between the Middle East and Europe (local effect) [29]. This slow 'wave of advance' of a population of early farmers with a high frequency of DQ2 and DQ8 could lead to progressive dilution of their genetic background by mixing with the local European populations.

(b) A positive selection of HLA CD-predisposing genotypes pushed by protection against deleterious conditions driven by the agricultural revolution (worldwide effect). An extensive search of the literature showed that only one disease is partially 'protected' by an HLA-DQ, CD-predisposing haplotype (DQ2), which is dental caries. A recent Brazilian study showed that adolescents positive for the HLA-DQ2 allele were less likely to have dental caries than their counterparts who were negative for this allele (OR = 0.33, CI 0.16–0.66) [30]. Nothing was found about disease protection induced by the HLA-DQ8 haplotype.

Dental caries is the typical Neolithic disease that dramatically increased after wheat carbohydrates acquired a primary role in human diet [31]. Interestingly, CD patients show a reduced prevalence of dental caries when compared to controls, despite high incidence of dental enamel hypoplasia [32]. *Streptococcus mutans*, the principal agent responsible for oral fermentation of sugars leading to dental caries, is less abundant in the intestinal mucosa of CD children, regardless of inflammatory status [33]. The consumption of wheat is positively correlated with the development of dental caries, whereas rice, the typical gluten-free cereal, shows less cariogenic potential. In the context of the ancestral wheat-consuming society, when cure and prevention of dental caries were basically nonexistent, some sort of genetically determined resistance to dental caries could well drive a positive selection of HLA-DQ2. It remains to be elucidated how DQ2 positivity protects from dental caries development, e.g. by accelerating the clearance of 'sticky' (and possibly cariogenic) gluten peptides from the mouth and teeth surface. The DQ2-dental caries protection hypothesis needs to find confirmation by further population studies.

Explanation b is more generalizable than a and could explain the high gluten/high DQ2 co-localization in different, apparently unrelated areas of the world such as Europe, Africa and India. Thus, the highest prevalence of DQ2 among wheat-consuming populations could be another example of evolutionary adaptation driven by the dietary changes imposed by the agricultural revolution, in analogy to lactase persistence in milk-drinking populations [34] and glucose-6-phosphate deficiency in Mediterranean populations consuming broad beans [35]. In this context, CD could simply represent the modern 'dark side' of a genetic structure (DQ2 positivity) conferring resistance to a negative consequence of a wheat-based diet.

Conclusions

CD is one of the commonest lifelong disorders in countries populated by individuals of European origin, affecting approximately 1% of the general population. This is a common disease also in North Africa, the Middle East and India. The huge prevalence of CD in the Saharawi people (5.6%) is an outlier finding probably related to strong genetic predisposition and abrupt dietary changes. CD in the Saharawi children as well as in other developing countries is sometimes a severe disease characterized by chronic diarrhea, stunting, anemia, and increased mortality. Further studies are needed to quantify the incidence of the celiac condition in apparently 'celiac-free' areas as Sub-Saharan Africa and the Far East. In many developing countries, the frequency of CD is likely to increase in the near future, given the diffuse tendency to adopt Western, gluten-rich dietary pattern. As most cases currently escape diagnosis all over the world, an effort should be made to increase the awareness of CD polymorphism. A cost-effective case-finding policy and new strategies of mass CD screening could significantly reduce the morbidity and mortality associated with untreated disease.

The current high prevalence of CD is just the last link in a chain of events started about 10,000 years ago after wheat domestication and diffusion from the Middle East. We hypothesize different mechanisms to explain the so-called evolutionary celiac paradox of co-localization of gluten consumption and HLA CD-predisposing genotypes. We suggest a primary role for: (a) a founder effect related to the demic diffusion of Middle East farmers into

Europe and (b) positive selection of the major CD-predisposing haplotype, that is HLA-DQ2, in wheat-consuming populations. The driving force of HLA-DQ2 selection could have been protection against dental caries, a disease that certainly had a tremendous negative impact on the health and reproductive fitness of ancient populations. The DQ2-dental caries protection hypothesis needs to find confirmation in further population studies.

Disclosure Statement

Carlo Catassi served as a consultant for Menarini Diagnostics s.r.l., for Dr. Shaer and for the Heinz Company. Elena Lionetti served as a consultant for the Heinz Company.

References

1 Fasano A, Catassi C: Clinical practice. Celiac disease. N Engl J Med 2012;367:2419–2426.
2 Catassi C, Gatti S, Fasano A: The new epidemiology of celiac disease. J Pediatr Gastroenterol Nutr 2014;59(suppl 1):S7–S9.
3 Mustalahti K, Catassi C, Reunanen A, et al: The prevalence of celiac disease in Europe: results of a centralized, international mass screening project. Ann Med 2010;42:587–595.
4 Fasano A, Berti I, Gerarduzzi T, et al: Prevalence of celiac disease in at-risk and not-at-risk groups in the United States: a large multicenter study. Arch Int Med 2003;163:286–292.
5 Ivarsson A, Myléus A, Norström F, et al: Prevalence of childhood celiac disease and changes in infant feeding. Pediatrics 2013;131:e687–e694.
6 White LE, Merrick VM, Bannerman E, et al: The rising incidence of celiac disease in Scotland. Pediatrics 2013;132:e924–e931.
7 Rubio-Tapia A, Ludvigsson JF, Brantner TL, et al: The prevalence of celiac disease in the United States. Am J Gastroenterol 2012;107:1538–1544.
8 Catassi C, Kryszak D, Bhatti B, et al: Natural history of celiac disease autoimmunity in a USA cohort followed since 1974. Ann Med 2010;42:530–538.
9 Bai JC, Fried M, Corazza GR, et al: World gastroenterology organization global guidelines on celiac disease. J Clin Gastroenterol 2013;47:121–126.
10 Israeli E, Hershcovici T, Grotto I, et al: Prevalence of celiac disease in an adult Jewish population in Israel. Isr Med Assoc J 2010;12:266–269.
11 Catassi C, Rätsch IM, Gandolfi L, et al: Why is coeliac disease endemic in the people of Sahara? Lancet 1999;354:647–648.
12 Catassi C, Doloretta Macis M, Rätsch IM, De Virgilis S, Cucca F: The distribution of DQ genes in the Saharawi population provides only a partial explanation for the high celiac disease prevalence. Tissue Antigens 2001;58:402–406.
13 Gupta R, Reddy DN, Makharia GK, et al: Indian task force for celiac disease: current status. World J Gastroenterol 2009;15:6028–6033.
14 Kochhar R, Dachdev S, Aggarwal A, et al: Prevalence of coeliac disease in healthy blood donors: a study from north India. Dig Liver Dis 2012;44:530–532.
15 Makharia GK, Verma AK, Amarchand R, et al: Prevalence of celiac disease in the northern part of India: a community based study. J Clin Gastroenterol 2011;26:894–900.
16 Yuan J, Gao J, Li X, Liu F, Wijmenga C, Chen H, Gilissen LJ: The tip of the 'celiac iceberg' in China. Systematic review and meta-analysis. PLoS One 2013;8:e81151.
17 Wang X, Liu W, Xu C, et al: Celiac disease in children with diarrhea in 4 cities of China. J Pediatr Gastroenterol Nutr 2011;53:368–370.
18 Catassi C, Lionetti E: Case finding for celiac disease is ok, but is it enough? J Pediatr Gastroenterol Nutr 2013;57:415–417.
19 Størdal K, Bakken IJ, Surén P, Stene LC: Epidemiology of coeliac disease and comorbidity in Norwegian children. J Pediatr Gastroenterol Nutr 2013;57:467–471.
20 Catassi C, Bai JC, Bonaz B, et al: Non-celiac gluten sensitivity: the new frontier of gluten-related disorders. Nutrients 2013;5:3839–3853.
21 Rosén A, Emmelin M, Carlsson A, Hammarroth S, Karlsson E, Ivarsson A: Mass screening for celiac disease from the perspective of newly diagnosed adolescents and their parents: a mixed-method study. BMC Public Health 2011;11:822.
22 Lionetti E, et al: Infant feeding pattern, HLA status, and prevalence of celiac disease, in press.
23 Alessandrini S, Giacomoni E, Muccioli F: Mass population screening for celiac disease in children: the experience in Republic of San Marino from 1993 to 2009. Ital J Pediatr 2013;39:67.
24 Catassi C, Fasano A: Coeliac disease: the debate on coeliac disease screening – are we there yet? Nat Rev Gastroenterol Hepatol 2014;11:457–458.
25 Lionetti E, Catassi C: Co-localization of gluten consumption and HLA-DQ2 and -DQ8 genotypes: a clue to the history of celiac disease. Dig Liver Dis 2014, Epub ahead of print.
26 Barada K, Abu Daya H, Rostami K, Catassi C: Celiac disease in the developing world. Gastrointest Endosc Clin N Am 2012;22:773–796.
27 Simoons FJ: Coeliac disease as a geographic problem; in Walcher DN, Kretchmer N (eds): Food, Nutrition and Evolution. New York, Masson, 1981, pp 179–199.
28 Catassi C, Anderson RP, Hill ID, et al: World perspective on celiac disease. J Pediatr Gastroenterol Nutr 2012;55:494–499.
29 Ammerman AJ, Cavalli-Sforza LL: The Neolithic Transition and the Genetics of Populations in Europe. Princeton, Princeton University Press, 1984, p 176.
30 Valarini N, Maciel SM, Moura SK, Poli-Frederico RC: Association of dental caries with HLA class II allele in Brazilian adolescents. Caries Res 2012;46:530–535.
31 Larsen CS: The agricultural revolution as environmental catastrophe: implications for health and lifestyle in the Holocene. Quat Int 2006;150:12–20.
32 Pastore L, Carroccio A, Compilato D, et al: Oral manifestations of celiac disease. J Clin Gastroenterol 2008;42:224–232.
33 Sánchez E, Donat E, Ribes-Koninckx C, Fernández-Murga L, Sanz Y: Duodenal-mucosal bacteria associated with celiac disease in children. Appl Environ Microbiol 2013;79:5472–5479.
34 Tishkoff SA, Reed FA, Ranciaro A, et al: Convergent adaptation of human lactase persistence in Africa and Europe. Nat Genet 2007;39:31–40.
35 Mehta A, Mason PJ, Vulliamy TJ: Glucose-6-phosphate dehydrogenase deficiency. Baillieres Best Pract Res Clin Haematol 2000;13:21–38.

Celiac Disease: Clinical Perspective

Dig Dis 2015;33:147–154
DOI: 10.1159/000369541

Extraintestinal Manifestations of Celiac Disease

María Inés Pinto-Sánchez[a] Premysl Bercik[a] Elena F. Verdu[a] Julio C. Bai[b, c]

[a]Farncombe Family Digestive Health Institute, McMaster University, Hamilton, Ont., Canada; [b]Gastroenterology, Universidad del Salvador, and [c]Dr. Carlos Bonorino Udaondo Gastroenterology Hospital, Buenos Aires, Argentina

Key Words
Celiac disease · Extraintestinal manifestations · Diagnosis

Abstract
Case finding for celiac disease (CD) is becoming increasingly common practice and is conducted in a wide range of clinical situations ranging from the presence of gastrointestinal symptoms to failure to thrive in children, prolonged fatigue, unexpected weight loss and anemia. Case finding is also performed in associated conditions, such as autoimmune thyroid disease, dermatitis herpetiformis and type 1 diabetes, as well as in patients with irritable bowel syndrome, unexplained neuropsychiatric disorders and first-degree relatives of patients with diagnosed CD. This aggressive active case finding has dramatically changed the clinical characteristics of newly diagnosed patients. For instance, higher numbers of patients who present with extraintestinal symptoms are now being diagnosed with CD. Current recommendations state that due to a high risk for complications if the disease remains undiagnosed, patients with extraintestinal symptoms due to CD require appropriate diagnosis and treatment. Despite criticism regarding the cost-effectiveness of case finding in CD, such an aggressive approach has been considered cost-effective for high-risk patients. The diagnosis of CD among patients with extraintestinal symptoms requires a high degree of awareness of the clinical conditions that carry a high risk for underlying CD. Also, understanding the correct use of specific serology and duodenal histology is key for an appropriate diagnostic approach. Both procedures combined are able to confirm diagnosis in the vast majority of cases. However, in certain circumstances, serology and even duodenal histology cannot confirm or rule out CD. A common cause of negative IgA serology is IgA deficiency. For such eventuality, IgG-based serological tests can help confirm the diagnosis. Importantly, some histologically diagnosed cases still remain seronegative despite exclusion of IgA deficiency. On the other hand, duodenal histology may be normal despite the presence of CD-specific antibodies and active CD. This has been clearly demonstrated in some cases of untreated dermatitis herpetiformis, but may also be due to the patchy condition of CD or lesions that are not adequately recognized by nonexpert endoscopists and/or pathologists. The effectiveness of agluten-free diet depends on the clinical end point addressed. A good example is the outcome of bone loss. While risk for fracture normalizes after the first year of dietary treatment, bone parameters measured by densitometry may not be normalized in the long-term follow-up. Moreover, it is still unclear how far an early gluten-free diet will positively affect associated autoimmune diseases like type 1 diabetes and autoimmune thyroiditis.

KARGER 125

© 2015 S. Karger AG, Basel
0257–2753/15/0332–0147$39.50/0

E-Mail karger@karger.com
www.karger.com/ddi

Prof. Julio C. Bai
Dr. Carlos Bonorino Udaondo Gastroenterology Hospital
Av. Caseros 2061
Buenos Aires 1264 (Argentina)
E-Mail jbai@intramed.net

Introduction

The 'Oslo consensus' has recently defined celiac disease (CD) as a chronic small intestinal immune-mediated enteropathy precipitated by exposure to dietary gluten in genetically predisposed individuals [1]. Traditionally, patients with CD presented with malabsorption dominated by diarrhea, steatorrhea, weight loss or failure to thrive ('classical CD'). However, the proportion of newly diagnosed patients with malabsorptive symptoms has decreased over time, and CD with 'non-classical' and even asymptomatic presentation is gaining prominence [2]. The current awareness of CD complications in combination with the advent of highly sensitive and specific serological tests has dramatically increased the identification of patients among subjects having a higher risk for the disorder [3]. Case finding is now becoming more common and is conducted in a wide range of clinical situations ranging from the presence of gastrointestinal symptoms (diarrhea, abdominal pain and distension), failure to thrive in children [4, 5], prolonged fatigue [6], unexpected weight loss, recurrent aphthous stomatitis, anemia [7], increased liver transaminases [8] and unexplained neuropsychiatric disorder [9]. Case finding is also recommended in conditions that associate with CD such as autoimmune thyroid disease, dermatitis herpetiformis (DH) and type 1 diabetes [7], and in patients with irritable bowel syndrome associated with diarrhea and first-degree relatives of celiacs [10, 11]. This aggressive active case finding introduced in the last decades has dramatically changed the clinical characteristics of newly diagnosed patients. In such context, increasing numbers of CD patients are now diagnosed who present with an extraintestinal phenotype and a diversity of symptoms affecting many different systems.

The present review aims to analyze the most common extraintestinal manifestations of CD and proposes an appropriate diagnostic workup. We also discuss the effect of the gluten-free diet (GFD) on these extraintestinal manifestations of CD.

Hematologic Manifestations of CD

CD is a common systemic disorder that can present with multiple hematologic manifestations prior to receiving a diagnosis of CD [12]. Iron deficiency anemia (IDA) without other clinical clues of intestinal malabsorption, is one of the most common extraintestinal manifestations of the disorder being encountered in around 50% of patients with subclinical phenotype [13]. This is considered the most frequent extraintestinal feature of the condition [14]. Evidence suggests that IDA, as the leading symptom, is more frequent in adults than in children [13, 14], and it is usually due to either increased iron loss or impaired absorption of iron, folate or vitamin B_{12}, although occult blood loss from the gastrointestinal tract may occur [13, 15]. Bergamaschi et al. [16] have suggested that anemia of chronic diseases is due to immune activation and defective production of endogenous erythropoietin in a significant proportion of patients at presentation. The treatment of anemia associated with CD is primarily a GFD. Iron supplementation is usually indicated for the treatment of IDA associated with CD until the iron stores have been restored, which could take up to 2 years [12].

Thrombocytosis is also frequently seen in CD, occurring in up to 60% of patients [12, 17, 18]. The presence of inflammatory mediators, iron deficiency and hyposplenism have all been proposed as contributing factors [12]. The thrombocytopenia associated with CD usually improves with specific treatment [12, 17].

Defective splenic function affects more than one third of adult patients with symptomatic CD, and it may predispose to a higher risk of infections by encapsulated bacteria and thromboembolic and autoimmune complications [19]. The prevalence of hyposplenism increases from 19% in CD to 80% in CD with premalignant or malignant complications, and it is associated with a poor prognosis factor in CD [19, 20]. However, the evaluation of splenic function is not considered as a regular procedure in the clinical management of patients with non-complicated CD, and in patients with a high degree of hyposplenism or splenic atrophy the prophylactic immunization with specific vaccines against the polysaccharide antigens of encapsulated bacteria remains controversial [19]. As demonstrated by Corazza et al. [20], the splenic hypofunction measured by pitted cells improves at least partially in some CD patients and even reverts to normal after 3–12 months of GFD.

IgA deficiency is the most common primary immunodeficiency in Caucasians that is strongly overrepresented among patients with CD accounting for ~5% (CD) [12, 21]. The importance of the association is due to the fact that IgA-deficient individuals are prone to other enteric conditions such as inflammatory bowel disease or chronic parasite infections, especially giardiasis, and even to developing anaphylactic transfusion reactions that may be life-threatening [12]. The diagnosis of CD could be challenging in this population that by definition will show false-negative IgA type CD-specific antibodies. IgG anti-

Table 1. Extraintestinal manifestations of CD

System affected	Extraintestinal manifestation	Estimated prevalence in CD	Comments	Ref.
Hematological	Anemia	~50%	Most commonly secondary to iron deficiency but may be multifactorial in etiology; low serum levels of folate and vitamin B_{12} without anemia are frequently seen	12
	Thrombocytosis	up to 60%	Possibly secondary to iron deficiency or hyposplenism	
	Hyposplenism	~19%	Possibly associated with increased risk for infections	
	IgA deficiency	~5–10%	CD patients have 10-fold increased risk for IgA deficiency; IgA deficiency predisposes to other enteric conditions	
	Leukopenia/neutropenia/ thrombocytopenia	<1%	Leukopenia possibly associated with deficit in folate and copper	
Mucocutaneous	DH	~15–25%	Proved association; skin manifestation of CD	24–26, 30
	Psoriasis	~4%	In CD, psoriasis responds to GFD	
	AA	~1%	Prevalence of CD is up to 41% in AA	
	Urticaria/atopic dermatitis	~5%	AD is 4 times more frequent in CD patients than in normal population	
	Chronic ulcerative stomatitis	~20%	Multifactorial; autoimmune and genetic factors play a role; does not always respond to GFD	
Bones	Osteopenia/osteoporosis	~50%	Affects 50% of nontreated CD; multifactorial etiology: malabsorption, inflammation, immunology and autoimmunity	45, 46
	Fractures	~50%	Multifactorial etiology; CD clinical presentation and gender influence	
Neurologic	Peripheral neuropathy	49%	Most common neurologic affection in CD	48–52
	Gluten ataxia	<1%	TTG6 prevalent in gluten ataxia. Sensitivity increases up to 85% if anti-gliadin antibodies are present	
	Epilepsy	~1–5%	Frequently associated with occipital calcifications	
	Migraines	~50%	Response to treatment with a GFD	
Psychological	Anxiety	~23%	State, but not trait anxiety might be associated with CD	62–69
	Depression	~50%	Response to GFD	70–72
	Chronic fatigue		Unclear response to GFD specific for CD	72–74
Liver	Hypertransaminasemia	6%	Associated with immunity and severity of duodenal affection	76–78
Gynecologic	Infertility	~15%	5-fold increased risk for CD	79–81
	Recurrent abortions	~15%	8-fold increased risk for CD	

bodies against tissue transglutaminase (tTG) and deamidated gliadin peptides (DGP) serve as serological markers for CD in IgA-deficient individuals, although the diagnostic value remains uncertain. Furthermore, the levels of IgG antibodies appear to decrease slowly in IgA-deficient CD patients despite being on a GFD for a long period [21]. This makes the follow-up of this population based on serological markers difficult. Leukopenia, neutropenia and thrombocytopenia have also been reported rarely in CD patients. Both have been related to folate and copper deficiency [22], and supplements containing these nutrients along with a GFD are proposed as treatment for these particular cases [12].

Mucocutaneous Manifestations of CD

Mucocutaneous diseases often accompany the diagnosis of CD. Among them, DH, psoriasis, atopic dermatitis (AD), urticaria, nodular prurigo, alopecia areata (AA) and chronic ulcerative stomatitis are the most frequently reported [23]. The most important skin disease closely associated with CD is DH, currently considered as the cutaneous manifestation of CD [24]. The condition was initially described by L. Duhring in 1983 and is considered an autoimmune disorder affecting more frequently adults and males [25]. It is clinically characterized by a polymorphism consisting of erythema, urticarial plaques, papules, grouped vesicles and blisters associated with intense itch and therefore followed by erosions, excoriations, and hyperpigmentation [24]. The lesions are distributed on the extensor areas of elbows and knees and over the buttocks and on the scalp [2]. The diagnosis of DH is based on physical examination, histopathology, immunofluorescence studies, and serologic testing. A biopsy of the skin in DH should be taken in the vicinity of the blister. Direct immunofluorescence of perilesional skin is considered the gold standard, with two typical patterns: (a) granular deposits of IgA in dermal papillae or (b) granular deposits of IgA along the basement membrane [24]. CD-specific serology performance varies according to the degree of enteropathy. The majority of tests available detect DH presenting with villous atrophy (VA). However, only 50% of DH cases without VA have positive serology. Evidence suggests that DGP antibodies are more sensitive and specific than tTG in detecting CD in patients with DH [26]. The first-line therapy of DH and CD is GFD that should continue even after lesions have disappeared. It usually takes several months to control the skin disease. For this reason, pharmacological treatment with dapsone, sulfasalazine, steroids and antihistamines could be used as adjuvant therapy [24].

A link between psoriasis and CD was proposed by early studies [27–30] and controverted by others [31]. The prevalence of CD increases 2–4-fold in the population with psoriasis. Psoriasis is a common chronic relapsing inflammatory disease of the skin, which affects about 2% of the general population and is characterized by scaling, erythema, and less commonly pustulation, and some patients even have affected nails and joints (psoriatic arthritis) [30]. Several mechanisms related to vitamin D deficiency [32], cross-reaction to gluten [33] and shared genetic factors [34]. The treatment of psoriasis is often difficult, and a subgroup of patients usually shows improvement only after adopting the GFD. This fact suggests pathogenic differences compared to nonceliac psoriatic patients [30].

AA is an autoimmune disorder affecting children and adults with an estimated prevalence in CD of 1/85 [30, 35]. The prevalence of CD in AA has been reported to be up to 41% [36], suggesting the need to screen for CD in AA. It is characterized by areas of hair loss that show a smooth nonscarred scalp with no obvious inflammation [35]. Although autoantibodies are postulated to play an integral role in the disease process, current research implicates a cell-mediated autoimmune mechanism as the underlying pathogenic mechanism [36]. The response of AA in CD patients to GFD is controversial. Some studies have reported a complete regrowth of scalp and other body hair in CD patients with AA [30, 37], while others did not find any response [38, 39].

AD is a multifactorial chronic inflammatory skin disease characterized by intense pruritus and relapsing eczematous skin lesions caused by congenital skin barrier defects, microbial colonization, and complex immune dysregulation [40]. Some earlier studies have demonstrated that atopic disorders are more common in CD than the general population, and the risk of CD was increased 4-fold in AD [40, 41]. Unfortunately, no data are available about the efficacy of GFD in atopic patients with CD.

Recurrent aphthous stomatitis (RAS) belongs to the group of chronic, inflammatory, ulcerative diseases of the oral mucosa. The etiopathogenesis of this condition is still unclear. It is, however, considered to be multifactorial [42]. The association between CD and RAS has been evaluated in different studies with controversial results. While some studies have reported an increased prevalence of CD in up to 31% of patients with RAS, others have failed to find this association [43]. The clinical response of RAS to a GFD in CD patients has been demonstrated in many different studies [43].

Osteopathy in CD

In the past two decades, the effect of CD on bone health has been extensively studied. CD predisposes to metabolic osteopathy, and bone loss may be detected in more than 50% of untreated CD patients. The pathogenesis of bone damage in CD is multifactorial, and both systemic and local mechanisms may play a role. Intestinal malabsorption secondary to mucosal lesions leads to calcium and vitamin D malabsorption which may produce secondary hyperparathyroidism [44]. Other local mechanisms, such as inflammation, IL-6 production and increased RANKL/OPG ratio may contribute to the pathogenesis of bone derangement [44]. Finally, an autoimmune pathogenesis involving tTG as autoantigen has been suggested.

Osteopenia or osteoporosis detected by bone mineral density measurements has been observed in >50% of patients at the time of their diagnosis of CD. Accumulating data show that low bone mineral density is more common in adults, and is present even when patients have atypical or asymptomatic CD at the time of diagnosis [45]. CD patients also have a higher risk of fractures compared with people without CD, as demonstrated by a recent meta-analysis [46]. The risk of fracture in CD is influenced by the type of clinical presentation and gender, with more fractures occurring in symptomatic cases and male patients [45].

As far as the need to measure bone mineral density in celiacs is concerned, several doubts are present. It is not clear which patients should undergo bone mass measurement, when the first and subsequent measurements should be performed, but also why measurement should be performed. For symptomatic CD, a bone mineral densitometry (BMD) should be done at diagnosis and after 1–2 years of a GFD; however, a baseline BMD seems unnecessary in subclinical CD [45].

Gluten restriction can significantly reverse the systemic and local physiological mechanisms of bone deterioration in CD patients. Although normalization of bone mass is unlikely in adult CD, significant remineralization of axial and peripheral skeleton has been demonstrated in several studies. However, reducing the risk of fracture does not solely depend on increasing bone mass and mineral density. Other risk factors, such as structural alteration of bones with impairment of the mechanical quality (stiffness of cortical bones), deterioration of body mass, fat and muscle compartments, and neuromuscular dysfunction, also contribute to bone weakness in CD patients. In this context, improving body mass and fat/muscle composition, nutritional status, and bone architecture through long-term GFD treatment have been shown to reduce the overall risk of fractures in CD patients [46].

Neurologic and Psychiatric Manifestations in CD

CD is associated with neurologic and psychiatric disorders including migraines, cerebellar ataxia, peripheral neuropathy, epilepsy, dementia, and depression, even though they do not present intestinal symptoms [47]. The prevalence of neurologic symptoms in CD has been estimated at around 7% [50]. Recently, peripheral neuropathy has been considered as the most common manifestation affecting up to 49% of patients with established CD, and the pathophysiological mechanism is not well known [47, 48], although a perivascular lymphocytic infiltration has been reported [48]. Chronic distal, symmetric, predominantly sensory neuropathy is described most commonly in patients with CD. However, pure motor neuropathy, mononeuritis multiplex, Guillain-Barré-like syndrome and autonomic neuropathy have also been reported [47]. The most common electrophysiologic finding is a mixed sensorimotor axonal peripheral neuropathy. Nevertheless, electrophysiologic studies can be normal or only mildly abnormal in many CD patients with neuropathy [47, 52]. The response of neuropathy to GFD remains unclear and controversial [47].

Cerebellar ataxia is one of the two most common neurological manifestations of gluten intolerance. Gluten ataxia, defined as ataxia associated with antigliadin antibodies, usually presents with pure cerebellar ataxia or, rarely, ataxia in combination with myoclonus, palatal tremor, opsoclonus, or chorea [48]. Often, it has an insidious onset and it is developed in adulthood. Interestingly, less than 10% of patients with gluten ataxia have gastrointestinal symptoms and a third will have evidence of enteropathy on biopsy [49]. Specific transglutaminase isoenzyme antibodies have been linked to particular gluten ataxia. Anti-TG2 or TG6 IgA antibodies are present in up to 38% of patients with gluten ataxia; however, the presence of these antibodies is increased up to 85% if antigliadin antibodies are also present. It is important to note that IgG class antibodies to TG2 in patients with gluten ataxia are more common than IgA [48]. MRI could also be used to test the previous cases, with cerebellar atrophy shown in up to 60% of patients with gluten ataxia [48]. Reports on the effect of GFD on ataxia have been inconsistent, and the outcome seems to depend on the duration of the neurologic affection [49].

The first report of an association between CD and epilepsy with occipital calcifications was performed in Italy more than 20 years ago [53]. CD with epilepsy and cerebral calcifications (CEC) is a neurological syndrome characterized by pharmacologically resistant occipital epilepsy [54, 55]. The prevalence of epilepsy in CD has been estimated at 1.2–5%. On the other hand, up to 77% of CEC are diagnosed with CD [56]. Previously, co-occurring folate deficiency in CEC has been thought to be contributory. The diagnosis is established based on clinical and serological findings as well as electroencephalography and neuroimaging. Clinically, seizures may consist of versive and/or visual seizures (simple hallucinations, amaurosis), visual seizures followed by complex seizures or secondary generalization. In the great majority of the patients, electroencephalography shows focal abnormalities (spike waves or slow waves), mainly localized to one or both occipital regions [56]. Specific serology, such as TG6 autoantibodies, has been suggested as a specific marker for the neurological manifestations, and they can also be found in CEC [55]. Typical CT features of CEC syndrome consist of bilaterally subcortical, roughly symmetrical or asymmetrical, occipital calcifications, absence of contrast enhancement, and absence of brain atrophy [56]. The treatment of epilepsy associated with CD is based on a GFD and supported by antiepileptic drugs. It has been demonstrated that the chances of seizure control after GFD seem to be significantly inversely related to the duration of epilepsy before diagnosis and to the age at the beginning of GFD [53]. Studies have suggested that headache is an atypical presentation of CD [57]. Migraine defined as a periodic, commonly unilateral, throbbing headache, with or without cerebral disturbance, with intervening periods free from headache and without evidence of primary structural abnormality, is the most frequent subtype of primary headache and might affect 15–18% of women and 6% of men in the general population [58]. The pathophysiology of migraine, as well as tension headache, involves personality and biochemical factors such as serotonin [59]. A study suggested that the 'aura phenomenon' is strictly associated with a reduction in regional cortical blood flow caused by ischemia, probably due to cerebral vasospasm [58]. It is possible that this phenomenon could explain the improvement in migraine symptoms after switching to a GFD [58, 59].

Psychological alterations, such as anxiety and depression, have also been described in CD patients. Although for more than 20 years several studies reported an increased prevalence of anxiety in CD patients [60–62], a recent meta-analysis with some limitations failed to confirm the association [63]. However, large studies on the topic are lacking, and most of them do not differentiate between state and trait anxiety. For instance, Addolorato et al. [61] suggested that a transitory 'state' anxiety, but not personality 'trait' anxiety, affected CD patients. The association of depression with CD has been described for more than 20 years [64, 65]. A recent study by our group [66] demonstrated an increased prevalence of depressive symptoms in untreated CD patients. Furthermore, the meta-analysis included 18 studies on depression that confirmed this condition is common in adult CD [63]. Different mechanisms have been proposed to explain the association of CD and psychological affection. Malabsorption of nutrients causing deficit of folate and hyperhomocysteinemia [67], and diseases such as hypothyroidism [68], and autoimmune disorders [69] may explain the association. The effect of a GFD on psychological affection is contradictory. While some studies support a beneficial effect of the GFD on anxiety and depression [66, 70], others suggested the contrary [61, 64, 65].

Fatigue is probably the most common presentation of CD, and conditions such as 'being tired all the time' have previously been underestimated [71]. However, there is now evidence from primary care of a surprisingly high frequency of unsuspected positive EMA tests in people with nonspecific symptoms, such as chronic fatigue. It has been recently suggested that patients with chronic fatigue should undergo case finding for CD [71]. There is some evidence that fatigue might respond to a GFD in the CD population [72, 73]. However, further evidence is required to understand whether the response is specific for CD since other disorders involving fatigue might benefit from this diet [74, 75].

Liver Affection in CD

CD is a relevant cause of hypertransaminasemia and also has been associated with other liver diseases, such as viral hepatitis, liver steatosis and primary sclerosing cholangitis [76]. In a recent meta-analysis, Sainsbury et al. [77] reported a pooled prevalence of a 6% yield of serologic testing and a 4% yield of biopsy-proven CD in patients with cryptogenic hypertransaminasemia. However, a prevalence up to 42% has been reported for hypertransaminasemia in the CD population. The mechanisms predisposing to hypertransaminasemia in CD have been associated with the clinical diagnosis of malabsorption and with the increasing severity of duodenal lesion [78]. Most of the evidence supports a beneficial effect of the GFD on the liver affection in CD [76–78].

Gynecological and Obstetric Disorders in CD

During the last decades, the association between CD and a wide range of reproductive disorders has been described in a growing number of papers, and it is now well recognized that the disorder may have implications on women's reproductive health [79]. Delayed menarche, early menopause, amenorrhea, infertility and spontaneous abortions have been frequently observed among CD patients [80]. A recent meta-analysis concluded that patients with unexplained infertility, recurrent miscarriage or intrauterine growth restriction have a nearly 5- to 8-fold increased risk of being affected by CD compared with the general population. The mechanisms proposed for impaired gynecological and obstetric health in CD are related to malabsorption of nutrients and autoimmunity [79]. Due to the increased prevalence and beneficial effect of the GFD on gynecological and obstetric health, serologic screening for CD is suggested in cases of unexplained infertility, recurrent miscarriage and intrauterine growth restriction [79, 81].

Conclusion

There is a clear increase in the occurrence of subclinical/silent CD, which currently is considered the most frequent clinical presentation of the disorder. Diagnosis of CD among patients with extraintestinal symptoms requires a high degree of awareness of clinical conditions that carry a high risk for underlying CD and the correct use of specific serology and duodenal histology. The GFD is an effective treatment for many of the extraintestinal manifestations of CD and is required to decrease the risk of complications associated with the celiac condition.

Acknowledgements

M.I.P.-S. received a CIHR-FHP Health Professional Award Fellowship. E.F.V. holds a CRC and is funded by a CIHR grant MOP No. 8-11836.

Disclosure Statement

The authors declare no conflict of interest.

References

1 Ludvigsson JF, Leffler DA, Bai JC, et al: The Oslo definitions for coeliac disease and related terms. Gut 2013;62:43–45.
2 Ludvigsson JF, Bai JC, Biagi F, et al: Diagnosis and management of adult coeliac disease: guidelines from the British Society of Gastroenterology. Gut 2014;63:1210–1228.
3 Rampertab SD, Pooran N, Brar P, et al: Trends in the presentation of celiac disease. Am J Med 2006;119:355.e9–e14.
4 Groll A, Candy DC, Preece MA, et al: Short stature as the primary manifestation of coeliac disease. Lancet 1980;ii:1097–1099.
5 Guandalini S, Assiri A: Celiac disease: a review. JAMA Pediatr 2014;168:272–278.
6 Sanders DS, Evans KE, Hadjivassiliou M: Fatigue in primary care. Test for coeliac disease first? BMJ 2010;341:c5161.
7 Rubio-Tapia A, Hill I, Ciaran PK, et al: ACG Clinical Guidelines: Diagnosis and Management of Celiac Disease. Am J Gastroenterol 2013;108:656–676.
8 Sainsbury A, Sanders DS, Ford AC: Meta-analysis: coeliac disease and hypertransaminasaemia. Aliment Pharmacol Ther 2012;34:33–40.
9 Addolorato G, Leggio L, D'Angelo C, et al: Affective and psychiatric disorders in celiac disease. Dig Dis 2008;26:140–148.
10 Rubio-Tapia A, Van Dyke CT, Lahr BD, et al: Predictors of family risk for celiac disease: a population-based study. Clin Gastroenterol Hepatol 2008;6:983–987.
11 Murray JA: Celiac disease in patients with an affected member, type 1 diabetes, iron-deficiency, or osteoporosis? Gastroenterology 2005;128:S52–S56.
12 Halfdanarson TR, Litzow MR, Murray JA: Hematologic manifestations of celiac disease Blood 2007;109:412–420.
13 Bottaro G, Cataldo F, Rotolo N, et al: The clinical pattern of subclinical/silent celiac disease: an analysis on 1026 consecutive cases. Am J Gastoenterol 1999;94:691–696.
14 Brandimarte G, Tursi A, Giorgetti GM: Changing trends in clinical form of celiac disease. Which is now the main form of celiac disease in clinical practice? Minerva Gastroenterol Dietol 2002;48:121–130.
15 Smukalla S, Lebwohl B, Mears JG, et al: How often do hematologists consider celiac disease in iron-deficiency anemia? Results of a national survey. Clin Adv Hematol Oncol 2014;12:100–105.
16 Bergamaschi G, Markopoulos K, Albertini R, et al: Anemia of chronic disease and defective erythropoietin production in patients with celiac disease. Haematologica 2008;93:1785–1791.
17 Nelson EW, Ertan A, Brooks FP, et al: Thrombocytosis in patients with celiac sprue. Gastroenterology 1976;70:1042–1044.
18 Caroccio A, Giannitrapani L, Di Prima L, et al: Extreme thrombocytosis as a sign of coeliac disease in the elderly; case report. Eur J Gastroenterol Hepatol 2002;14:897–900.
19 Di Sabatino A, Rosado MM, Cazzola P, et al: Splenic hypo function and the spectrum of autoimmune and malignant complications in celiac disease. Clin Gastroenterol Hepatol 2006;4:179–186.
20 Corazza GR, Frisoni M, Vaira D, et al: Effect of gluten-free diet on splenic hypofunction of adult coeliac disease. Gut 1983;24:228–230.
21 Wang N, Truedsson L, Elvin K, et al: Serological assessment for celiac disease in IgA deficient adults. PLoS One 2014;9:e93180.
22 Jameson B, Hollsing K, Magnusson S: Copper malabsorption in coeliac disease. Sci Total Environ 1985;42:29–36.
23 Bonciolini V, Antiga E, Fabbri P, et al: Skin manifestations of celiac disease: not always dermatitis herpetiformis. Int J Dermatol 2014;53:e352–e353.
24 Caproni M, Bonciolini V, D'Errico A, et al: Celiac disease and dermatologic manifestations: many skin clue to unfold gluten-sensitive enteropathy. Gastroenterol Res Pract 2012;2012:952753.
25 Bolotin D, Petronic-Rosic V: Dermatitis herpetiformis. 1. Epidemiology, pathogenesis and clinical presentation. J Am Acad Dermatol 2011;64:4–11.
26 Sugai E, Esmecuol E, Niveloni S, et al: Celiac disease serology in dermatitis herpetiformis. Which is the best option for detecting gluten sensitivity? Acta Gastroenterol Latinoam 2006;36:197–201.
27 Michaelsson G, Gerden B, Ottosson M, et al: Patients with psoriasis often have increased serum levels of IgA antibodies to gliadin. Br J Dermatol 1993;129:667–673.
28 Michaelsson G, Gerden B, Hagforsen E, et al: Psoriasis patients with antibodies to gliadin can be improved by a gluten-free diet. Br J Dermatol 2000;142:44–51.
29 Ojetti V, Aguilar Sanchez J, Guerriero C, et al: High prevalence of celiac disease in psoriasis. Am J Gastroenterol 2003;98:2574–2575.
30 Ludvigsson JF, Lindelof B, Zingone F, et al: Psoriasis in a nationwide cohort study of patients with celiac disease. J Invest Dermatol 2011;131:2010–2016.
31 Collin P, Reunala T: Recognition and management of the cutaneous manifestations of celiac disease: a guide for dermatologists. Am J Clin Dermatol 2000;4:13–20.
32 Lehmann B: Role of the vitamin D_3 pathway in healthy and diseased skin – facts, contradictions and hypotheses. Exp Dermatol 2009;18:97–108.
33 Monteleone G, Pallone F, MacDonald TT, et al: Psoriasis: from pathogenesis to novel therapeutic approaches. Clin Sci (Lond) 2010;120:1–11.
34 Liu Y, Helms C, Liao W, et al: A genome-wide association study of psoriasis and psoriatic arthritis identifies new disease loci. PLoS Genet 2008;4:e1000041.
35 Corazza GR, Andreani ML, Venturo N, et al: Celiac disease and alopecia areata: report of a new association. Gastroenterology 1995;109:1333–1337.

36 Ertekin V, Tosun MS, Erdem T: Screening of celiac disease in children with alopecia areata. Indian J Dermatol 2014;59:317.

37 Fessatou S, Kostaki M, Karpathios T: Celiac disease and alopecia areata in childhood. J Pediatr Child Health 2003;39:152–154.

38 Bardella MT, Marino R, Barbareschi M, et al: Alopecia areata and coeliac disease: no effect of a gluten-free diet on hair growth. Dermatology 2000;200:108–110.

39 Bondavalli P, Quadri G, Parodi A, et al: Failure of gluten-free diet in celiac disease-associated alopecia areata. Acta Derm Venereol 1998;78:319.

40 Ress K, Annus T, Putnik U, et al: Celiac disease in children with atopic dermatitis. Pediatr Dermatol 2014;31:483–488.

41 Ciacci C, Cavallaro R, Iovino P, et al: Allergy prevalence in adult celiac disease. J Allergy Clin Immunol 2004;113:1199–1203.

42 Slebioda Z, Szponar E, Kowalska A: Etiopathogenesis of recurrent aphthous stomatitis and the role of immunologic aspects: literature review. Arch Immunol Ther Exp (Warsz) 2014;62:205–215.

43 Yaşar S, Yaşar B, Abut E, et al: Clinical importance of celiac disease in patients with recurrent aphthous stomatitis. Turk J Gastroenterol 2012;23:14–18.

44 Corazza GR, Di Stefano M, Mauriño E, et al: Bones in coeliac disease: diagnosis and treatment. Best Pract Res Clin Gastroenterol 2005; 19:453–465.

45 Sánchez MI, Mohaidle A, Baistrocchi A, et al: Risk of fracture in celiac disease: gender, dietary compliance, or both? World J Gastroenterol 2011;17:3035–3042.

46 Olmos M, Antelo M, Vazquez H, et al: Systematic review and meta-analysis of observational studies on the prevalence of fractures in coeliac disease. Dig Liver Dis 2008;40:46–53.

47 Bushara KO, et al: Neurologic presentation of celiac disease. Gastroenterology 2005; 128:S92–S97.

48 Hadjivassiliou M, Sanders DS, Grünewald RA, et al: Gluten sensitivity: from gut to brain. Lancet Neurol 2010;9:318–330.

49 Hadjivassiliou M, Sanders DS, Woodroofe N, et al: Gluten ataxia. Cerebellum 2008;7:494–498.

50 Luostarinen L, Pirttila T, Collin P: Coeliac disease presenting with neurological disorders. Eur Neurol 1999;42:132–135.

51 Luostarinen L, Himanen SL, Luostarinen M, et al: Neuromuscular and sensory disturbances in patients with well treated celiac disease. J Neurol Neurosurg Psychiatry 2003;74:490–494.

52 Kaplan JG, Pack D, Horoupian D, et al: Distal axonopathy associated with chronic gluten enteropathy: a treatable disorder. Neurology 1988;38:642–645.

53 Gobbi G, Furio B, et al: Coeliac disease, epilepsy, and cerebral calcifications. Lancet 1992; 340;439–443.

54 Molteni N, Bardella MT, Baldassarri AR, et al: Celiac disease associated with epilepsy and intracranial calcifications: report of two patients. Am J Gastroenterol 1988;83:992–994.

55 Johnson A, Dale R, Wienholt L, et al: Coeliac disease, epilepsy, and cerebral calcifications: association with TG6 autoantibodies. Develop Med Child Neurol 2013;55:90–93.

56 Gobbi G: Celiac disease, epilepsy and cerebral calcifications. Brain Dev 2005;27:189–200.

57 Dimitrova AK, Ungaro RC, Lebwohl B, et al: Prevalence of migraine in patients with celiac disease and inflammatory bowel disease. Headache 2013;53:344–355.

58 Gabrielli M, Cremonini F, Fiore G, et al: Association between migraine and celiac disease: results from a preliminary case-control and therapeutic study. Am J Gastroenterol 2003;98:625–629.

59 Roche Herrero MC, Arcas Martínez J, Martínez-Bermejo A, et al: The prevalence of headache in a population of patients with coeliac disease. Rev Neurol 2001;32:301–309.

60 Goldberg D: A psychiatric study of patients with diseases of the small intestine. Gut 1970; 11:459–465.

61 Addolorato G, Stefanini GF, Capristo E, et al: Anxiety and depression in adult untreated celiac subjects and in patients affected by inflammatory bowel disease: a personality 'trait' or a reactive illness? Hepatogastroenterology 1996;43:1513–1517.

62 Häuser W, Janke KH, Klump B, et al: Anxiety and depression in adult patients with celiac disease on a gluten-free diet. World J Gastroenterol 2010;16:2780.

63 Smith D, Gerdes L: Meta-analysis on anxiety and depression in adult celiac disease. Acta Psychiatr Scand 2012;125:183–193.

64 Zingone F, Siniscalchi M, Capone P, et al: The quality of sleep in patients with coeliac disease. Aliment Pharmacol Ther 2010;32:1031–1036.

65 Siniscalchi M, Iovino P, Tortora R, et al: Fatigue in adult coeliac disease. Aliment Pharmacol Ther 2005;22:489–494.

66 Nachman F, del Campo MP, González A, et al: Long-term deterioration of quality of life in adult patients with celiac disease is associated with treatment noncompliance. Dig Liver Dis 2010;42:685–691.

67 Ferretti A, Parisi P, Villa MP: The role of hyperhomocysteinemia in neurological features associated with coeliac disease. Med Hypotheses 2013;81:524–531.

68 Carta MG, Hardoy MC, Boi MF, et al: Association between panic disorder, major depressive disorder and celiac disease: a possible role of thyroid autoimmunity. J Psychosom Res 2002;53:789–793.

69 Garud S, Leffler D, Dennis M, et al: Interaction between psychiatric and autoimmune disorders in coeliac disease patients in the Northeastern United States. Aliment Pharmacol Ther 2009;29:898–905.

70 Van Hees NJ, Van der Does W, Giltay EJ: Coeliac disease, diet adherence and depressive symptoms. J Psychosom Res 2013;74: 155–160.

71 Skowera A, Peakman M, Cleare A, et al: High prevalence of serum markers of coeliac disease in patients with chronic fatigue syndrome. J Clin Pathol 2001;54:335–336.

72 Barratt SM, Leeds JS, Sanders DS: Factors influencing the type, timing and severity of symptomatic responses to dietary gluten in patients with biopsy-proven coeliac disease. J Gastrointest Liver Dis 2013;22:391–396.

73 Pulido O, Zarkadas M, Dubois S, et al: Clinical features and symptom recovery on a gluten-free diet in Canadian adults with celiac disease. Can J Gastroenterol 2013;27:449–453.

74 Rodrigo L, Blanco I, Bobes J, et al: Effect of one year of a gluten-free diet on the clinical evolution of irritable bowel syndrome plus fibromyalgia in patients with associated lymphocytic enteritis: a case-control study. Arthritis Res Ther 2014;16:421.

75 Herfarth HH, Martin CF, Sandler RS, et al: Prevalence of a gluten-free diet and improvement of clinical symptoms in patients with inflammatory bowel diseases. Inflamm Bowel Dis 2014;20:1194–1197.

76 Ludvigsson JF, Elfström P, Broomé U: Celiac disease and risk of liver disease: a general population-based study. Clin Gastroenterol Hepatol 2007;5:63–69.

77 Sainsbury A, Sanders DS, Ford AC, et al: Meta-analysis: coeliac disease and hypertransaminasemia. Aliment Pharmacol Ther 2011;34:33–34.

78 Zanini B, Baschè R, Ferraresi A, et al: Factors that contribute to hypertransaminasemia in patients with celiac disease or functional gastrointestinal syndromes. Clin Gastroenterol Hepatol 2014;12:804–810.

79 Tersigni C, Castellani R, de Waure C, et al: Celiac disease and reproductive disorders: meta-analysis of epidemiologic associations and potential pathogenic mechanisms. Hum Reprod Update 2014;20:582–593.

80 Smecuol E, Mauriño E, Vazquez H, et al: Gynaecological and obstetric disorders in coeliac disease: frequent clinical onset during pregnancy or the puerperium. Eur J Gastroenterol Hepatol 1996;8:63–69.

81 Lasa JS, Zubiaurre I, Soifer LO: Risk of infertility in patients with celiac disease: a meta-analysis of observational studies. Arq Gastroenterol 2014;51:144–150.

Dig Dis 2015;33:155–161
DOI: 10.1159/000369535

Celiac Disease and Endocrine Autoimmunity

George J. Kahaly[a] Detlef Schuppan[b–d]

[a]Department of Medicine I, and [b]Institute for Translational Immunology and Research Center for Immunotherapy, Johannes Gutenberg University Medical Center, Mainz, Germany; [c]Division of Gastroenterology, Beth Israel Deaconess Medical Center, and [d]Harvard Medical School, Boston, Mass., USA

Key Words

Celiac disease · Autoimmune thyroid disease · Endocrine autoimmunity · Polyglandular autoimmune syndrome · Type 1 diabetes

Abstract

Background: Celiac disease (CD) is a small-intestinal inflammatory disease that is triggered by the ingestion of the storage proteins (gluten) of wheat, barley and rye. ***Key Messages:*** Endocrine autoimmunity is prevalent in patients with CD and their relatives. The genes that predispose to endocrine autoimmune diseases, e.g. type 1 diabetes, autoimmune thyroid diseases, and Addison's disease, i.e. DR3-DQ2 and DR4-DQ8, are also the major genetic determinants of CD, which is the best understood HLA-linked disease. Thus, up to 30% of first-degree relatives both of patients with CD and/or endocrine autoimmunity are affected by the other disease. In CD, certain gluten proteins bind with high affinity to HLA-DQ2 or -DQ8 in the small-intestinal mucosa, to activate gluten-specific T cells which are instrumental in the destruction of the resorptive villi. Here, the autoantigen tissue transglutaminase increases the T cell response by generating deamidated gluten peptides that bind more strongly to DQ2 or DQ8. Classical symptoms such as diarrhea and consequences of malabsorption like anemia and osteoporosis are often absent in patients with (screening-detected) CD, but this absence does not significantly affect these patients' incidence of endocrine autoimmunity. Moreover, once autoimmunity is established, a gluten-free diet is not able to induce remission. However, ongoing studies attempt to address how far a gluten-free diet may prevent or retard the development of CD and endocrine autoimmunity in children at risk. ***Conclusions:*** The close relationship between CD and endocrine autoimmunity warrants a broader immune genetic and endocrine screening of CD patients and their relatives.

Celiac Disease

Celiac disease (CD) is defined as a lifelong intolerance to dietary gluten that results in small-intestinal inflammation, villous atrophy, crypt hyperplasia and often malabsorption. The ingestion of certain cereal grains, mainly wheat, rye and barley drives this T cell-driven autodestructive process within the small-intestinal mucosa which usually recovers when these cereals are rigorously withdrawn from the diet. Both endoscopic-histological diagnosis and the presence of circulating IgA antibodies (Ab) to tissue transglutaminase (TG2) confirm the diagnosis. These Ab ultimately disappear in most patients with CD who follow a gluten-free diet. Susceptibility to CD is determined to a significant extent by genetic factors

KARGER 125

© 2015 S. Karger AG, Basel
0257–2753/15/0332–0155$39.50/0

E-Mail karger@karger.com
www.karger.com/ddi

Prof. George J. Kahaly
Johannes Gutenberg University Medical Center
Langenbeckstrasse 1
DE–55101 Mainz (Germany)
E-Mail Kahaly@ukmainz.de

Table 1. Autoantigens in patients with CD and autoimmune endocrine syndromes

Autoantigens	Autoimmune disease
TG2	CD
TPO, Tg	HT
TSH receptor, TPO	GD
Islet cells, GAD, IA2, insulin	T1D
P450 cytochromes: 21-OH, 17-OH, SCC	AD
17-OH	Hypogonadism
Calcium-sensing receptor	Hypoparathyroidism

17-OH and 21-OH = 17- and 21-α-hydroxylase (steroid P450 enzymes); SCC = side chain cleavage enzyme (steroidogenic P450 enzyme); Tg = thyroglobulin.

localized within the HLA region. Approximately 90–95% of CD patients share the HLA DR3/DQ2, mainly HLA DQA1*0501-DQB1*0201, the rest carries HLA DR4/DQ8, or both haplotypes. However, HLA DR4/DQ8 can be the prevalent predisposition in e.g. indigenous populations of South America. The prevalence of HLA DQ2 in most populations is 25–30%, but only a minority of these will ever develop CD. This implies the involvement of additional, non-HLA-linked genes and environmental triggers in the pathogenesis of CD. The ubiquitous enzyme TG2, the CD autoantigen, is central to the pathogenesis of CD since it can deamidate specific glutamine residues in certain gluten peptides that reach the subepithelial small-intestinal lamina propria, thereby increasing their affinity to DQ2 or DQ8 on antigen-presenting cells like dendritic and B cells, favoring the subsequent gluten-specific destructive T cell response.

The coexistence of CD and endocrine autoimmune diseases, e.g. type 1 diabetes (T1D), could be explained by sharing a common genetic factor in the HLA region, such as DR3 or DR4 (in association with DQ2 and DQ8, respectively), or by molecular mimicry by which gliadin or TG2 would activate T cells that are cross-reactive with autoantigens relevant to T1D. During active β-cell destruction, TG2, which is expressed in pancreatic islets, might be presented in an immunogenic form. In view of the high frequency of CD in patients with the HLA DQA1*0501-DQB1*0201 haplotype, this presentation may be facilitated by these alleles. Such inflammatory responses may have the capacity to persist in genetically susceptible hosts and lead to chronic organ-specific autoimmune disease. Furthermore, it has been suggested that in the development of autoimmunity in T1D the failure to achieve tolerance to autoantigens derives from the gut.

The prevalence of CD in Western countries is estimated at 0.5% in Germany and 2.5% in elderly Fins. It ranges between 3 and 8% in patients with T1D. Conversely, between 3 and 12% of patients with CD have T1D. Also, at least 5% of patients with CD have autoimmune thyroid disease (AITD), and between 2 and 4% of patients with AITD are affected by CD. In more than 50% of today's newly detected patients with CD, clinical features are subtle, with mild abdominal discomfort and bloating, weight loss, fatigue, but also growth abnormalities mimicking constitutional growth delay, infertility, recurrent aphthous stomatitis, low bone mineralization and hypocalcemia with vitamin D deficiency and compensatory hyperparathyroidism. Late complications like refractory CD type II, a premalignant condition and overt enteropathy-associated T-cell lymphoma are rare. Iron or folic acid deficiency with or without anemia is the most common laboratory finding. Hypoglycemia, a reduction of insulin requirements and brittle diabetes may indicate the presence of CD in T1D (table 1). CD is considered sufficiently prevalent, and the benefits of diagnosis and treatment by gluten withdrawal are such that it is advocated to screen all T1D patients for this disorder. When serological screening is used, most cases of CD will be detected within 1 year after onset of T1D. Current recommendations for screening subjects with T1D and AITD are to measure TG2 autoantibodies at diagnosis and with symptoms of CD. When positive, subjects should have a small-intestinal biopsy to confirm diagnosis [1–7].

Autoimmune Thyroid Diseases

AITD include Hashimoto's thyroiditis (HT) and Graves' disease (GD). HT is the most prevalent autoimmune disease associated with other autoimmune endocrinopathies and is defined by the presence of thyroid peroxidase (TPO) or thyroglobulin Ab and either normal or elevated TSH concentrations in the absence of medications. Although many subjects with HT are hypothyroid, there is a subgroup of thyroid Ab-positive cases who are euthyroid. It may take years for those subjects to develop thyroid dysfunction. TPO-Ab are predictive of thyroid failure with an annual incidence of 4.3% in subjects with an initial elevated TSH level (>5.0 mU/l). TSH alone predicts thyroid failure since at a TSH level of 5 mU/l, the probability of hypothyroidism is 0.5% per year, and rates of progression increase with higher initial serum TSH or thyroid Ab concentrations. TPO-Ab are present in 15–30% of adults and in 5–22% of children with T1D, compared with 2–10% and 1–4%, respectively, in matched controls. The prevalence of subclinical hypothyroidism in T1D patients is estimated at 13–20% compared with 3–6% in a nondiabetic population, with preponderance for older female patients. Up to 50% of TPO-Ab-positive T1D patients progress to overt AITD. Cross-sectional analysis has shown that hypothyroidism is present in 4–18% of subjects with T1D. Long-term follow-up suggests that as many as 30% of patients with T1D will develop AITD. T1D subjects with glutamate decarboxylase (GAD) Ab positivity, in contrast to tyrosine phosphatase (IA2) Ab-positive patients, are more prone to have TPO-Ab. T1D patients with persisting islet cell Ab positivity for more than 3 years or with GAD-Ab-positivity are at increased risk of thyroid autoimmunity. Other factors such as age, T1D duration, and gender (female preponderance) influence the link between T1D and AITD. At-risk haplotypes for HT are the HLA DQA1*0301 (linked to DR4), DQB1*0301 (linked to DR5) and DQB1*0201 (linked to DR3). The HLA haplotype DR3-DQB1*0201 contributes to the genetic susceptibility to T1D, AITD and the polyglandular autoimmune syndrome (PAS). Other loci may also contribute to the clustering and may influence disease phenotype and severity.

A symmetric, painless goiter is usually the first presentation in HT, although about 10% of patients have atrophic thyroid glands. Treatment of hypothyroidism is important because the decrease in basal metabolism may cause weight gain, hyperlipidemia, atherosclerotic heart disease, and may affect diabetes control, growth, menses, and increase the risk of adverse pregnancy outcome. Even more, the presence of Ab may be associated with an increased likelihood of spontaneous abortion, even in the absence of overt disease. Although thyroid lymphoma is very rare, the risk of this disease is increased ~67-fold in patients with HT. Treatment of HT-induced hypothyroidism consists of supplementation of levothyroxine sodium. The goal of replacement therapy is to normalize serum TSH levels. Current recommendations are to screen T1D patients for dysthyroidism using TSH after stabilization at onset of T1D, or in case of symptoms of hypothyroidism or hyperthyroidism, and every 1–2 years thereafter. Since patients who are TPO-Ab positive have an 18-fold increased risk of developing thyroid disease compared with patients who are TPO-Ab negative, it is suggested to screen T1D patients using TPO-Ab, TSH and T4 levels at onset of T1D and yearly thereafter.

Autoimmune hyperthyroidism is less common. Graves' hyperthyroidism is caused by thyroid-stimulating Ab that bind to and activate the TSH receptor (TSH-R) on thyroid cells. These Ab not only cause hypersecretion of thyroid hormone but also promote hypertrophy and hyperplasia of thyroid follicles, resulting in a goiter. GD shares many immunological features with HT, including high serum concentrations of Ab against thyroglobulin and TPO. Thyroid function tests reveal a suppressed TSH level, elevated levels of serum T4 and T3, and positive TSH-R-Ab. GD affects approximately 1% of the general population and is the underlying cause of 50–80% of cases of hyperthyroidism. Subclinical hyperthyroidism can be diagnosed in 6–10% of T1D patients, compared with 0.1–2% in the nondiabetic population. The incidence of overt hyperthyroidism in persons with a suppressed serum TSH is calculated at 2–4% per year. Women are 5–10 times more at risk of developing GD than men. Stress may trigger the disease. At-risk haplotypes for GD are DQA1*0501 (linked to DR3 and to DR5) and DQB1*0302 (linked to DR4). The severity and duration of GD and the age of the patient determine the manifestations of hyperthyroidism: nervousness, emotional lability, disturbed sleep, fatigue, palpitations and atrial fibrillation, heat intolerance, weight loss, and orbitopathy. Among T1D patients treated with insulin, hyperthyroidism increases insulin requirements. Hyperthyroidism may aggravate glucose intolerance by mechanisms which include increased hexose intestinal absorption, increased glucose production (gluconeogenesis and glycogenolysis), and decreased responsiveness to insulin. Current treatment of GD consists of antithyroid drugs (ATD), radioactive iodine, and surgery. ATD inhibit thyroid hormone production and decrease the levels of TSH-R-Ab. In older subjects, consensus exists regarding the treatment of subclinical hyperthyroidism with ATD to prevent atrial fibrillation [8–20].

Type 1 Diabetes

T1D is a T cell-mediated autoimmune disease that develops in genetically susceptible individuals and results in destruction of insulin-producing β-cells. In up to one third of patients, the autoimmune attack is not limited to β-cells, but expands into a PAS. Of T1D subjects, 15–30% have AITD, 0.5% have Addison's disease (AD), and 3–12% present with CD. The association between T1D and organ-specific autoimmune disease can be explained by sharing a common genetic background, but also by a defective immunoregulation. T1D is characterized by the appearance of insulitis and the presence of β-cell Ab. Several lines of evidence support the autoimmune nature of the β-cell destructive process: (a) infiltration of the pancreatic islets by lymphocytes and macrophages (insulitis), (b) presence of Ab to islet cell antigens (ICA), IA2, glutamic acid decarboxylase-65 (GAD), insulin (IAA), and zinc transporter ZnT8 (Slc30A8), (c) a preferential occurrence of T1D in persons carrying specific allelic combinations at immune response loci within the HLA gene complex, (d) increased prevalence of organ-specific autoimmune disorders in T1D, (e) the disease can be transferred by spleen or bone marrow cells, and finally (f) animal models of T1D that show a defect in immunoregulation contributing to the onset of disease.

One or more β-cell Ab are present in approximately 90% of new-onset patients with T1D. They appear to develop sequentially. Insulin-Ab are often the first expressed, especially in younger children. GAD-Ab positivity is suggested to represent a propensity for general autoimmunity, while IA2-Ab positivity may be a more specific marker of β-cell destruction. β-Cell Ab also represents important preclinical markers of the disease as they may be present for years before T1D diagnosis. The risk of T1D for a first-degree relative depends on the number and type of Ab that are present. Family members who express insulin, GAD and IA2-Ab have a 75% risk of developing T1D within the next 5 years, as compared with a 10–25% 5-year risk in those expressing only one of the Ab. The general 5-year risk for T1D is 34% in subjects positive for ≥3 Ab. Progression to T1D amounted to 12% within 5 years among siblings positive for IAA, 20% for ICA, 19% for GAD but 59% for IA-2-Ab. IA-2-Ab were detected in 1.7% of all siblings and in 56% of the prediabetic subjects on first sampling. Among genes associated with T1D, the HLA gene complex on chromosome 6p21 is the genetic factor with the strongest association. Another gene located on chromosome 11p15 in the upstream region of the insulin gene also confers susceptibility to T1D. Multiple additional genes also contribute to T1D susceptibility. One of these is IDDM12 on chromosome 2q33, which contains two autoimmune disease candidate genes: CTLA-4 (cytotoxic T-lymphocyte-associated protein 4) and CD28, encoding for T-cell receptors involved in controlling T-cell proliferation. Other important genes include the MHC I-related gene A (MIC-A) and the protein IA2 nonreceptor type 22 (PTPN22). Ninety percent of Caucasian T1D patients express the HLA DR3 and/or DR4 alleles. These HLA alleles are expressed in 30–40% of the general white population. Expression of HLA DR2 is decreased in persons with T1D. Certain combinations of HLA alleles are found with a frequency greater than expected and are thus not randomly distributed within the general population. This phenomenon is called linkage disequilibrium. Particularly, HLA DQA1*0301-DQB1*0302 (in linkage disequilibrium with DR4) and DQA1*0501-B1*0201 (in linkage disequilibrium with DR3) haplotypes confer a high diabetogenic risk. The absolute risk of a child with this DR3/DR4 genotype developing T1D from the general population is similar to a first-degree relative of a T1D patient (1 in 20). DQB1*0602 and DQA1*0102 alleles are associated with dominant protection.

The model of T1D as a chronic autoimmune disorder begins with environmental triggers in genetically susceptible persons, progressing to autoimmunity with appearance of β-cell Ab, further evolving towards metabolic dysregulation with loss of first-phase insulin response, increasing HbA1c within the normal range, impaired fasting glycemia or impaired glucose tolerance, and finally resulting in overt T1D and loss of C-peptide. The first-phase insulin response measured by i.v. glucose tolerance testing is the sum of insulin levels at the 1st and 3rd min after administration of an i.v. glucose load. Many subjects with T1D had a low first phase before the diagnosis of T1D, and this may persist for years before clinical disease onset. These data suggest that subjects go through a phase of decreasing β-cell mass. The exact β-cell mass at diagnosis is poorly defined. For patients with long-term T1D, it is usually decreased to less than 1% of normal. Residual β-cell function can also be analyzed according to the measurement of C-peptide release as induced by a hyperglycemic clamp procedure. Low first-phase C-peptide response specifically predicts impending T1D, while a low second-phase response probably reflects an earlier disease stage. A typical de novo T1D patient presents with hyperglycemia and polyuria, polydipsia and weight loss. Ketoacidosis is common and Ab status at the moment of T1D diagnosis should be verified [21–30].

Addison's Disease

AD is the most frequent cause of primary adrenal insufficiency. It results from destruction of the adrenal cortex with an ensuing deficiency of cortisol, aldosterone, and in females of adrenal androgens. AD affects 1 in 10,000 in the general population and results from destruction of the adrenal cortex by cytotoxic T lymphocytes. In the active phase of the disease, there is a widespread mononuclear cell infiltrate. There is loss of normal three-layer structure of the adrenal cortex, and adrenocortical cells show necrosis and pleomorphism. The cytochrome P450 enzyme steroid 21-hydroxylase (21-OH) has been identified as a major antigen for the Ab. Also in AD, screening for 21-OH-Ab identifies subjects who are at risk to develop AD before clinical presentation. Clinical disease can either present as isolated AD or in combination with other autoimmune diseases as part of the PAS. In T1D, the prevalence of 21-OH-Ab ranges between 1 and 3%, compared with 1 and 0.5% in first-degree relatives and controls, respectively. A small number of Ab-positive subjects have been followed for the development of AD, and a yearly incidence of AD of approximately 20% has been observed. Adrenal-Ab are more frequent in female subjects and in T1D patients with persisting islet cell Ab. Furthermore, AD is frequently associated with other autoimmune endocrinopathies, particularly with HT. In patients with AD, as many as 70% with 21-OH-Ab also expressed thyroid autoimmunity. Genetic susceptibility for AD has also been linked to the MHC complex on chromosome 6, as CD, AITD and T1D. The HLA DRB1*0404/DQ8-DRB1*0301/DQ2 genotype occurs at an increased frequency in individuals with isolated AD and in those with AD and T1D. A second locus within the MHC, the MHC class I-related MIC-A, has been linked to AD. Homozygosity for MICA5.1 (allele 5.1) was associated with an 18-fold increased risk for AD.

Adrenal insufficiency may cause persistent vomiting, anorexia, hypoglycemia, and unexplained weight loss in an adult, malaise, ill-defined fatigue, muscular weakness, hypotension, and craving for salt. The most specific sign of primary AD is generalized hyperpigmentation of the skin and mucosal surfaces, which is due to the high plasma concentrations of melanocyte-stimulating activity of β-lipotropin, which derives from the same precursor as ACTH. Laboratory tests can aid in the diagnosis: hyponatremia, hyperkalemia, and acidosis. In addition, hypocorticism may, by reducing the insulin needs, cause frequent attacks of hypoglycemia.

Patients with symptomatic AD should be treated with hydrocortisone and with fludrocortisone as a substitute for aldosterone. Patients with suspected AD and hypothyroidism should be evaluated and treated for adrenal insufficiency prior to replacement of thyroid hormone to avoid an Addison crisis, since thyroxine may increase hepatic corticosteroid metabolism. The natural history of the progression of the disease follows a typical pattern (different stages) which can be correlated with clinical symptoms. One discriminates a potential phase (genetic susceptibility and/or 21-OH-Ab), a latent phase [elevated plasma renin activity (PRA) and normal basal cortisol and ACTH levels], and a clinical phase (a diminished basal cortisol and elevated ACTH concentration). These parameters constitute the endocrine evaluation of adrenal function: PRA, ACTH, cortisol and corticotropin stimulation testing. Screening for 21-OH-Ab at diagnosis of T1D and then every 2 years seems to be a good practice. If Ab are positive, one has to evaluate morning baseline ACTH, cortisol and PRA levels (supine position) and perform a corticotropin stimulation test. However, in the absence of symptoms, an annual basal cortisol and ACTH may be sufficient [31–34].

Polyglandular Autoimmune Syndromes

PAS form different clusters of autoimmune disorders and are rare endocrinopathies characterized by the coexistence of at least two glandular autoimmune-mediated diseases. Two major subtypes of PAS, types I and II, are distinguished according to age at presentation, characteristic patterns of disease combinations, and different modes of inheritance. PAS I, also known as autoimmune polyendocrinopathy, candidiasis and ectodermal dystrophy or multiple endocrine deficiency autoimmune candidiasis syndromes, usually manifests in infancy or childhood at age 3–5 years or in early adolescence and, therefore, is also called juvenile autoimmune polyendocrinopathy. It is defined by a persistent fungal infection (chronic mucocutaneous candidiasis), the presence of acquired hypoparathyroidism, and AD. In most patients, mucocutaneous candidiasis precedes the other immune disorders, usually followed by hypoparathyroidism. The female-to-male ratio varies from 0.8:1 to 2.4:1. The highest prevalences of PAS I have been found in populations characterized by high degree of consanguinity or descendant of small founder populations, particularly in Iranian Jews and Finns. PAS I is a monogenic disease with autosomal recessive inheritance caused by mutations in the autoimmune regulatory gene on chromosome 21.

PAS II is more common and occurs in adulthood, mainly in the third or fourth decade (table 2). It is characterized by AD with AITD and/or T1D. AD may precede other endocrinopathies. Vitiligo and gonadal failure are more rarely associated with PAS II than with type I. Especially in adults, the presence of one autoimmune endocrine disease is associated with an increased risk of developing autoimmunity to other tissues. Each of these disorders is characterized by several stages beginning with

Table 2. Characteristics of the PAS

	PAS type I	PAS type II
Incidence	<1:100,000/year	1–2:100,000/year
Male:female ratio	3:4	1:3
Age at onset	Childhood	Adulthood
Autoimmune Endocrine Diseases	Hypoparathyroidism (80–85%) AD (60–70%) T1D (<20%) Hypogonadism (12%) Thyroid disease (10%)	Thyroid disease (70–75%) T1D (50–60%) AD (40–50%) Hypoparathyroidism (0–5%) Hypopituitarism (0–2%)
Concomitant Disease	Mucocutaneous candidiasis (70–80%)	No candidiasis

Nonendocrine autoimmune disorders: vitiligo, alopecia areata, autoimmune gastritis, pernicious anemia, autoimmune hepatitis, malabsorption, Sjögren's syndrome, myasthenia gravis.

active autoimmunity and followed by metabolic abnormalities with overt disease. The prevalence of PAS II is estimated to be 1:20,000, and females are affected three times more frequently than males. In contrast to type I, family members of PAS II patients are often affected. PAS II is believed to be polygenic, characterized by autosomal dominant inheritance [35–40].

Conclusions

In view of the possible long time interval between the manifestations of CD and the first and further autoimmune endocrinopathies, regular and long-term observation of patients with CD and autoimmune endocrine disorders is warranted. Moreover, if a patient has one endocrinopathy and a family member has another, it is likely that they also have Ab against other endocrine tissues. In view of the tendency of autoimmune diseases to associate with other disorders, of the metachronous manifestations of the component diseases, and of the often subclinical initial course, it is necessary to suspect in all patients with CD and/or one immune endocrinopathy the existence of a further autoimmune disorder, particularly in patients with positive family histories. Approximately 1 in 7 first-degree relatives of patients with endocrine autoimmunity has an unrecognized endocrine disorder, and we recommend regular screening in this high-risk population. Thus, for patients with CD and/or monoglandular autoimmune endocrinopathy and/or in subjects at risk, regular serological screening with measurement of organ-specific Ab is recommended every 2 years. If pathological findings, e.g. occurrence of a second autoimmune endocrine disease, are noted, functional screening is warranted (table 3). Furthermore, serological screening for autoimmune endocrine diseases of the first-degree relatives of these patients should follow. Especially in the offspring of patients with T1D, serological testing for the presence of diabetes as well as CD-specific Ab should be considered. Genetic screening is currently useful in PAS I only.

Table 3. Diagnostic investigation for patients with CD and/or autoimmune endocrine disorders

Serological testing Autoantibodies to – Islet cells, GAD, optional IA2 – TPO, TSH receptor – Cytochrome P450 enzymes (especially 21-OH) – H^+-K^+-ATPase of the parietal cells, intrinsic factor – TG2, optional gliadin
Functional testing – TSH, FSH, LH, fT4, testosterone, estradiol, glucose, fasting morning cortisol – ACTH stimulation test (when adrenal antibodies are present) – Serum Na^+, K^+, Ca^+, blood cell count
Molecular analysis of the AIRE gene for PAS type I, only HLA typing and subtyping (optional and for scientific purpose)

AIRE gene = Autoimmune regulatory gene.

Disclosure Statement

The authors have nothing to disclose.

References

1 Dieterich W, Ehnis T, Bauer M, et al: Identification of tissue transglutaminase as the autoantigen of celiac disease. Nat Med 1997;3:797–801.
2 Green PH, Cellier C: Celiac disease. N Engl J Med 2007;357:1731–1743.
3 Schuppan D, Junker Y, Barisani D: Celiac disease: from pathogenesis to novel therapies. Gastroenterology 2009;137:1912–1933.
4 Fasano A, Catassi C: Clinical practice. Celiac disease. N Engl J Med 2012;367:2419–2426.
5 Leffler DA, Schuppan D: Update on serologic testing in celiac disease. Am J Gastroenterol 2010;105:2520–2524.
6 Sollid LM, Jabri B: Triggers and drivers of autoimmunity: lessons from coeliac disease. Nat Rev Immunol 2013;13:294–302.
7 Koning F: Pathophysiology of celiac disease. J Pediatr Gastroenterol Nutr 2014;59(suppl 1):S1–S4.
8 Badenhoop K, Dieterich W, Segni M, Hofmann S, Hufner M, Usadel KH, Schuppan D: HLA DQ2 and/or DQ8 is associated with celiac disease-specific autoantibodies to tissue transglutaminase in families with thyroid autoimmunity. Am J Gastroenterol 2001;96:1648–1649.
9 Frohlich-Reiterer EE, Hofer S, Kaspers S, Herbst A, Kordonouri O, Schwarz HP, et al: Screening frequency for celiac disease and autoimmune thyroiditis in children and adolescents with type 1 diabetes mellitus – data from a German/Austrian multicentre survey. Pediatr Diabetes 2008;9:546–553.
10 Boelaert K, Newby PR, Simmonds MJ, Holder RL, Carr-Smith JD, Heward JM, et al: Prevalence and relative risk of other autoimmune diseases in subjects with autoimmune thyroid disease. Am J Med 2010;123:183.e1–e9.
11 Dittmar M, Libich C, Brenzel T, Kahaly GJ: Increased familial clustering of autoimmune thyroid diseases. Horm Metab Res 2011;43:200–204.
12 Dittmar M, Kahaly GJ: Immunoregulatory and susceptibility genes in thyroid and polyglandular autoimmunity. Thyroid 2005;15:239–250.
13 Villano MJ, Huber AK, Greenberg DA, Golden BK, Concepcion E, Tomer Y: Autoimmune thyroiditis and diabetes: dissecting the joint genetic susceptibility in a large cohort of multiplex families. J Clin Endocrinol Metab 2009;94:1458–1466.
14 Dultz G, Matheis N, Dittmar M, Bender K, Kahaly GJ: CTLA-4 CT60 polymorphism in thyroid and polyglandular autoimmunity. Horm Metab Res 2009;41:426–429.
15 Dultz G, Matheis N, Dittmar M, Rohrig B, Bender K, Kahaly GJ: The protein tyrosine phosphatase non-receptor type 22 C1858T polymorphism is a joint susceptibility locus for immunthyroiditis and autoimmune diabetes. Thyroid 2009;19:143–148.
16 Ban Y, Davies TF, Greenberg DA, Concepcion ES, Tomer Y: The influence of human leucocyte antigen (HLA) genes on autoimmune thyroid disease (AITD): results of studies in HLA-DR3 positive AITD families. Clin Endocrinol 2002;57:81–88.
17 Ide M, Dittmar M, Wurm M, Kanitz M, Kahaly GJ: Polymorphisms of MICA microsatellites in thyroidal autoimmunity. Med Klin 2007;102:11–15.
18 Tomer Y, Menconi F: Type 1 diabetes and autoimmune thyroiditis: the genetic connection. Thyroid 2009;19:99–102.
19 Kordonouri O, Klinghammer A, Lang EB, Gruters-Kieslich A, Grabert M, Holl RW: Thyroid autoimmunity in children and adolescents with type 1 diabetes: a multicenter survey. Diabetes Care 2002;25:1346–1350.
20 Denzer C, Karges B, Nake A, Rosenbauer J, Schober E, Schwab KO, et al: Subclinical hypothyroidism and dyslipidemia in children and adolescents with type 1 diabetes mellitus. Eur J Endocrinol 2013;168:601–608.
21 Kordonouri O, Dieterich W, Schuppan D, Webert G, Müller C, Sarioglu N, Becker M, Danne T: Autoantibodies to tissue transglutaminase are sensitive serological parameters for detecting silent coeliac disease in patients with type 1 diabetes mellitus. Diabet Med 2000;17:441–444.
22 Pociot F, McDermott MF: Genetics of type 1 diabetes mellitus. Genes Immun 2002;3:235–249.
23 Todd JA: Etiology of type 1 diabetes. Immunity 2010;32:457–467.
24 Bluestone JA, Herold K, Eisenbarth G: Genetics, pathogenesis and clinical interventions in type 1 diabetes. Nature 2010;464:1293–1300.
25 Tuomilehto J: The emerging global epidemic of type 1 diabetes. Curr Diab Rep 2013;13:795–804.
26 Morahan G: Insights into type 1 diabetes provided by genetic analyses. Curr Opin Endocrinol Diabetes Obes 2012;19:263–270.
27 Steck AK, Rewers MJ: Genetics of type 1 diabetes. Clin Chem 2011;57:176–185.
28 Atkinson MA, Eisenbarth GS, Michels AW: Type 1 diabetes. Lancet 2014;383:69–82.
29 Barker JM: Clinical review: type 1 diabetes-associated autoimmunity: natural history, genetic associations, and screening. J Clin Endocrinol Metab 2006;91:1210–1217.
30 Perros P, McCrimmon RJ, Shaw G, Frier BM: Frequency of thyroid dysfunction in diabetic patients: value of annual screening. Diabet Med 1995;12:622–627.
31 Triolo TM, Armstrong TK, McFann K, Yu L, Rewers MJ, Klingensmith GJ, et al: Additional autoimmune disease found in 33% of patients at type 1 diabetes onset. Diabetes Care 2011;34:1211–1213.
32 Arlt W, Allolio B: Adrenal insufficiency. Lancet 2003;361:1881–1893.
33 Mitchell AL, Pearce SH: Autoimmune Addison disease: pathophysiology and genetic complexity. Nat Rev Endocrinol 2012;8:306–316.
34 Erichsen MM, Løvås K, Skinningsrud B, et al: Clinical, immunological, and genetic features of autoimmune primary adrenal insufficiency: observations from a Norwegian registry. J Clin Endocrinol Metab 2009;94:4882–4890.
35 Kahaly GJ: Polyglandular autoimmune syndromes. Eur J Endocrinol 2009;161:11–20.
36 Dittmar M, Kahaly GJ: Polyglandular autoimmune syndromes: immunogenetics and long-term follow-up. J Clin Endocrinol Metab 2003;88:2983–2992.
37 Weinstock C, Matheis N, Barkia S, Haager MC, Janson A, Markovic A, et al: Autoimmune polyglandular syndrome type 2 shows the same HLA class II pattern as type 1 diabetes. Tissue Antigens 2011;77:317–324.
38 Selmi C: Autoimmunity in 2011. Clin Rev Allergy Immunol 2012;43:194–206.
39 Anaya JM: The diagnosis and clinical significance of polyautoimmunity. Autoimmun Rev 2014;13:423–426.
40 Cutolo M: Autoimmune polyendocrine syndromes. Autoimmun Rev 2014;13:85–89.

Dig Dis 2015;33:162–166
DOI: 10.1159/000369539

Celiac Disease: Prevention in Children

M. Luisa Mearin

Department of Pediatrics, Leiden University Medical Center, Leiden, The Netherlands

Key Words
Celiac disease · Gluten · Early nutrition · Breastfeeding · Prevention

Abstract
Several studies have suggested a protective role of breastfeeding and/or the timing and quantity of gluten introduction in the subsequent development of celiac disease. Especially, prolonged breastfeeding during the introduction of gluten-containing feeding has been associated with a reduced risk of developing celiac disease in infancy. The mentioned results suggest the existence of a 'window of opportunity' between 4 and 6 months of age in which gluten can be introduced in small amounts. Therefore, the European Society for Pediatric Gastroenterology Hepatology and Nutrition recommends avoiding gluten introduction before the age of 4 months and after the age of 7 months and that gluten should be preferably introduced during ongoing breastfeeding. However, the influence of breastfeeding in the development of celiac disease is not clear, since some studies report prevention and others do not, and the studies reporting a protective effect of breastfeeding do not make clear if it concerns prevention of the disease or delays the onset of symptoms. In addition, most of the studies on this topic have been observational and retrospective. For these reasons, prospective studies are needed to understand the relationship between early nutrition in particular and environmental factors in general, concerning the development and possible prevention of celiac disease. Some of these studies are ongoing. One example is the European multicenter PreventCD project (www.preventcoeliacdisease.com) among infants with a first-degree family member with celiac disease carrying HLA-DQ2 and/or -DQ8, randomized to a double-blind dietary intervention with 100 mg of gluten daily or placebo between the age of 4–6 months. All included children are already 3 years old, and the first analyses are being prepared (http://www.trialregister.nl).

Introduction

Celiac disease (CD) is a common but frequently unrecognized disease, in part because of its variable clinical presentation and symptoms [1]. Screening studies have shown that CD is severely underdiagnosed, with a frequency of about 1–3% among the European population [2–4]. This frequency corresponds to about 5 million people in the European Community, and it is possibly the most common food intolerance in Europe [5]. CD increases the overall mortality risk [6], reduces quality of life [7] and has extensive negative economic consequences [8]. According to an estimate by the Dutch Celiac Dis-

KARGER 125

E-Mail karger@karger.com
www.karger.com/ddi

0257–2753/15/0332–0162$39.50/0

M. Luisa Mearin
Department of Pediatrics
Leiden University Medical Center
PO Box 9600, NL–2300 RC Leiden (The Netherlands)
E-Mail M.L.Mearin_Manrique@lumc.nl

ease Society (www.glutenvrij.nl), the necessary gluten-free diet gives extra costs of EUR 1,200–1,300 per patient a year, which corresponds to a European financial burden of EUR 6.0–6.6 billion, when considering all 5 million CD cases (www.CDEUSA.com). The health status of the patients improves with a gluten-free diet, but primary prevention would be even more beneficial [9].

Prevention is usually defined as any activity which reduces the burden of mortality or morbidity from disease, which takes place at primary, secondary or tertiary level. The aim of tertiary prevention is to reduce the negative impact of an already established disease by restoring function and reducing disease-related complications. Secondary prevention activities are aimed at early disease detection, thereby increasing opportunities for interventions to prevent progression of the disease and emergence of symptoms. Primary prevention avoids the development of a disease [10].

Tertiary Prevention in CD

Since adherence to a gluten-free diet might reduce the long-term complications of CD, like chronic anemia, infertility, autoimmune disorders, malignancy and osteoporosis [11], adherence to the diet may be considered as a tertiary preventive measurement. However, adherence to the gluten-free diet has a negative impact on quality of life [12], stressing the need to develop adjunctive or alternative therapies [13].

Secondary Prevention in CD

Early diagnosis and treatment of CD represents secondary prevention, but it may only be achieved on a large scale by mass screening in the general population since the majority of screening-detected CD cases have no associated symptoms or conditions [2, 14, 15]. Screening for CD can be done by measuring specific antibodies against the enzyme transglutaminase type 2, endomysium or against deamidated gliadin peptides [16]. However, it is not clear if mass screening for CD should be performed since CD does not comply with all the 10 principles for early disease detection elaborated by Wilson and Jungner [17]. Especially, the lack of information on the natural history of CD in patients with none or subtle symptoms identified by mass screening, having or not the same health risks and long-term complications as these with clinically diagnosed CD, has been a traditional argument against mass screening for CD. However, recent prospective studies have shown that undiagnosed CD in woman is associated with reduced fetal growth and birth weight [18], and in children with reduced bone mineral density and delayed growth at age 6 years [19]. In addition, prospective studies also show that treatment of CD patients detected by mass screening with a gluten-free diet results in health improvement, both in children [20] and adults [21]. These results support active screening for CD, and the discussion on mass screening for CD may be reopened in the future.

Primary Prevention in CD

In CD, primary prevention would mean that the tolerance for gluten has to be maintained or acquired since patients with CD do not develop it early in life or they lose their gluten tolerance later [22]. The potentiality for primary prevention of CD has been suggested based on: (a) the possibility to improve tolerance for (food) allergens, and (b) the existence of environmental factors involved in CD.

The intestinal immune system has adaptive defenses to avoid systemic and peripheral inflammatory immune responses by activation of regulatory T cells to tolerate innocuous antigens, such as food proteins and commensal bacteria. This hyporesponsiveness to dietary protein antigens in the intestine is a phenomenon termed 'oral tolerance' [23]. Oral tolerance experimentally studied in rodents has revealed an overwhelming complexity, including genetics, age, feeding dose and timing, antigenic structure, epithelial barrier integrity, maturation state of mucosal antigen-presenting cells and the microenvironmental cytokine profiles [24]. Experiments in animal models have suggested possibilities for induction of tolerance for gluten: intravenous or intranasal administration of multiple doses of gliadin to mice was able to downregulate the specific immune response [25]. Breastfeeding protected young AVN rats from CD-like lesions [26]. The development of a gluten peptide or a T-cell vaccination could enable specific interference with T-cell function in CD, as it has been proposed for another autoimmune disorder, namely rheumatoid arthritis. In this aspect, the development of the Nexvax2 vaccine to be used as immunotherapy to induce tolerance to gluten is underway and in phase 1 trials (ImmusanT, Cambridge, Mass., USA).

The indispensable environmental factor in CD is exposure to gluten ingestion. Theoretically, CD could be prevented by not introducing gluten in the diet of genetically predisposed infants. However, the strongest genetic factors in CD, HLA-DQ2 and DQ8, are present in about 40% of the general population, and other preventive possibilities have been sought in the timing and quantity of gluten introduction. The development of oral tolerance for gluten is initiated early in life, and the question is whether the age at first introduction of gluten in predisposed individuals could influence the onset of CD. However, until recently all studies investigating early nutrition and CD were observational and retrospective. Much knowledge about gluten introduction and CD has been obtained from the Swedish epidemic of symptomatic CD in the mid-1980s [27]. The start of the epidemic was related to new dietary recommendations, delaying the introduction of all gluten-containing food to infants until 6 months of age. Results from other retrospective studies have shown different results, from protection by early introduction (<4 months to >4 months) [28] to no effect at all [29]. A prospective observational study in children genetically predisposed to CD and type 1 diabetes mellitus showed that both early (<3 months) and late (>7 months) introduction of gluten was associated with an increased development of CD autoimmunity, but in this study the gluten ingested was not quantified, and the diagnosis of CD was not confirmed by small bowel biopsies [30]. Recently, a prospective birth cohort study found an increased risk of CD in children introduced to gluten after 6 months (OR 1.27; 95% CI: 1.01–1.65, p = 0.045) [31]. Altogether, these results suggest the existence of a 'window of opportunity' between 4 and 6 months of age in which gluten can be introduced in small amounts. Therefore, the European Society for Pediatric Gastroenterology Hepatology and Nutrition recommends that complementary feeding should not be introduced before 17 weeks and not later than 26 weeks, and that it is prudent to avoid gluten introduction before the age of 4 months and after the age of 7 months, and gluten should be preferably introduced during ongoing breastfeeding [32].

The Swedish epidemic of CD suggests also that the amount of gluten introduced in the food of young children plays a role in the development of the disease [27]. Later analysis of the epidemic revealed that in children under the age of 2 years, the risk of CD was greater when gluten was introduced in large amounts than when introduced in small or medium amounts [33]. Follow-up studies of Swedish children born during the CD epidemic have recently shown that 12-year-old children born after the Swedish epidemic, and thus exposed to a favorable way of gluten introduction, have a significantly lower risk of CD (2%) compared with those born during the epidemic (3%), suggesting that early infant feeding practices affect CD risk also later in life [4].

Breastfeeding is another environmental factor that has been associated with the induction of tolerance in young children [34]. Many studies have evaluated the role of breastfeeding and the risk of CD [4, 28–31, 33, 35–37]. A systemic review and meta-analysis including all the studies published on this topic between 1966 and 2004 found that children being breastfed had a 52% risk reduction of developing CD compared to those who were not breastfed at the time of gluten introduction (pooled OR 0.48; 95% CI: 0.40–0.59) [36]. However, the influence of breastfeeding on the development of CD is not well understood since some studies report prevention [4, 28, 29, 36, 38] and others do not [30, 31, 39]. A recent prospective study in a big cohort of Norwegian children shows an even higher risk of CD in children breastfed after 12 months of age [31]. A systematic review published by the PreventCD group (www.preventcd.com) shows that the most important difficulties in interpreting and comparing studies investigating the effect of early nutrition on the development of CD are caused by the inability to randomize and blind such studies, the retrospective design of many of them and their associated parental recall bias [37].

Infections have also been related to the development of CD, and a seasonal variation in the risk for the disease has been reported, suggesting causal environmental exposure(s) with a seasonal pattern [38]. The finding of rod-shaped bacteria attached to the small intestinal epithelium of some untreated and treated CD patients, but not to the epithelium of healthy controls, suggested that bacteria may be involved in the pathogenesis of CD and may trigger the aberrant innate immunity [40]. Repeated infection with rotavirus, the most common cause of acute gastroenteritis in children worldwide, has been reported to correlate with the development of CD [41]. An imbalance in the composition of the gut microbiome has also been suggested to be associated with the pathogenesis of CD [42], but the results of studies comparing intestinal microbiome in children with and without CD are contradictory [43, 44].

The optimal method to investigate the effect of environmental factors, both nutritional and others, in the development of CD is to perform prospective, randomized, placebo-controlled interventions in newborns with long-term follow-up. Some of these studies are ongoing and are presented below.

PreventCD (Prevent Coeliac Disease) is an international, prospective, randomized, placebo-controlled intervention study among infants with a first-degree family member with CD and carrying HLA-DQ2 and/or -DQ8 [45]. From 2007 to 2010, soon after birth, and after parental informed consent, the children were randomized to a double-blind dietary intervention with 100 mg of gluten daily or placebo given between the age of 4 and 6 months. The children are repeatedly screened for CD. Breastfeeding for at least 6 months was explicitly encouraged. The gluten intake is quantified and the breastfeeding is analyzed. All included children are already 3 years old, and the first analyses are being prepared (http://www.trialregister.nl).

The Environmental Determinants of Diabetes in the Young (TEDDY) is a multinational study that follows children at high genetic risk for type 1 diabetes, with the development of CD as a secondary outcome. TEDDY studies prospectively from birth 6,403 children with genetic predisposition to CD (HLA DQ2 or DQ8) in the United States, Finland, Germany, and Sweden. The risk of CD autoimmunity and CD by the age of 5 years was 11 and 3%, respectively, among children with a single DR3-DQ2 haplotype, and 26 and 11%, respectively, among those with two copies (DR3-DQ2 homozygosity). Residence in Sweden was also independently associated with an increased risk of CD autoimmunity (hazard ratio, 1.90; 95% CI: 1.61–2.25), highlighting again the importance of studying environmental factors associated with CD [46].

The Generation R study, a population-based prospective cohort study from fetal life until young adulthood in Rotterdam, the Netherlands, suggests that early gluten introduction (<6 months) provides a trigger for functional constipation in a subset of children. Results concerning effect of time of gluten introduction and other environmental factors in the development of CD are expected [18].

The Italian Baby study on weaning and CD is a prospective, multicenter, intervention trial in a cohort of 707 children at family risk for CD followed from birth and randomized to gluten introduction at 6 or 12 months of age. The results show that introduction at 12 months did not prevent CD, but delayed the onset, and that breastfeeding duration was irrelevant for the development of CD [47].

The Norwegian Mother and Child Cohort Study is a prospective population-based pregnancy cohort study conducted by the Norwegian Institute of Public Health. Participants were recruited from all over Norway from 1999 to 2008, and 38.7% of invited women consented to participate. In 107,000 children, CD is identified by questionnaires and by linkage to the Norwegian Patient Register [31].

Conclusion

In order to reduce the mortality and morbidity rates caused by CD, the (pediatric) gastroenterologist can be active at the secondary and tertiary levels of prevention. Therefore, the current available diagnostic procedures have to be used adequately to avoid underdiagnosis of the disease, and adherence and good compliance with the gluten-free diet should be encouraged. More research is needed to fully explore the field of primary prevention of the disease. Future prospective studies should investigate the effect of different intervention strategies, including nutrition, immunomodulation and the role of the microbiome. Especially, large, multicenter, dietary and nondietary interventional studies with long-term follow-up in different countries and continents should be carried out.

Disclosure Statement

The author declares no conflicts of interest.

References

1 Steens RFR, Csizmadia CGDS, George EK, Ninaber MK, Hira Sing RA, Mearin ML: Better recognition of childhood celiac disease in the Netherlands and its changing clinical picture: a national prospective study 1993–2000. J Pediatr 2005;147:239–243.

2 Csizmadia CGDS, Mearin ML, von Blomberg BME, Brand R, Verloove-Vanhorick SP: An iceberg of childhood coeliac disease in the Netherlands. Lancet 1999;353:813–814.

3 Schweizer JJ, von Blomberg ME, Bueno-de Mesquita HB, Mearin ML: Coeliac disease in the Netherlands. Scand J Gastroenterol 2004; 39:359–364.

4 Ivarsson A, Myleus A, Norström F, van der Pals M, Rosén A, Högberg L, Danielsson L, Halvarsson B, Hammarroth S, Hernell O, Karlsson E, Stenhammar L, Webb C, Sandström O, Carlsson A: Prevalence of childhood celiac disease and changes in infant feeding. Pediatrics 2013;131:e687–e694.

5 Mearin ML: Celiac disease among children and adolescents. Curr Probl Pediatr Adolesc Health Care 2007;37:86–105.

6 Biagi F, Corazza GR: Mortality in celiac disease. Nat Rev Gastroenterol Hepatol 2010;7: 158–162.

7 van Doorn RK, Winkler LM, Zwinderman KH, Mearin ML, Koopman HM: CDDUX: a disease-specific health-related quality-of-life questionnaire for children with celiac disease. J Pediatr Gastroenterol Nutr 2008;47:147–152.

8 Shamir R, Hernell O, Leshno M: Cost-effectiveness analysis of screening for celiac disease in the adult population. Med Decis Making 2006;26:282–293.
9 Hogen Esch CE, Kiefte-de Jong JC, Hopman GD, Koning F, Mearin ML: Strategies for prevention of celiac disease; in Fasano A, Troncone R, Branski D (eds): Frontiers in Celiac Disease. Pediatr Adolesc Med. Basel, Karger, 2008, vol 12, pp 188–197.
10 Maars van der PJ, Mackenbach JP: Volksgezondheid en gezondheidszorg, tweede druk. Amsterdam, Elsevier/Bunge, 1999.
11 Green PHR, Jabri B: Coeliac disease. Lancet 2003;362:383–391.
12 Hopman EG, Koopman HM, Wit JM, Mearin ML: Dietary compliance and health-related quality of life in patients with coeliac disease. Eur J Gastroenterol Hepatol 2009;21:1056–1061.
13 Maki M: Celiac disease treatment: gluten-free diet and beyond. J Pediatr Gastroenterol Nutr 2014;59(suppl 1):S15–S17.
14 Mearin ML, Ivarsson A, Dickey W: Coeliac disease: is it time for mass screening? Best Pract Res Clin Gastroenterol 2005;19:441–452.
15 Rosén A, Sandström O, Carlsson A, Högberg L, Olén O, Stenlund H, Ivarsson A: Usefulness of symptoms to screen for celiac disease. Pediatrics 2014;133:211–218.
16 Husby S, Koletzko S, Korponay-Szabo IR, Mearin ML, Phillips A, Shamir R, Troncone R, Giersiepen K, Branski D, Catassi C, Lelgeman M, Maki M, Ribes-Koninckx C, Ventura A, Zimmer KP: European Society for Pediatric Gastroenterology, Hepatology, and Nutrition guidelines for the diagnosis of coeliac disease. J Pediatr Gastroenterol Nutr 2012;54:136–160.
17 Wilson JM, Jungner G: Principles and Practice of Screening for Disease. Geneva, World Health Organisation, 1968.
18 Kiefte-de Jong J, Escher JC, Arends LR, Jaddoe VWV, Hofman A, Raat H, Moll HA: Infant nutritional factors and functional constipation in childhood: the Generation R study. Am J Gastroenterol 2010;105:940–945.
19 Jansen M, Kiefte-de Jong J, Gaillard R, Jaddoe V, Hofman A, Escher H, Hooijkaas H, Moll H: Coeliac disease antibodies are associated with reduced bone mineral density in subclinical children: the generation R study. JPGN 2014;58:S1.
20 Van Koppen EJ, Schweizer JJ, Csizmadia CGDS, Krom Y, Hylkema HB, Van Geel AM, Koopman HM, Mearin ML: Long-term health and quality-of-life consequences of mass screening for childhood celiac disease: a 10-year follow-up study. Pediatrics 2009;123:582–588.
21 Kurppa K, Paavola A, Collin P, Sievänen H, Laurila K, Huhtala H, Saavalainen P, Mäki M, Kaukinen K: Benefits of a gluten-free diet for asymptomatic patients with serologic markers of celiac disease. Gastroenterology 2014;147:610–617.
22 Schaart MW, Mearin ML: Early nutrition: prevention of celiac disease? J Pediatr Gastroenterol Nutr 2014;59(suppl 1):S18–S20.
23 Strobel S, Mowat AM: Oral tolerance and allergic response to food proteins. Curr Opin Allergy Clin Immunol 2006;6:207–213.
24 Mowat AM: Anatomical basis of tolerance and immunity to intestinal antigens. Nat Rev Immunol 2003;3:331–341.
25 Rossi M, Maurano F, Caputo N, Auricchio S, Sette A, Capparelli R, Troncone R: Intravenous or intranasal administration of gliadin is able to down-regulate the specific immune response in mice. Scand J Immunol 1999;50:177–182.
26 Stepankova R, Kofronova O, Tuckova L, Kozakova H, Cebra JJ, Tlaskalova- Hogenova H: Experimentally induced gluten enteropathy and protective effect of epidermal growth factor in artificially fed neonatal rats. J Pediatr Gastroenterol Nutr 2003;36:96–104.
27 Ivarsson A, Persson LA, Nystrom L, Ascher H, Cavell B, Danielsson L, Dannaeus A, Lindberg T, Lindquist B, Stenhammar L, Hernell O: Epidemic of coeliac disease in Swedish children. Acta Paediatr 2000;89:165–171.
28 Peters U, Schneeweiss S, Trautwein EA, Erbersdobler HF: A case-control study of the effect of infant feeding on celiac disease. Ann Nutr Metab 2001;45:135–142.
29 Falth-Magnusson K, Franzen L, Jansson G, Laurin P, Stenhammar L: Infant feeding history shows distinct differences between Swedish celiac and reference children. Pediatr Allergy Immunol 1996;7:1–5.
30 Norris JM, Barriga K, Hoffenberg EJ, Taki I, Miao D, Haas JE, Emery LM, Sokol RJ, Erlich HA, Eisenbarth GS, Rewers M: Risk of celiac disease autoimmunity and timing of gluten introduction in the diet of infants at increased risk of disease. JAMA 2005;293:2343–2351.
31 Stordal K, White RA, Eggesbo M: Early feeding and risk of celiac disease in a prospective birth cohort. Pediatrics 2013;132:e1202–e1209.
32 Agostoni C, Decsi T, Fewtrell M, Goulet O, Kolacek S, Koletzko B, Michaelsen KF, Moreno L, Puntis J, Rigo J, Shamir R, Szajewska H, Turck D, van Goudoever J: Complementary feeding: a commentary by the ESPGHAN Committee on Nutrition. J Pediatr Gastroenterol Nutr 2008;46:99–110.
33 Ivarsson A, Hernell O, Stenlund H, Persson LA: Breast-feeding protects against celiac disease. Am J Clin Nutr 2002;75:914–921.
34 Brandtzaeg PE: Mucosal immunity: integration between mother and the breast-fed infant. Vaccine 2003;21:3382–3388.
35 Ascher H, Krantz I, Rydberg L, Nordin P, Kristiansson B: Influence of infant feeding and gluten intake on coeliac disease. Arch Dis Child 1997;76:113–117.
36 Akobeng AK, Ramanan AV, Buchan I, Heller RF: Effect of breast feeding on risk of coeliac disease: a systematic review and meta-analysis of observational studies. Arch Dis Child 2006;91:39–43.
37 Szajewska H, Chmielewska A, Pieścik-Lech M, Ivarsson A, Kolacek S, Koletzko S, Mearin ML, Shamir R, Auricchio R, Troncone R; PREVENTCD Study Group: Systematic review: early infant feeding and the prevention of coeliac disease. Aliment Pharmacol Ther 2012;36:607–618.
38 Ivarsson A, Hernell O, Nystrom L, Persson LA: Children born in the summer have increased risk for coeliac disease. J Epidemiol Community Health 2003;57:36–39.
39 Welander A, Montgomery SM, Ludvigsson J, Ludvigsson JF: Infectious disease at gluten introduction and risk of childhood diabetes mellitus. J Pediatr 2014;165:326–331.
40 Forsberg G, Fahlgren A, Horstedt P, Hammarstorm S, Hernell O, Hammarstrom ML: Presence of bacteria and innate immunity of intestinal epithelium in childhood celiac disease. Am J Gastroenterol 2004;99:894–904.
41 Stene LC, Honeyman MC, Hoffenberg EJ, Haas JE, Sokol RJ, Emery L, Taki I, Norris JM, Erlich HA, Eisenbarth GS, Rewers M: Rotavirus infection frequency and risk of celiac disease autoimmunity in early childhood: a longitudinal study. Am J Gastroenterol 2006;101:2333–2340.
42 Schippa S, Iebba V, Barbato M, Di Nardo G, Totino V, Checchi MP, Longhi C, Maiella G, Cucchiara S, Conte MP: A distinctive 'microbial signature' in celiac pediatric patients. BMC Microbiol 2010;10:175.
43 Collado MC, Donat E, Ribes-Koninckx C, Calabuig M, Sanz Y: Specific duodenal and faecal bacterial groups associated with paediatric coeliac disease. J Clin Pathol 2009;62:264–269.
44 Meij T, Budding A, Grasman M, Kneepkens F, Savelkoul P, Mearin ML: Composition and diversity of the duodenal mucosa-associated microbiome in children with untreated coeliac disease. Scand J Gastroenterol 2013;48:530–536.
45 Hogen Esch CE, Rosen A, Auricchio R, Romanos J, Chmielewska A, Putter H, Ivarsson A, Szajewska H, Koning F, Wijmenga C, Troncone R, Mearin ML; PreventCD Study Group: The PreventCD Study design: towards new strategies for the prevention of coeliac disease. Eur J Gastroenterol Hepatol 2010;22:1424–1430.
46 Liu E, Lee H, Aronsson CA, Hagopian WA, Koletzko S, Rewers MJ, Eisenbarth GS, Bingley PJ, Bonifacio E, Ville V, Agardh D, for the TEDDY Study Group: Risk of pediatric celiac disease according to HLA haplotype and country. N Engl J Med 2014;371:42–49.
47 Tonutti E, Maggiore G, Francavilla R, Catassi C; Italian Working Group of Weaning and Coeliac Disease Risk: Age at gluten introduction and risk of coeliac disease: final results on a prospective, nutritional intervention study on infants at family risk. JPGN 2014;58:S1.

Dig Dis 2015;33:167–174
DOI: 10.1159/000369537

Celiac Disease Screening in Southern and East Asia

Govind K. Makharia

Departments of Gastroenterology and Human Nutrition, All India Institute of Medical Sciences, New Delhi, India

Key Words
Celiac disease · Epidemiology · India

Abstract
Until 1970s, celiac disease (CD) was considered to be an uncommon disease except in Western Europe. The global epidemiology of CD continues to evolve with improvement in the diagnostic tests, simplification of the diagnostic criteria and increase in awareness about the disease. The Asian region is currently at the crossroads of the frontier of knowledge and awareness of CD. In many Asian nations, CD is still considered to be either nonexistent or very rare. A notable exception is India, where CD has been well recognized, especially in the northern part, and 2 population-based studies have revealed a prevalence of 0.3–1.04%. Initial reports from Malaysia, China, Japan and Singapore suggest the existence of CD in these countries. Furthermore, a meta-analysis of the predisposing factors predicts a high probability of occurrence of CD in fair numbers in China. There are no formal reports on CD from Malaysia, Indonesia, Korea, Taiwan and many other nations in this region. With the impending CD epidemic in Asia, there are many challenges. Some of the efforts which are required include determination of prevalence of CD across the region, spreading of awareness among physicians and patients, training of dieticians for proper counseling and supervision of patients, creation of gluten-free food infrastructure in the food supply and creation of patient advocacy organizations. Although the absolute number of patients with CD at present is not very large, this number is expected to increase over the next few years/decades. It is thus appropriate that the medical community across Asia define the extent of the problem and get prepared to handle the impending CD epidemic.

Introduction

Until 1970s, celiac disease (CD) was considered to be an uncommon disease, mostly affecting individuals of European origin and characterized usually by the onset of the disease during early years of life [1–3]. The global epidemiology of CD continues to evolve with improvement in the diagnostic tests, simplification of the diagnostic criteria and increase in awareness about the disease amongst health care professionals. Over the past two decades, CD has been recognized as a major public health issue in many countries. In Europe and North America, the prevalence of CD in the general population is approximately

KARGER 125

© 2015 S. Karger AG, Basel
0257–2753/15/0332–0167$39.50/0

E-Mail karger@karger.com
www.karger.com/ddi

Prof. Govind K. Makharia
Departments of Gastroenterology and Human Nutrition
All India Institute of Medical Sciences
Ansari Nagar, New Delhi 110 029 (India)
E-Mail govindmakharia@gmail.com

1% [4]. However, there is a large intercountry variation in prevalence; for example, the prevalence of CD is as high as 2–3% in Finland and Sweden, while it is only 0.2% in Germany [5]. Despite sharing similar causal factors in these countries (level of gluten intake and frequency of HLA CD-predisposing genotypes HLA-DQ2 and -DQ8), reasons for such heterogeneity are unknown.

Asia is currently at the crossroads of the frontier of knowledge and awareness of CD. Although there has been an increase in the number of publications on CD from the Asian region, there is a paucity of literature on its prevalence in most Asian nations, with the exception of India [6–14]. Additionally, few case reports and short reports are available from China, Pakistan and Japan [15–20]. In many Asian nations, CD is still considered to be either nonexistent or very rare [21, 22].

Celiac Disease in Asia

Asia is a continent of diverse population, and Asians differ significantly in their ethnicity, genetic make-up, eating practices, cultural practices and economic standards, and thus susceptibility to many diseases. Realizing the emergence of an epidemic of CD in Asia, the World Gastroenterology Organization and Asia Pacific Association of Gastroenterology highlighted the issues specific to this region and have suggested a few steps to handle the impending epidemic of CD in this region [22].

Population-Based Studies from Asia

India is a country with a large (1.2 billion) but diverse population. The people of India vary in their languages, eating practices and cultural practices from one region to another. Until now, CD has been more prevalent in the northern part of India, and it is believed to be uncommon in the southern and northeastern part of India. There are 2 published studies on the prevalence of CD in the general population, and both studies have come from the northern part of India. In a questionnaire-based survey of 4,347 schoolchildren (3–17 years of age) from Ludhiana, Sood et al. [13] have reported the prevalence of CD to be 1 in 310. In another recent study done in the Ballabhgarh District of Haryana State, we applied a three-step clinical/serological screening procedure. With a large population sample (n = 2,879), the prevalence of CD was 1.04% (1 in 96) and of positive anti-transglutaminase antibodies (anti-tTG) was 1.44% (1 in 69) [14]. Based on these 2 community-based studies, 5–8 millions of Indians are expected to have CD. Of such a large pool of patients, only a few thousands of patients have been diagnosed as having CD and the majority still remains undiagnosed. Therefore, the prevalence of CD in an Indian community is nearly the same as that reported from the European nations and United States, and CD is a much greater problem in India than has been previously thought [13–14].

Hospital-Based Studies from Asia

Despite the belief that CD was rare in India, Walia et al. [23] in children and Misra et al. [24] in adults described CD in India as early as in 1960s. Most of the subsequent reports on CD came from the northern part of India (States of Punjab, Haryana, Delhi, Rajasthan, Uttar Pradesh), where wheat is the staple dietary cereal [6–14, 25–28].

During the past 5 years, a few small case series and case reports on CD have been published from China [15, 16]. These reports are of great importance and confirm occurrence of CD in China, a country where CD is thought to be nonexistent [15, 16]. In a recently published systematic review and meta-analysis, Yuan et al. [17] have predicted that CD should not be uncommon in China.

While there are a few case reports on CD from Japan, Watanabe et al. [18] have reported a positive anti-tTG Ab and anti-deamidated gliadin peptide antibody (anti-DGP Ab) in 22 (12.8%) and 23 (13.4%), respectively, of 172 patients with inflammatory bowel disease and 3 (1.6%) and 1 (0.5%), respectively of 172 controls. While many had increased levels of intraepithelial lymphocytes, none had villous atrophy. Interestingly, in a subset of patients who were put on gluten-restricted diet, not only did the serum antibody titers decrease, an improvement in inflammatory bowel disease activity score was also observed. In another recently published study from Singapore, Lu et al. [19] reported evidence of a positive IgA DGP Ab in 34 (18%) of 186 patients with irritable bowel syndrome. Although small, the abovementioned studies highlight the existence of CD in certain nations of Southern and East Asia.

CD in Migrant Population

CD has been described in South Asian patients who had immigrated to Europe or to North America [29–32]. A recent Italian multicenter study on immigrant children with CD showed that 3 of the children that migrated to Italy were native to Pakistan and 1 to Sri Lanka [32]. Ten and 13 children of Punjabi descent were reported to have CD in the UK [33]. Recently, 3 patients with CD were observed in Canada among descendants of Japanese and Chinese immigrants [30]. With population mixing now becoming more common, it should not be inappropriate to consider the whole world as a global village for CD [34].

Regional Variations in the Prevalence of CD

CD in India has mostly been reported from the northern part of India, and there are only occasional reports from the southern part of India. Although rice is the staple cereal in the southern states of India, there certainly has been a change in the dietary behavior, and wheat and wheat products are often included in their diet [35–36]. In order to study the differences in the prevalence of CD in different regions of India, we have just completed a study to estimate the prevalence of CD in the three regions of India including the northern and southern parts and the northeastern region. The result of this study is expected to be released by 2015.

The Absolute Number of Patients with CD Is Likely to Increase in Asia

There are phases of evolution of disease in a particular region. In the initial years, a disease is considered uncommon/rare in a region, and this phase is based generally on beliefs and is not evidence based. In subsequent years, while a few foci/individuals start recognizing the existence of the disease, many others still refuse to accept it. With further increase in the awareness, the availability of diagnostic tests and therapeutic strategies start increasing. Ultimately, physicians even at the level of secondary and primary health care appreciate the existence of the disease, and thus the absolute number of patients starts increasing exponentially. CD has gone through such phases in the recent past in many parts of Europe and North America. CD is going through such phases in many Asian countries. While it is well recognized in the northern part of India, in other regions including China, Japan, Malaysia and Philippines, CD is still considered uncommon [22]. There are no systematic studies to confirm that CD is uncommon in these regions.

Risk Factors in CD

CD occurs because of the interaction between both environmental (gluten) and genetic factors (HLA and non-HLA genes), and the distribution of these two components can guide to identify the areas of the world at risk for CD [37]. During the very early part of the evolution, humans led a nomadic life and obtained food by hunting or collecting fruits and vegetables. One can infer, there was no CD in that era. Due to the special environmental conditions created by flooding, the cultivation first started approximately 10,000 years ago in a small region of southwestern Asia (Turkey, Lebanon, Syria, Palestine and Iraq) called the 'Fertile Crescent'. In the Fertile Crescent, some tribes changed their lifestyle from nomadic to more stable settlement because land cultivation allowed them to store food [37]. The progressive spread of agriculture from the East to Europe took place through the migration of farmers. The successfully domesticated wheat varieties initially were einkorn and emmer wheat [1]. Based on the overall archaeological picture of the spread of agriculture in Europe, the population migrated at a rate of 1 km/year, reaching the Atlantic side of Europe (e.g. UK and Ireland) about 4,000 years ago [38–39]. There might have been patients with CD after the cultivation started; this, however, was originally described in the 19th century, principally in children, by Samuel Gee in England and by Christian Herter in the United States [40]. In the modern era, population migration is rather rapid, and there is a constant mixing of different ethnic groups all over the world.

Wheat as a Preferred Cereal

Wheat is a preferred cereal as it has a high protein content (8–17% by weight), and 78–85% of the total wheat endosperm protein is gluten. When wheat flour is washed with water, the insoluble protein fraction forms a viscoelastic protein mass called gluten [41–42]. Gluten is a very large protein complex composed mainly of polymeric (multiple polypeptide chains linked by disulphide bonds) and monomeric (single-chain polypeptides) proteins known as glutenins and gliadins, respectively. Glutenins confer elasticity, while gliadins mainly confer viscous flow and extensibility to the gluten complex. Because of the viscoelastic properties of wheat flour dough, wheat is commonly used in home-made food (flat breads) and food industry (varieties of bread and pasta making) [41–42].

Wheat Consumption Pattern

India and China are the largest cultivators of wheat grains. The per capita consumption of wheat in India is approximately 48 kg/year [43]. Wheat consumption is higher in the northern and central parts of India and considerably less in the southern and northeastern parts of India [43]. Similarly, the national annual consumption of wheat in China is over 100 million metric tons for over 1.370 billion population [17]. Overall, the consumption of wheat (or wheat flour) is higher in the northern than in the southern part of China. In 2009, according to the wheat consumption pattern in China, the per capita annual consumption of wheat in rural households and of wheat flour in urban households was 59.6 and 12.5 kg, respectively [44, 45].

Furthermore, the consumption of gluten-containing convenience foods (such as breads, instant noodles, pasta, biscuits) is also increasing in many Asian countries including both India and China. This accompanies the gradually improving quality and accelerating pace of urban life. Even in some southern cities of India and China, people are increasingly using wheat-based foods (breads, biscuits, steamed stuffed bun, noodles). Furthermore, people from the rural areas migrate to urban areas, big cities and metro cities and adopt urban-type lifestyle including frequent eating in fast-food restaurants [17]. The rapidly changing diet, from rice to wheat based, may imply that genetically predisposed individuals are increasingly vulnerable to becoming overt CD patients [17].

Predisposing Genetic Factors

HLA Genes

CD is a multigenic disorder, in which the most dominant genetic risk factors are the genotypes encoding the HLA class II molecules HLA-DQ2 (encoded by *HLA-DQA1*0501* and *HLA-DQB1*0201*) and HLA-DQ8 (encoded by *HLA-DQA1*0301* and *HLA-DQB1*0302*) [46–50]. Approximately 90% of individuals with CD carry the HLA-DQ2 heterodimer encoded either in *cis* or in *trans*, and practically all of the remaining patients express HLA-DQ8 [48]. Deamidated gliadin peptides have a high binding affinity to HLA-DQ2 and HLA-DQ8 molecules, but not to other HLA class II molecules, which explains the immunogenicity of gluten in carriers of HLA-DQ2 and HLA-DQ8 [49]. These HLA-encoding genes are associated with approximately 40% of the heritable risk of developing CD [50–51]. Furthermore, a correlation has been found between homozygosity for the genes encoding the HLA-DQ2 molecule and the development of serious complications of CD, in particular refractory CD and enteropathy-associated T cell lymphoma, which implies a gene-dose effect [50–51]. The HLA-DQ2 heterodimer is frequently found in white populations in Western Europe (20–30%), North and West Africa, the Middle East and Central Asia, whereas HLA-DQ8 is more prevalent in Latin America and Northern Europe [52–53]. One of the highest prevalences of CD that is found in the Saharawi population of the Arab-Berber origin has been attributed to higher frequencies of HLA-DQ2 in this population [52–54].

With the second largest population in the world, India is known for its vast ethnic and cultural variability. The distribution of the genetic and environmental determinants of CD in India shows distinctive features. Recently, a case series from New Delhi showed that 38/38 local children with CD had HLA-DQ2, similar to the strength of the association found in Europe [55].

In a meta-analysis of HLA-DQ2 and -DQ8 haplotype and antigens in China, Yuan et al. [17] have reported that HLA-DQ2 antigen is more common in the northwestern than in the southeastern populations. The DQB1*0201 allele also appeared at a much higher frequency in northern China than in southern China, not only in the Han subgroups but also in the ethnic minorities. If one looks at the regional variations in China, the DQB1*0201 allele is reported to be highly prevalent in Xinjiang Uygur Autonomous Region in northwest China (22.04%), whereas this allele was least common in people living in the Yunnan province in southwest China (2.89%) [17]. Studies on the frequency of various genetic loci and on anthropological characteristics clearly show the geographical and genetic boundary between Europeans and Asians runs through northwestern China [17, 56, 57]. Additionally, the population in northwest China is related more closely to Europeans than the other populations in southern China [17, 56, 57]. Anthropological data suggest that Caucasian genes flowed particularly into northern China from the West to the East and then from the East to the South. This migratory route would explain why the DQB1*02 allele is more common in the northern populations than southern populations [17].

In other Asian countries such as Japan, Taiwan, Korea, Indonesia the frequency of predisposing HLA allele is lower (<5%) [21].

Non-HLA Genes

Currently, several other susceptibility loci, not related to HLA, have also been identified by genome-wide association studies, each of which is estimated to be associated with only a small risk of developing CD [58–64]. The proteins encoded by these genes include integrins, chemokines, cytokines and their receptors, and proteins involved in several signaling pathways in regulating B-cell and T-cell activation and in maintaining cell adhesion and motility. Most of these loci contain immune-related genes, in particular genes implicated in the control of the adaptive immune response. Genetic variation in all currently known non-HLA genes together accounts for less than 10% of the familial risk of CD. Further research is needed to determine the functions of the proteins that these genes encode and their involvement in the pathogenesis of CD [58–64].

Screening for CD in Asia

CD is not recognized in many Asian nations and even in nations where CD is recognized, only the most apparent patients are being diagnosed [22]. The available data suggest that CD is much more common in some Asian region than previously appreciated. Looking at the population of India and China, the absolute number of patients with CD can even exceed the total number of patients in Europe and North America combined together [22, 65]. The foremost among the possible explanations for underdiagnosis of CD is the mistaken belief that CD is rare/uncommon in this part of the world. Just an increased awareness about the disease, its wide clinical spectrum and the availability of highly sensitive and specific serologic tests have led to an increase in recognition of CD in India. Furthermore, CD was thought to be a disease of children, and most medical professionals dealing with adult patients did not recognize this disease to be relevant in their practice. Additionally, those children with CD in whom diagnosis is missed or those that remain undiagnosed will present in adulthood with either classical (chronic diarrhea) or nonclassical manifestations [4, 22, 65, 66].

How to Increase Recognition of CD in Asia

There are three broad strategies to increase recognition of CD in Asia, namely estimation of the burden of the disease, increase in education about the disease and creation of an infrastructure for the diagnosis and management of the disease.

Estimation of the Burden of the Disease across the Region

In order to increase the recognition of CD, it is essential to establish the burden of the disease in Asian countries. While population-based studies are ideal for estimating the prevalence of CD in a particular country/region, this is labor-intensive and expensive. An alternative is conducting pilot studies to estimate the prevalence of CD in some of the high-risk patient groups, for instance patients with type 1 diabetes, chronic diarrhea, anemia, or short stature, where prevalence of CD is severalfold higher than in the general population. If the existence of CD is confirmed by these pilot studies, population-based studies can be conducted. Furthermore, a multicenter epidemiological effort aimed to measure the relevant parameters (level of gluten intake, frequency and pattern of CD-predisposing genotypes) could help clarify the complex interplay between genetic and environmental factors leading to CD development [22].

Increase in Awareness and Education about the Disease

It is essential that the awareness of and knowledge about CD and its disease associations increase in medical practitioners and population at large. The obvious groups to target are pediatricians, family physicians, gastroenterologists and histopathologists. However, it should be emphasized that other medical specialists may come in contact with CD. Patients with CD present to endocrinologists with short stature or type 1 diabetes, to hematologists with anemia, to rheumatologists with metabolic bone diseases, and to gynecologists with delay in menarche, secondary amenorrhea or infertility [22].

Very often, histopathologists are not conversant with the handling and reporting of mucosal biopsies from patients suspected to have CD. While specialist gastrointestinal pathologists may be consulted or slides sent for review, it is necessary for all pathologists to be trained in handling such biopsies and at least providing a preliminary report to the attending physician. With the estimated prevalence of CD in Asia, it is very unlikely that there would be a commensurate increase in gastrointestinal pathologists [22]. Hence, general histopathologists in these countries would screen biopsies, and referrals would be limited to difficult cases. Furthermore, histopathologists would be required to train and supervise technical staff handling such specimens. This could be done by ensuring appropriate training during residency, postgraduation and fellowships, and through continuing medical educational programs.

Currently, a due emphasis is not placed on CD in the undergraduate and postgraduate medical curriculum. In the majority of the undergraduate and postgraduate textbooks of medicine, CD is generally dealt with in the chapters on malabsorption and only limited information about CD is provided. A due emphasis should be put on CD during undergraduate and postgraduate medical education. Furthermore, a constant reminder should be provided to physicians, internists, gastroenterologists, hematologists, and endocrinologists through continuing medical education programs.

Focus on Primary Care Physician

The first contact of CD patients is generally with primary care physicians and family physicians. Empowering primary care physicians and family physicians should play a key role in increasing CD detection. It is clear from a study in Northern Ireland that the primary care physician is the most likely source of the increase in the rate of diagnosis of CD in that country [68]. Gastroenterologists in Asian countries can play an immense role in increasing awareness in their own countries about CD and can educate the referring doctors about the prevalence, diverse clinical manifestations of the disease, and availability of the serologic tests.

Development of the Infrastructure for the Diagnosis and Management of CD

Increase in Funding

Government and nongovernmental funding agencies should prioritize and allocate funds for CD research (epidemiological and basic research) [22].

Widespread Availability of Serological Tests

Currently, most celiac-specific serological assay kits in Asia are imported from Europe. Their diagnostic cutoff values of antibody concentrations have been determined based on Caucasian populations. With the difference and diversity in gluten ingestion and genetic background, the cutoff values for a positive test in Asia may not be similar to those reported in the Caucasians. Therefore, there is a real need for the estimation of population-specific cutoff values of serological tests especially for anti-tTG Ab, and anti-DGP Ab. The other diagnostic aspects of serological tests such as specificity, sensitivity, positive predictive values and negative predictive values should also be determined in Asian populations [22].

Training of Dietitians

Management of CD is very different from that of other gastrointestinal diseases in that the core of the treatment is dietary and nonmedicinal [69–70]. Prescribing gluten-free diet (GFD) after diagnosis is easy, but its institution and maintenance of adherence pose real challenges. Most physicians may not have enough expertise in counseling for GFD. In Western countries, dietitians play a pivotal role in the management of patients with CD. However, there is a lack of trained dietitians in most Asian nations; and even if they are there, most do not have sufficient expertise in the management of CD.

Creation of Gluten-Free Infrastructure in the Food Supply

Because of the perception that CD is uncommon in Asia and a low absolute number of patients with CD in Asia, the need for making a GFD available has not been perceived. At present, there is neither an organized sector nor industry for gluten-free products in Asia, and gluten-free food products are not readily available. Gluten is ubiquitous in the food industry and often used in a variety of food items. More importantly, there is no gluten labeling in the available food products. The patient cannot judge the safety of an over-the-counter food product. There is an urgent need for legislation to enforce gluten labeling of the marketed food products.

Patient Advocacy Organizations

The importance of excellent written information in the local language and with relevance to the local food supply cannot be overstated. This has been facilitated in many countries by patient advocacy organizations. They have also provided a collective voice for patients to exert political pressure.

Conclusion

In conclusion, although the absolute number of patients with CD at present is not very large, this number is expected to increase over the next few years/decades. It is thus appropriate that the medical community across Asia define the extent of the problem and get prepared to handle the impending CD epidemic.

Disclosure Statement

The author declares no conflict of interest.

References

1 Rewers M: Epidemiology of CeD: what are the prevalence, incidence, and progression of CeD? Gastroenterology 2005;128(suppl 1): S47–S51.

2 Catassi C, Rätsch IM, Fabiani E, Rossini M, Bordicchia F, Candela F, Coppa GV, Giorgi PL: Coeliac disease in the year 2000: exploring the iceberg. Lancet 1994;343:200–203.

3 Tack GJ, Verbeek WH, Schreurs MW, Mulder CJ: The spectrum of CeD: epidemiology, clinical aspects and treatment. Nat Rev Gastroenterol Hepatol 2010;7:204–213.
4 Fasano A, Catassi C: Clinical practice. Celiac disease. N Engl J Med 2012;367:2419–2426.
5 Mustalahti K, Catassi C, Reunanen A, Fabiani E, Heier M, McMillan S, Murray L, Metzger MH, Gasparin M, Bravi E, Mäki M; Coeliac EU Cluster, Project Epidemiology: The prevalence of celiac disease in Europe: results of a centralized, international mass screening project. Ann Med 2010;42:587–595.
6 Khoshoo V, Bhan MK, Jain R, Phillips AD, Walker-Smith JA, Unsworth DJ, Stintzing G: Coeliac disease as cause of protracted diarrhoea in Indian children. Lancet 1988;1:126–127.
7 Poddar U, Thapa BR, Nain CK, Prasad A, Singh K: Celiac disease in India: are they true cases of celiac disease? J Pediatr Gastroenterol Nutr 2002;35:508–512.
8 Mohindra S, Yachha SK, Srivastava A, Krishnani N, Aggarwal R, Ghoshal UC, Prasad KK, Naik SR: Coeliac disease in Indian children: assessment of clinical, nutritional and pathologic characteristics. J Health Popul Nutr 2001;19:204–208.
9 Bhattacharya M, Kapoor S, Dubey AP: Celiac disease presentation in a tertiary referral centre in India: current scenario. Indian J Gastroenterol 2013;32:98–102.
10 Makharia GK, Baba CS, Khadgawat R, Lal S, Tevatia MS, Madan K, Dattagupta S: Celiac disease: variations of presentations in adults. Indian J Gastroenterol 2007;26:162–166.
11 Nijhawan S, Katiyar P, Nagaich N, Saradava V, Nijhawan M, Gupta G, Mathur A, Sharma R, Nepalia S: Prevalence of associated disorders in Indian patients with celiac disease. Indian J Gastroenterol 2013;32:330–334.
12 Rastogi A, Bhadada SK, Bhansali A, Kochhar R, Santosh R: Celiac disease: a missed cause of metabolic bone disease. Indian J Endocrinol Metab 2012;16:780–785.
13 Sood A, Midha V, Sood N, Avasthi G, Sehgal A: Prevalence of celiac disease among school children in Punjab, North India. J Gastroenterol Hepatol 2006;21:1622–1625.
14 Makharia GK, Verma AK, Amarchand R, Bhatnagar S, Das P, Goswami A, Bhatia V, Ahuja V, Datta Gupta S, Anand K: Prevalence of celiac disease in the northern part of India: a community based study. J Gastroenterol Hepatol 2011;26:894–900.
15 Wu J, Xia B, von Blomberg BM, Zhao C, Yang XW, Crusius JB, Peña AS: Coeliac disease: emerging in China? Gut 2010;59:418–419.
16 Wang XQ, Liu W, Xu CD, Mei H, Gao Y, Peng HM, Yuan L, Xu JJ: Celiac disease in children with diarrhea in 4 cities in China. J Pediatr Gastroenterol Nutr 2011;53:368–370.
17 Yuan J, Gao J, Li X, Liu F, Wijmenga C, Chen H, Gilissen LJ: The tip of the 'celiac iceberg' in China: a systematic review and meta-analysis. PLoS One 20134;8:e81151.
18 Watanabe C, Komoto S, Hokari R, Kurihara C, Okada Y, Hozumi H, Higashiyama M, Sakuraba A, Tomita K, Tsuzuki Y, Kawaguchi A, Nagao S, Ogata S, Miura S: Prevalence of serum celiac antibody in patients with IBD in Japan. J Gastroenterol 2014;49:825–834.
19 Lu W, Gwee KA, Siah KT, Kang JY, Lee R, Ngan CC: Prevalence of anti-deamidated gliadin peptide antibodies in Asian patients with irritable bowel syndrome. J Neurogastroenterol Motil 2014;20:236–241.
20 Ikram MA, Sajid A, Hameed S, Arshad K, Irshad-ul-Haq: Coeliac disease in children presenting with failure to thrive. J Ayub Med Coll Abbottabad 2011;23:6–9.
21 Cummins AG, Roberts-Thomson IC: Prevalence of celiac disease in the Asia-Pacific region. J Gastroenterol Hepatol 2009;24:1347–1351.
22 Makharia GK, Mulder CJ, Goh KL, Ahuja V, Bai JC, Catassi C, Green PH, Gupta SD, Lundin KE, Ramakrishna BS, Rawat R, Sharma H, Sood A, Watanabe C, Gibson PR; World Gastroenterology Organization-Asia Pacific Association of Gastroenterology Working Party on Celiac Disease: Issues associated with the emergence of coeliac disease in the Asia-Pacific region: a working party report of the World Gastroenterology Organization and the Asian Pacific Association of Gastroenterology. J Gastroenterol Hepatol 2014;29:666–677.
23 Walia BN, Sidhu JK, Tandon BN, Ghai OP, Bhargava S: Coeliac disease in North Indian children. BMJ 1966;2:1233–1234.
24 Misra RC, Kasturi D, Chuttani HK: Adult celiac disease in tropics. BMJ 1966;2:1230–1232.
25 Khoshoo V, Bhan MK: Celiac disease in Indian children. Indian Pediatr 1989;26:627–629.
26 Sood A, Midha V, Sood N, Malhotra V: Adult celiac disease in northern India. Indian J Gastroenterol 2003;22:124–126.
27 Sood A, Midha V, Sood N, Kaushal V, Puri H: Increasing incidence of celiac disease in India. Am J Gastroenterol 2001;96:2804–2805.
28 Agarwal N, Monga R, Puri AS: Adult celiac disease in northern India. Indian J Gastroenterol 2003;22:238.
29 Butterworth JR, Iqbal TH, Cooper BT: Coeliac disease in South Asians resident in Britain: comparison with white Caucasian coeliac patients. Eur J Gastroenterol Hepatol 2005;17:541–545.
30 Freeman HJ: Biopsy-defined adult CeD in Asian-Canadians. Can J Gastroenterol 2003;17:433–436.
31 Cataldo F, Accomando S, Fragapane ML, Montaperto D; SIGENP and GLNBI Working Groups on Food Intolerances: Are food intolerances and allergies increasing in immigrant children coming from developing countries? Pediatr Allergy Immunol 2006;17:364–369.
32 Cataldo F, Pitarresi N, Accomando S, Greco L; SIGENP; GLNBI Working Group on Coeliac Disease: Epidemiological and clinical features in immigrant children with coeliac disease: an Italian multicentre study. Dig Liver Dis 2004;36:722–729.
33 Sher KS, Fraser RC, Wicks AC, Mayberry JF: High risk of coeliac disease in Punjabis. Epidemiological study in the south Asian and European populations of Leicestershire. Digestion 1993;54:178–182.
34 Accomando S, Cataldo F: The global village of CeD. Dig Liver Dis 2004;36:492–498.
35 Gupta R, Reddy DN, Makharia GK, Sood A, Ramakrishna BS, Yachha SK, Thapa BR, Banerjee R, Anuradha S, Datta U, Puri AS, Jain AK, Mulder CJJ, Kumar A, Boindala S: Indian task force for celiac disease: current status. World J Gastroenterol 2009;15:6028–6033.
36 Ramakrishna BS: Celiac disease: can we avert the impending epidemic in India? Indian J Med Res 2011;133:5–8.
37 Cataldo F, Montalto G: Celiac disease in the developing countries: a new and challenging public health problem. World J Gastroenterol 2007;13:2153–2159.
38 Rostami K, Malekzadeh R, Shahbazkhani B, Akbari MR, Catassi C: Coeliac disease in Middle Eastern countries: a challenge for the evolutionary history of this complex disorder? Dig Liver Dis 2004;36:694–697.
39 Abu-Zekry M, Kryszak D, Diab M, Catassi C, Fasano A: Prevalence of celiac disease in Egyptian children disputes the east-west agriculture-dependent spread of the disease. J Pediatr Gastroenterol Nutr 2008;47:136–140.
40 Gee SJ: On the celiac affection. St Bartholomews Hosp Rep 1888;24:17–20.
41 Carroccio A, Di Prima L, Noto D, Fayer F, Ambrosiano G, Villanacci V, et al: Searching for wheat plants with low toxicity in celiac disease: between direct toxicity and immunologic activation. Dig Liver Dis 2011;43:34–39.
42 Matsuoka Y: Evolution of polyploid triticum wheats under cultivation: the role of domestication, natural hybridization and allopolyploid speciation in their diversification. Plant Cell Physiol 2011;52:750–764.
43 Kumar P, Joshi PK, Birthal PS: Demand projections for foodgrains in India. Agric Econ Res Rev 2009;22:237–243.
44 Zhang SY, Wan DH, Zhao JH, Xu ZQ, Wang PP, et al (eds): China Yearbook Rural Household Survey – 2010. Beijing, China Statistics Press, 2010, p 327.
45 Chen XJ, Wang QQ, Que XQ, Shuai R, Xu FJ, et al (eds): China Urban Life and Price Yearbook – 2010. Beijing, China Statistics Press, 2010, p 46.
46 Sollid L, Thorsby E: HLA susceptibility genes in CeD: genetic mapping and role in pathogenesis. Gastroenterology 1993;105:910–922.
47 Kaukinen K, Partanen J, Mäki M, Collin P: HLA-DQ typing in the diagnosis of celiac disease. Am J Gastroenterol 2002;97:695–699.

48 Lundin KE, Sollid LM, Qvigstad E, Markussen G, Gjertsen HA, Ek J, Thorsby E: T lymphocyte recognition of a CeD-associated cis- or trans-encoded HLA-DQ alpha/beta-heterodimer. J Immunol 1990;145:136–139.

49 Tollefsen S, Arentz-Hansen H, Fleckenstein B, Molberg O, Ráki M, Kwok WW, Jung G, Lundin KE, Sollid LM: HLA-DQ2 and -DQ8 signatures of gluten T cell epitopes in CeD. J Clin Invest 2006;116:2226–2236.

50 Tjon JM, van Bergen J, Koning F: CeD: How complicated can it get? Immunogenetics 2010;62:641–651.

51 Stepniak D, Koning F: Celiac disease sandwiched between innate and adaptive immunity. Hum Immunol 2006;67:460–468.

52 Lindfors K, Koskinen O, Kaukinen K: An update on the diagnostics of celiac disease. Int Rev Immunol 2011;30:185–196.

53 Abadie V, Sollid LM, Barreiro LB, Jabri B: Integration of genetic and immunological insights into a model of celiac disease pathogenesis. Annu Rev Immunol 2011;29:493–525.

54 Catassi C, Doloretta Macis M, Rätsch IM, De Virgiliis S, Cucca F: The distribution of DQ genes in the Saharawi population provides only a partial explanation for the high celiac disease prevalence. Tissue Antigens 2001;58: 402–406.

55 Kaur G, Sarkar N, Bhatnagar S, Kumar S, Rapthap CC, Bhan MK, Mehra NK: Pediatric CeD in India is associated with multiple DR3-DQ2 haplotypes. Hum Immunol 2002;63:677–682.

56 Xiao CJ, Cavalli-Sforza LL, Minch E, Du RF: Principal component analysis of gene frequencies of Chinese populations. Sci China C Life Sci 2000;43:472–481.

57 Xue F, Wang J, Hu P, Ma D, Liu J, et al: Identification of spatial genetic boundaries using a multifractal model in human population genetics. Hum Biol 2005;77:577–617.

58 Garner CP, Murray JA, Ding YC, Tien Z, van Heel DA, Neuhausen SL: Replication of celiac disease UK genome-wide association study results in a US population. Hum Mol Genet 2009;18:4219–4225.

59 Adamovic S, Amundsen SS, Lie BA, Gudjónsdóttir AH, Ascher H, Ek J, van Heel DA, Nilsson S, Sollid LM, Torinsson Naluai A: Association study of IL2/IL21 and FcgRIIa: significant association with the IL2/IL21 region in Scandinavian coeliac disease families. Genes Immun 2008;9:364–367.

60 Romanos J, Barisani D, Trynka G, Zhernakova A, Bardella MT, Wijmenga C: Six new coeliac disease loci replicated in an Italian population confirm association with coeliac disease. J Med Genet 2009;46:60–63.

61 Trynka G, Zhernakova A, Romanos J, Franke L, Hunt KA, Turner G, Bruinenberg M, Heap GA, Platteel M, Ryan AW, de Kovel C, Holmes GK, Howdle PD, Walters JR, Sanders DS, Mulder CJ, Mearin ML, Verbeek WH, Trimble V, Stevens FM, Kelleher D, Barisani D, Bardella MT, McManus R, van Heel DA, Wijmenga C: Coeliac disease-associated risk variants in TNFAIP3 and REL implicate altered NF-kappaB signalling. Gut 2009;58: 1078–1083.

62 Forabosco P, Neuhausen SL, Greco L, Naluai AT, Wijmenga C, Saavalainen P, Houlston RS, Ciclitira PJ, Babron MC, Lewis CM: Meta-analysis of genome-wide linkage studies in CeD. Hum Hered 2009;68:223–230.

63 Dubois PC, Trynka G, Franke L, Hunt KA, et al: Multiple common variants for celiac disease influencing immune gene expression. Nat Genet 2010;42:295–302.

64 Zhernakova A, Stahl EA, Trynka G, Raychaudhuri S, et al: Meta-analysis of genome-wide association studies in celiac disease and rheumatoid arthritis identifies fourteen non-HLA shared loci. PLoS Genet 2011;7:e1002004.

65 Makharia G: Where are Indian adult celiacs? Trop Gastroenterol 2006;27:1–3.

66 Ludvigsson JF, Leffler DA, Bai JC, Biagi F, Fasano A, Green PH, Hadjivassiliou M, Kaukinen K, Kelly CP, Leonard JN, Lundin KE, Murray JA, Sanders DS, Walker MM, Zingone F, Ciacci C: The Oslo definitions for coeliac disease and related terms. Gut 2013; 62:43–52.

67 Theethira TG, Kelly CP: Coeliac disease. Missing villi? The search for coeliac disease in the Asia-Pacific region. Nat Rev Gastroenterol Hepatol 2014;11:204–205.

68 Dickey W, McMillan SA: Increasing numbers at a specialist coeliac clinic: contribution of serological testing in primary care. Dig Liver Dis 2005;37:928–933.

69 See J, Murray JA: Gluten-free diet: the medical and nutrition management of celiac disease. Nutr Clin Pract 2006;21:1–15.

70 García-Manzanares A, Lucendo AJ: Nutritional and dietary aspects of celiac disease. Nutr Clin Pract 2011;26:163–173.

Dig Dis 2015;33:175–182
DOI: 10.1159/000369504

Celiac Disease and the Gluten-Free Diet: Consequences and Recommendations for Improvement

Thimmaiah G. Theethira   Melinda Dennis

Division of Gastroenterology, Celiac Center, Beth Israel Deaconess Medical Center, Boston, Mass., USA

Key Words

Celiac disease · Gluten-free diet · Micronutrients · Macronutrients · Nutritional deficiency

Abstract

Background: Celiac disease (CD) is a chronic small intestinal immune-mediated enteropathy precipitated by exposure to dietary gluten in genetically susceptible individuals. CD-related enteropathy leads to multiple nutritional deficiencies involving macro- and micronutrients. Currently, medical nutrition therapy consisting of the gluten-free diet (GFD) is the only accepted treatment for CD. ***Key Messages:*** The GFD is the cornerstone of treatment for CD. Prior published studies have concluded that maintenance of the GFD results in improvement of the majority of nutritional deficiencies. In the past, counseling for CD focused mainly on the elimination of gluten in the diet. However, the GFD is not without its inadequacies; compliance to the GFD may result in certain deficiencies such as fiber, B vitamins, iron, and trace minerals. Paucity of fortified gluten-free foods may be responsible for certain deficiencies which develop on the GFD. Weight gain and obesity have been added to the list of nutritional consequences while on the GFD and have been partially attributed to hypercaloric content of commercially available gluten-free foods. Follow-up of patients diagnosed with CD after starting the GFD has been reported to be irregular and, hence, less than ideal. ***Conclusions:*** Monitoring of the nutritional status using blood tests and use of appropriate gluten-free supplementation are integral components in the management of CD. The ideal GFD should be nutrient-dense with naturally gluten-free foods, balanced with macro- and micronutrients, reasonably priced, and easily accessible. Rotation of the pseudo-cereals provides a good source of complex carbohydrates, protein, fiber, fatty acids, vitamins and minerals. Fortification/enrichment of commonly consumed gluten-free commercial grain products should be encouraged. Dietitians specializing in CD play a critical role in the education and maintenance of the GFD for patients with CD.

Introduction

Celiac disease (CD) is defined as a chronic small intestinal immune-mediated enteropathy precipitated by exposure to dietary gluten in genetically predisposed individuals [1]. CD has been reported around the globe with a prevalence of 1–2% of the population in North and South America, North Africa, the Middle East and India [2, 3]. There is a paucity of reliable data regarding the

KARGER 125

© 2015 S. Karger AG, Basel
0257–2753/15/0332–0175$39.50/0

E-Mail karger@karger.com
www.karger.com/ddi

Melinda Dennis, MS, RD, LDN
Nutrition Coordinator, Celiac Center
Beth Israel Deaconess Medical Center
Dana 603, 330 Brookline Avenue, Boston, MA 02215 (USA)
E-Mail mdennis@bidmc.harvard.edu

prevalence in Sub-Saharan Africa and in the Asia-Pacific region [4]. The prevalence of CD has been increasing in the US as noted by a recent study which showed a 5-fold increase since 1975 [5]. Though the reasons for these changes are unclear, they may have to do with the environmental components of CD (changes in the quantity and quality of ingested gluten, infant feeding patterns, the spectrum of intestinal infections, gut microbiota colonization, etc.) [6]. Some of the increase in prevalence can also be attributed to increased awareness and improved diagnostic and epidemiologic tools. The economic burden of undiagnosed CD over 10 years was estimated to be EUR 4 billion in the Mediterranean region alone [7].

Gluten is the alcohol-soluble fraction of wheat protein which is consumed in large quantities (10–20 g per day) as part of the normal food intake in Western countries [8]. It includes a group of prolamines found in the wheat (gliadins and glutenins), rye (secalin), barley (hordein) and other closely related grains [9, 10]. In individuals carrying the haplotype DQ2/DQ8, gluten intake results in activation of a cellular immune response which leads to different degrees of small bowel mucosal injury, ranging from mild intraepithelial lymphocytosis to total villous atrophy [11]. Villous atrophy in the small bowel leads to chronic malabsorption of macro- and micronutrients, which is the hallmark of untreated CD.

Gluten-Free Diet

CD is unique amongst chronic immune-mediated disorders in that diet is the only recognized treatment. Currently, initiation and lifelong maintenance of the gluten-free diet (GFD) remains the cornerstone of therapy in CD. The National Institute of Health guidelines on CD emphasize consultation with a skilled registered dietitian (RD) as being a key feature in adhering to the GFD [12]. Learning to follow the GFD often involves major changes in lifelong dietary patterns [13]. Wheat, rye and barley serve as the primary grains in most cereal-based foods in North America and Europe, including breads, cakes, cookies, pastries, pasta, breakfast cereals and many snack foods. In addition, wheat is frequently used as a binder in many soups, sauces and dressings, deli meats, sausages, meat patties and artificial seafood, and as a coating on meat, poultry and fish. Most soy sauce is wheat-based and barley malt is used in the preparation of beer [14].

Adherence to the GFD leads to regression of symptoms, normalization of histological and laboratory findings and reduction in the risk of CD-related complications in most individuals with CD [15]. Zarkadas et al. [16] reported improvement of symptoms in 83% of the respondents with CD on the GFD in a mail-out survey.

It was generally assumed that patients with CD adhering to a strict GFD for years would consume a diet that was nutritionally adequate [17]. However, in the last two decades, multiple studies have shown that patients on the GFD need to be monitored for certain nutritional deficiencies which may complicate the GFD [18–20]. It is well established that the nutritional impact of CD depends on the duration of the untreated disease, extent and location of mucosal injury, and the degree of malabsorption of certain nutrients [21]. In the last 20 years, an additional factor has come into the picture – 'quality of the GFD'. It is the objective of this paper to highlight the nutritional imbalances of the GFD and suggest measures to overcome them (fig. 1).

Macronutrient Imbalances in the GFD

Often, patients with CD overcome the restriction of the GFD by substituting foods with high fat, sugar and calorie content [22]. Gluten-free products often contain a greater carbohydrate and lipid content than their gluten-containing equivalents. Segura and colleagues reported that the nutritional composition of a range of gluten-free breads had a high glycemic index, with low protein and high fat content. Caponio et al. [23] showed that commercially available gluten-free biscuits were richer in saturated fatty acids compared to the gluten-containing equivalents. Mariani et al. [22] reported in a study involving adolescents with CD that these subjects had a higher fat and protein intake than recommended. In their study, it was proposed that patients following a strict GFD preferred food with the higher amount of protein (meat, eggs, legumes) and snacks with a high content of lipids. The authors also speculated that these dietetic habits in adolescents could cause a disturbance in the growth pattern. Wild et al. [24] in a British study reported that the dietary intake of British female patients with CD contained more energy across all macronutrients as compared to the local population. This was attributed to a higher intake of nonmilk extrinsic sugar present in sugary snacks. The authors cautioned that maintaining available carbohydrate intake using naturally occurring products like beans, pulses and starchy

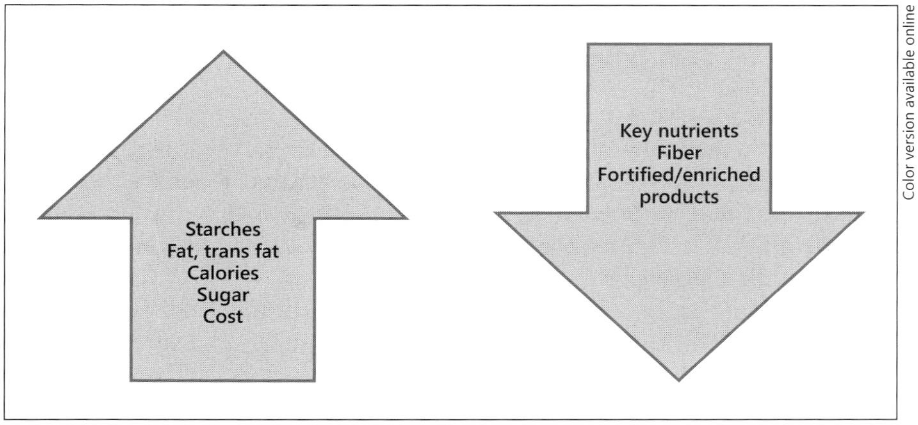

Color version available online

Fig. 1. Negative factors affecting quality of gluten-free products [19, 33, 37, 48, 52, 53].

vegetables such as a potato or alternative grains should be done without resorting to processed gluten-free sugary foods. Ohlund et al. [25] reported in a Swedish study involving children with CD that dietary fat intake was relatively high when compared to the Nordic nutrition recommendations (NNR 2004). It was observed that Swedish children with CD had a mean intake of 14% saturated fatty acids and less than 4% polyunsaturated fatty acids [25, 26]. The Nordic Nutrition recommendations suggest saturated fatty acids should contribute less than 10% of the total caloric intake and polyunsaturated fatty acid should contribute at least 5–10% of the total caloric intake [26].

Fiber Intake and the GFD

Chronic constipation is a common and significant symptom in patients with CD [27]. Hence, adequate intake of fiber is important for patients with the above presentation. Dietary fiber is a complex mixture of plant materials and molecules that are resistant to digestion. The beneficial effect of a high-fiber diet in preventing diseases like coronary heart disease, diabetes, and colon cancer has been studied in the past [28]. Some studies have reported that the GFD is associated with a lower intake of dietary fiber. Thompson et al. [19] reported in a 2005 study that less than half of the female survey respondents consumed daily recommended amounts of fiber. Nearly 15% of the US adult daily intake of fiber comes from gluten-containing yeast bread. Unfortunately, the vast majority of gluten-free commercial grain-based products (made from refined gluten-free grains and/or starches) contain significantly less fiber than their gluten-containing counterparts. Two other studies from the UK also reported similar results. In a British study done by Kinsey et al. [29], a reduced intake of dietary fiber was observed in adult patients with CD with similar results in the general population. Wild et al. [24] reported an inadequate intake of dietary fiber in British individuals consuming a strict GFD.

Micronutrient Imbalances in the GFD

Vitamins

Prior studies have documented deficiencies of both fat- and water-soluble vitamins in patients with newly diagnosed CD [30–32]. Logic dictates that once the GFD is instituted, villous atrophy improves and leads to resolution of malabsorption correcting vitamin deficiencies. However, in the last two decades nutritional studies have indicated that some vitamin deficiencies tend to persist years after institution of the GFD [20, 33]. In a study reported from Australia, inadequate intake of folate and thiamine was documented in patients with CD who had been on the GFD for at least 2 years. This discrepancy was attributed to the fact that (1) very few gluten-free breakfast cereals were fortified with folate as compared to the common practice of fortification in wheat-based cereals, and (2) in the case of thiamine, there was mandatory fortification of thiamine in the wheat flour for regular bread which was not the case for gluten-free equivalents [33]. Hallert et al. [20] in a study conducted in Sweden reported that over 50% of the patients with CD had low vitamin levels (vitamin B_6 and folate), and that these patients had been adhering to a strict GFD for years. An additional finding of this study was an elevated plasma homocysteine level in adult patients with CD, which could imply an independent increased risk for cardiovascular disease like hypertension and hyperlipidemia. In Sweden, neither gluten-free products nor their gluten-containing counterparts are folate enriched and, hence, it was concluded that the major determinant of the poor vitamin status of patients with CD may be their choice of foods.

This finding again emphasizes the importance of the 'quality' of the GFD in the treatment of patients with CD. The same author conducted a double-blind placebo-controlled multicenter trial where patients with CD on a strict GFD for several years were randomized to a daily vitamin supplementation consisting of pyridoxine, vitamin B_{12}, and folic acid for 6 months. Researchers noted that total homocysteine levels dropped 34% in patients with CD on daily vitamin supplementation and were accompanied by significant improvement in well-being [34].

Martin et al. [35] analyzed the dietary intake of 88 German patients with CD on the GFD and found suboptimal intake of vitamins B_1, B_2, B_6 and folic acid. Similar findings have been published from studies in the US. Thompson [36] in a study published in 1999 observed that only 35 of the 368 gluten-free flours, breads, pastas and cereals were enriched with thiamine, riboflavin and/or niacin. As a result of the findings, a concern was raised about the long-term GFD being deficient in the above nutrients. In a similar study in 2005, Thompson et al. [19] noted that of the 58 gluten-free breads, pastas, and cold cereals, only 3 cold cereals were fortified with folic acid. None of the bread products or pastas was enriched with folic acid.

In addition to inadequate intake of B complex vitamins, reduced intake of vitamin D has been documented in two European studies. Ohlund et al. [25] reported reduced intake of vitamin D in Swedish children on the GFD. Similarly, a British study in adult patients with CD showed reduced intake of vitamin D while adhering to the GFD [29].

Minerals and Trace Elements in the GFD

Iron deficiency is highly prevalent in patients with newly diagnosed CD [30]. Correction of this deficiency is likely to improve some of the related symptoms seen in patients with CD, such as fatigue. Some studies have reported decreased iron intake while following the GFD. Thompson [37] noted that 64 of the 83 gluten-free cereal products had lower amounts of iron as compared to their gluten-containing counterparts. Only 9 of the 58 gluten-free breads, pastas, and cold cereals were fortified with iron. In a recently published study from Australia, the majority of the female patients with CD on the GFD for at least 2 years were consuming inadequate intakes of iron in relation to recommended daily intake [33]. Reduced calcium intake has also been reported in patients following the GFD. Thompson et al. [19] noted that less than one third of the female survey respondents consumed daily recommended amounts of calcium during the recording period. Similar findings of reduced calcium intake while on the GFD have also been reported in other countries [29, 33]. Reduced milk intake secondary to temporary lactose intolerance in patients with active CD is one of the mechanisms which could explain reduced calcium intake [38].

Other minerals and trace elements which have been documented to be inadequate in intake while on the GFD include magnesium, zinc and selenium [24, 33, 35].

Weight Gain on the GFD

In contrast to the 'classic' celiac presentation of malabsorption and weight loss, overweight and obese patients presenting with CD are becoming increasingly prevalent [39]. A retrospective study published in 2006 reported that nearly 40% of patients with CD were overweight at diagnosis with 13% of them falling in the obese range [39].

Recent studies in the last decade have raised concern that initiation and maintenance of the GFD result in weight gain further compounding the above problem. Valletta et al. [40] reported increased body mass index (BMI) after initiation of the GFD, and the percentage of overweight subjects almost doubled while on the GFD. A proposed theory put forward by the authors was incorrect dietary habits induced by unpalatable, expensive commercial gluten-free products and availability of high-fat commercial gluten-free snacks and biscuits. Kabbani et al. [41] reported significant increase in BMI after the GFD initiation. Nearly 22% of patients who were overweight at diagnosis gained weight while on the GFD.

Enhancing Nutrition of the GFD

Avoiding gluten is the single most important step in the management of CD. Emphasis should be placed on selecting naturally gluten-free foods and avoiding overreliance on gluten-free processed foods which tend to be low in fiber, vitamins, and minerals, and higher in sugar, fat, and calories. A naturally healthy GFD is rich in fruits and vegetables, labeled gluten-free whole grains and products made from them, legumes and dried beans, lean protein sources, nuts and seeds, low-fat dairy or nondairy alternatives rich in calcium and vitamin D, and healthy fats, including omega-3 fatty acids. The importance of eating a wide variety of colorful fruits and vegetables for their vitamins and minerals, and phytonutrient and antioxidant compounds cannot be overemphasized.

When initiating the GFD, a protein- and energy-rich diet should be encouraged, particularly if the patient has significant weight loss and deficiencies caused by malabsorption. In most patients, a 6-month period is adequate for malabsorption to improve [42]. Thereafter, a more balanced approach is warranted to avoid increased intake of unhealthy fats which is implicated in obesity and cardiovascular disease.

Weight Gain on the GFD

Weight gain, although a sign of improving absorption, is not always welcome, particularly in patients who are overweight at diagnosis. Weight gain following the diagnosis of CD can be attributed to several factors including the healing of the intestines and changes in diet [43]. Dickey and Kearney [39] reported that 55 of the 67 patients who were overweight at diagnosis gained weight at the end of 2 years on the GFD. The problem of excessive weight gain in patients with CD needs to be addressed by all members of the patient's healthcare team including the RD, gastroenterologist, and primary care physician [44].

Some weight loss tips include replacing at least half of the low fiber, highly refined grains and commercially prepared grain foods eaten daily with gluten-free whole grains and products and eating small, healthy meals and snacks at intervals during the day to avoid strong hunger and cravings. Consulting with an RD to create a healthy eating plan that promotes weight loss and engaging in appropriate regular physical activity are highly recommended [43].

Balanced Food Groups

In patients with CD and the general population, recommendations for food groups and caloric intake are similar and should be individualized as needed. For adults 19 years and older, complex and simple carbohydrates should represent 45–65% of total calories; dietary protein should contribute 10–35% of total calories [45]. Good protein choices include dried beans and legumes, nuts and seeds, fish, lean cuts of poultry, beef, and pork, fat-free or low-fat dairy, and pseudo-grains such as amaranth and quinoa. Total fat intake should represent 20–35% [45], and saturated fatty acid intake should comprise less than 10% of daily total calories, respectively, replaced primarily by monounsaturated and polyunsaturated fatty acids [46]. Trans fats, which are implicated in atherosclerosis, should be consumed as little as possible and be limited to less than 1% of the total caloric intake (5 g/day) [21]. While these acceptable macronutrient distribution ranges take into account intake of essential nutrients and reduction of chronic disease risk, there is wide variability in these proportions among individuals.

Micronutrient and Fiber Intake

Many gluten-free foods are made with refined flour and/or starches which are low in fiber due to processing. It is recommended that patients with CD consume labeled gluten-free whole grains and pseudo-cereals and fortified/enriched products made from them to increase the fiber content of the GFD [47]. These include brown rice, wild rice, buckwheat, quinoa, oats, amaranth, millet, sorghum, and teff. It is recommended to choose 6–11 servings of gluten-free grains daily depending on the caloric content of the patient's diet [19]. At least half of these daily grain servings should come from whole-grain sources. Recommendations for adult fiber intake range from 21 to 38 g per day based on age, gender, and health status [46].

In addition to fiber, the gluten-free grains and pseudo-cereals also provide key vitamins and minerals. In a study by Lee et al. [48], three servings of whole/enriched cereals and pseudo-cereals (oats, brown rice, and quinoa) positively impacted the nutrient profile (thiamin, riboflavin, niacin, folate, iron and fiber) of the grain portion of the diet and were more cost-effective than processed gluten-free grain products. In women of childbearing age, special effort should be made to include nongrain sources of iron and B vitamins during pregnancy and lactation.

The importance of calcium and vitamin D cannot be overemphasized, especially considering the prevalence of metabolic bone disease in the celiac population. It is recommended to select three servings/day of low-fat or nonfat dairy or calcium- and vitamin D-fortified non-

Table 1. Recommended nutritional management in patients with CD[a]

Nutrient	Epidemiology	Testing recommendation	Treatment recommendation
Iron	Deficiency present in 28–50% patients at diagnosis One of the most common extraintestinal manifestations	Serum iron and ferritin at diagnosis Repeat every 3–6 months until ferritin is normal Then every 1–2 years or for symptoms	Iron supplements (325 mg) 1–3 tablets based on initial ferritin level until iron stores are restored Consider i.v. iron for severe symptomatic iron deficiency anemia or intolerance of oral iron
Vitamin D	Low levels are seen in 20–66% of patients at diagnosis Recent reports of deficiency even in regions with high number of days of sunshine	Vitamin D (25 OH) level at diagnosis Repeat every 3 months until vitamin D level is normal Then every 1–2 years or for symptoms	Vitamin D (1,000 U or more per day) based on vitamin D level Vitamin D_2 (50,000 U weekly) if level <20 ng/ml
Folic acid	Reported to be deficient in 18–42% of patients at diagnosis Deficiency rare in North America	Serum folate levels at diagnosis in at-risk populations Check in all women planning pregnancy	Folic acid (1 mg/day) for 3 months Once diarrhea improves 400–800 μg/day
Vitamin B_{12}	Deficiency comparatively less common and seen in 8–41% of patients at diagnosis Suspected to be secondary to bacterial overgrowth	Serum B_{12} at diagnosis Then every 1–2 years or for symptoms	Vitamin B_{12} (1,000 μg) orally until B_{12} level is normal Thereafter daily gluten-free multi-vitamin/ mineral supplement
Zinc	Seen in 54–67% of newly diagnosed patients with CD Most common deficiency seen amongst the trace elements	Serum zinc level at diagnosis; repeat after 3 months until the level is normal Then every 1–2 years or for symptoms	Zinc supplement containing at least 25–40 mg/ day until zinc level is normal Thereafter gluten-free daily multivitamin/ mineral supplement
Calcium	More than 50% of patients consume less than the recommended daily intake of calcium	Regular dietary assessment by the dietitian	Recommended intake of calcium, including supplementation, for patients with CD is 1,200–1,500 mg/day[b]
Dietary fiber	Deficient intake reported while on the GFD causes constipation Deficiency reported in both genders and in Europe as well as the US	Regular dietary assessment by the dietitian	25–35 g/day based on age and gender Encourage intake of 'alternative grains' with high fiber content and adequate water

Reproduced with permission from Theethira et al. [44]. [a] All supplements must be labeled gluten free. [b] Calcium needs vary by age and medical condition. Supplemental, in addition to dietary calcium, may be needed to meet calcium needs (adapted from original chart).

dairy foods [19] for those with lactose intolerance, a dairy allergy, or a preference to avoid dairy. Additional supplementation of calcium and particularly of Vitamin D may be needed.

Iron deficiency is highly prevalent at diagnosis in individuals with CD [30]. The GFD can restore dietary iron absorption and resolve anemia in the majority of patients with CD [49]; however, additional supplementation is frequently required [44]. Iron-rich foods include, but are not limited to, animal protein, most kinds of seafood, quinoa, amaranth, teff, leafy greens, nuts and seeds, and gluten-free pasta, cereal, or breads that have been fortified with iron [21, 37, 50]. The daily iron needs should be discussed with the doctor or RD as they vary by gender, age, and medical condition.

The RD should advise individuals with CD to consume a daily gluten-free age- and sex-specific multivitamin/mineral supplement if the usual food intake shows nutritional inadequacies that cannot be alleviated through improved eating habits [47]. Nutritional management of patients with CD should also include diagnosis and treatment of specific micronutrient deficiencies with periodic blood tests and appropriate dietary supplementation, such as iron, zinc, B vitamins, vitamin D and/or calcium (table 1).

The NIH guidelines suggest a consultation with an RD with expertise in CD as one of the six main principles in the management of CD [51]. An RD with expertise in CD can help coordinate care including instruction on balancing a healthy GFD, understanding label reading, recommending GF supplements, managing symptoms through dietary interventions, and providing reliable resources. It is important to have regular follow-up visits and lab work to detect and treat nutritional deficiencies after initiation of the GFD [27, 51]. Indisputably, the GFD is the cornerstone of treatment for CD. Keeping these nutritional concerns in mind, a patient with CD can enjoy a healthy, well-rounded diet that improves and maximizes overall health and well-being.

Disclosure Statement

Thimmaiah G. Theethira has no conflict of interest to declare. Melinda Dennis, MS, RD, LDN, is co-author of *Real Life with Celiac Disease: Troubleshooting and Thriving Gluten-Free* published by AGA Press (2010).

References

1 Ludvigsson JF, Leffler DA, Bai JC, et al: The Oslo definitions for coeliac disease and related terms. Gut 2013;62:43–52.
2 Leffler DA, Schuppan D: Update on serologic testing in celiac disease. Am J Gastroenterol 2010;105:2520–2524.
3 Accomando S, Cataldo F: The global village of celiac disease. Dig Liver Dis 2004;36:492–498.
4 Makharia GK, Mulder CJ, Goh KL, et al: Issues associated with the emergence of coeliac disease in the Asia-Pacific region: a working party report of the World Gastroenterology Organization and the Asian Pacific Association of Gastroenterology. J Gastroenterol Hepatol 2014;29:666–677.
5 Catassi C, Kryszak D, Bhatti B, et al: Natural history of celiac disease autoimmunity in a USA cohort followed since 1974. Ann Med 2010;42:530–538.
6 Catassi C, Gatti S, Fasano A: The new epidemiology of celiac disease. J Pediatr Gastroenterol Nutr 2014;59(suppl 1):S7–S9.
7 Greco L, Timpone L, Abkari A, et al: Burden of celiac disease in the Mediterranean area. World J Gastroenterol 2011;17:4971–4978.
8 Schuppan D, Zimmer KP: The diagnosis and treatment of celiac disease. Dtsch Ärztebl Int 2013;110:835–846.
9 Rostom A, Murray JA, Kagnoff MF: American Gastroenterological Association (AGA) Institute technical review on the diagnosis and management of celiac disease. Gastroenterology 2006;131:1981–2002.
10 Platt SG, Kasarda DD: Separation and characterization of α-gliadin fractions. Biochim Biophys Acta 1971;243:407–415.
11 Marsh MN: Gluten, major histocompatibility complex, and the small intestine. A molecular and immunobiologic approach to the spectrum of gluten sensitivity ('celiac sprue'). Gastroenterology 1992;102:330–354.
12 National Institutes of Health Consensus Development Conference Statement on Celiac Disease, June 28–30, 2004. Gastroenterology 2005;128(suppl 1):S1–S9.
13 Hallert C, Granno C, Grant C, et al: Quality of life of adult coeliac patients treated for 10 years. Scand J Gastroenterol 1998;33:933–938.
14 Zarkadas M, Case S: Celiac disease and the gluten free diet-an overview. Top Clin Nutr 2005;20:127–138.
15 Ciacci C, Cirillo M, Cavallaro R, Mazzacca G: Long-term follow-up of celiac adults on gluten-free diet: prevalence and correlates of intestinal damage. Digestion 2002;66:178–185.
16 Zarkadas M, Cranney A, Case S, et al: The impact of a gluten-free diet on adults with coeliac disease: results of a national survey. J Hum Nutr Diet 2006;19:41–49.
17 Parnell ND, Ciclitira PJ: Review article: coeliac disease and its management. Aliment Pharmacol Ther 1999;13:1–13.
18 Penagini F, Dilillo D, Meneghin F, Mameli C, Fabiano V, Zuccotti GV: Gluten-free diet in children: an approach to a nutritionally adequate and balanced diet. Nutrients 2013;5:4553–4565.
19 Thompson T, Dennis M, Higgins LA, Lee AR, Sharrett MK: Gluten-free diet survey: are Americans with coeliac disease consuming recommended amounts of fibre, iron, calcium and grain foods? J Hum Nutr Diet 2005;18:163–169.
20 Hallert C, Grant C, Grehn S, et al: Evidence of poor vitamin status in coeliac patients on a gluten-free diet for 10 years. Aliment Pharmacol Ther 2002;16:1333–1339.
21 Saturni L, Ferretti G, Bacchetti T: The gluten-free diet: safety and nutritional quality. Nutrients 2010;2:16–34.
22 Mariani P, Viti MG, Montuori M, et al: The gluten-free diet: a nutritional risk factor for adolescents with celiac disease? J Pediatr Gastroenterol Nutr 1998;27:519–523.
23 Caponio f, Summo C, Clodoveo ML, Pasqualone A: Evaluation of the nutritional quality of the lipid fraction of gluten-free biscuits. Eur Food Res Technol 2008;43:198.
24 Wild D, Robins GG, Burley VJ, Howdle PD: Evidence of high sugar intake, and low fibre and mineral intake, in the gluten-free diet. Aliment Pharmacol Ther 2010;32:573–581.
25 Ohlund K, Olsson C, Hernell O, Ohlund I: Dietary shortcomings in children on a gluten-free diet. J Hum Nutr Diet 2010;23:294–300.
26 Becker W: New Nordic nutrition recommendations 2004. Physical activity as important as good nourishing food. Lakartidningen 2005;102:2757–2758, 2760–2762.
27 Rubio-Tapia A, Hill ID, Kelly CP, Calderwood AH, Murray JA, American College of Gastroenterology: ACG clinical guidelines: diagnosis and management of celiac disease. Am J Gastroenterol 2013;108:656–676; quiz 677.
28 Anderson JW, Baird P, Davis RH Jr, et al: Health benefits of dietary fiber. Nutr Rev 2009;67:188–205.
29 Kinsey L, Burden ST, Bannerman E: A dietary survey to determine if patients with coeliac disease are meeting current healthy eating guidelines and how their diet compares to that of the British general population. Eur J Clin Nutr 2008;62:1333–1342.
30 Wierdsma NJ, van Bokhorst-de van der Schueren MA, Berkenpas M, Mulder CJ, van Bodegraven AA: Vitamin and mineral deficiencies are highly prevalent in newly diagnosed celiac disease patients. Nutrients 2013;5:3975–3992.
31 Kemppainen TA, Kosma VM, Janatuinen EK, Julkunen RJ, Pikkarainen PH, Uusitupa MI: Nutritional status of newly diagnosed celiac disease patients before and after the institution of a celiac disease diet – association with the grade of mucosal villous atrophy. Am J Clin Nutr 1998;67:482–487.
32 Lerner A, Shapira Y, Agmon-Levin N, et al: The clinical significance of 25OH-vitamin D status in celiac disease. Clin Rev Allergy Immunol 2012;42:322–330.
33 Shepherd SJ, Gibson PR: Nutritional inadequacies of the gluten-free diet in both recently-diagnosed and long-term patients with coeliac disease. J Hum Nutr Diet 2013;26:349–358.
34 Hallert C, Svensson M, Tholstrup J, Hultberg B: Clinical trial: B vitamins improve health in patients with coeliac disease living on a gluten-free diet. Aliment Pharmacol Ther 2009;29:811–816.
35 Martin J, Geisel T, Maresch C, Krieger K, Stein J: Inadequate nutrient intake in patients with celiac disease: results from a German dietary survey. Digestion 2013;87:240–246.
36 Thompson T: Thiamin, riboflavin, and niacin contents of the gluten-free diet: is there cause for concern? J Am Diet Assoc 1999;99:858–862.
37 Thompson T: Folate, iron, and dietary fiber contents of the gluten-free diet. J Am Diet Assoc 2000;100:1389–1396.
38 Farrell RJ, Kelly CP: Celiac sprue. N Engl J Med 2002;346:180–188.
39 Dickey W, Kearney N: Overweight in celiac disease: prevalence, clinical characteristics, and effect of a gluten-free diet. Am J Gastroenterol 2006;101:2356–2359.

40 Valletta E, Fornaro M, Cipolli M, Conte S, Bissolo F, Danchielli C: Celiac disease and obesity: need for nutritional follow-up after diagnosis. Eur J Clin Nutr 2010;64:1371–1372.

41 Kabbani TA, Goldberg A, Kelly CP, et al: Body mass index and the risk of obesity in coeliac disease treated with the gluten-free diet. Aliment Pharmacol Ther 2012;35:723–729.

42 Garcia-Manzanares A, Lucendo AJ: Nutritional and dietary aspects of celiac disease. Nutr Clin Pract 2011;26:163–173.

43 Dennis MD: Weight Gain: A common and sometimes unwelcome, measure of healing; in Dennis M (ed): Real Life with Celiac Disease. Bethesda, AGA Press, 2010, pp 131–138.

44 Theethira TG, Dennis M, Leffler DA: Nutritional consequences of celiac disease and the gluten-free diet. Expert Rev Gastroenterol Hepatol 2014;8:123–129.

45 Trumbo P, Schlicker S, Yates AA, Poos M; Food and Nutrition Board of the Institute of Medicine, The National Academies: Dietary reference intakes for energy, carbohydrate, fiber, fat, fatty acids, cholesterol, protein, and amino acids. J Am Diet Assoc 2002;102:1621–1630.

46 US Department of Agriculture and Department of Health and Human Services: Dietary Guidelines for Americans 2010. Washington, US Government Printing Office, 2010.

47 Dennis MD, Kupper CR, Lee AR, Sharrett MK, Thompson T: Celiac Disease Toolkit. Chicago, American Dietetic Association, 2011.

48 Lee AR, Ng DL, Dave E, Ciaccio EJ, Green PH: The effect of substituting alternative grains in the diet on the nutritional profile of the gluten-free diet. J Hum Nutr Diet 2009;22:359–363.

49 Annibale B, Severi C, Chistolini A, et al: Efficacy of gluten-free diet alone on recovery from iron deficiency anemia in adult celiac patients. Am J Gastroenterol 2001;96:132–137.

50 Decher N, Parrish CR: Balanced and delicious: a healthy gluten-free diet; in Dennis M (ed): Real Life with Celiac Disease. Bethesda, AGA Press, 2010, p 77.

51 NIH Consensus Development Conference on Celiac Disease. NIH Consens State Sci Statements 2004;21:1–23.

52 Miranda J, Lasa A, Bustamante MA, Churruca I, Simon E: Nutritional differences between a gluten-free diet and a diet containing equivalent products with gluten. Plant Foods Hum Nutr 2014;69:182–187.

53 Kupper C: Dietary guidelines and implementation for celiac disease. Gastroenterology 2005;128(suppl 1):S121–S127.

Dig Dis 2015;33:183–189
DOI: 10.1159/000369540

Eosinophilic Enteritis

Guillaume Pineton de Chambrun[a–c] Pierre Desreumaux[b] Antoine Cortot[a]

[a]Clinique des maladies de l'appareil digestif et de la nutrition, Hôpital Claude Huriez, [b]Université Lille 2 Droit et Santé, Inserm U995, team 1, maladies inflammatoires digestives: physiopathologie et développement de cibles thérapeutiques, Faculté de Médecine, Pôle recherche, Laboratoire J&K, Lille, and [c]Service d'Hépato-Gastro-Entérologie, Hôpital Saint-Eloi, CHU Montpellier, Montpellier, France

Key Words
Eosinophils · Gastroenteritis · Intestinal mucosa · Corticosteroids · Natural history

Abstract
Background: Eosinophilic enteritis, also known as eosinophilic gastroenteritis, is a rare primary eosinophilic gastrointestinal disorder (EGID) of unknown etiology characterized by the presence of an intense eosinophilic infiltrate on histopathology of the intestinal mucosa. ***Key Messages:*** The etiology of eosinophilic enteritis remains obscure. There is growing evidence to support the role of aeroallergens and food allergens in the pathogenesis of this disorder as children and adults with EGIDs often have positive skin testing for food allergens and a familial history of allergic diseases. Moreover, significant progress has been made in elucidating that EGIDs involve mechanisms that fall between pure IgE-mediated and delayed Th2 type responses. Preclinical studies have identified a contributory role for the cytokine IL-5 and eotaxin chemokines, providing a rationale for specific disease therapy. Eosinophilic enteritis causes a wide array of gastrointestinal symptoms such as abdominal pain, diarrhea, nausea, vomiting, bloating or ascites, and its diagnosis requires a high degree of clinical likelihood given the nonspecific presentation and physical examination findings. The Klein classification arbitrarily divided patients with eosinophilic enteritis into those with predominantly mucosal, muscle layer or subserosal disease relying on the concept that clinical presentation is dependent on the predominant involved layer of the gastrointestinal tract. Main therapeutic options are represented by oral corticosteroids for a short period with good efficacy. Antihistaminic drugs and sodium cromoglycate have also been used to treat patients with eosinophilic enteritis. ***Conclusion:*** Eosinophilic enteritis is generally considered as a benign disease with no relapse, but half of the patients may present a more complex natural history characterized by unpredictable relapses and a chronic course.

Introduction

Eosinophilic enteritis, also known as eosinophilic gastroenteritis, is a rare gastrointestinal disorder of unknown etiology characterized by an intense infiltration of the intestinal wall by eosinophils [1, 2]. It is part of the primary eosinophil-associated gastrointestinal disorders (EGIDs) which also include eosinophilic esophagitis and allergic eosinophilic colitis (table 1). Described for the first time by Kaijser in 1937 [3], eosinophilic enteritis is defined by the presence of gastrointestinal symptoms associated with an eosinophil-rich infiltration of the intestinal mu-

KARGER 125
© 2015 S. Karger AG, Basel
0257–2753/15/0332–0183$39.50/0
E-Mail karger@karger.com
www.karger.com/ddi

Dr. Guillaume Pineton de Chambrun
Gastroenterology Department
Claude Huriez Hospital, Lille University Hospital
1 place de Verdun, FR–59000 Lille (France)
E-Mail gpinetondechambrun@yahoo.fr

Table 1. Primary EGIDs

Forms	Definition	Main clinical characteristics
Eosinophilic esophagitis		
Atopic Nonatopic Familial	Eosinophilic infiltration of the esophagus mucosa without other intestinal segments involved	Dysphagia Vomiting Food impaction
Eosinophilic gastroenteritis		
Mucosal Muscular Suberosal	Gastrointestinal symptoms Eosinophilic infiltration of one or more intestinal segments	Abdominal pain Diarrhea Obstruction Ascites
Eosinophilic colitis		
Atopic Nonatopic	Children Eosinophilic infiltration of the colon Atopy or cow milk protein allergy	Diarrhea Rectal bleeding

cosa without causes of secondary intestinal eosinophilia [4]. Eosinophilic enteritis may affect the entire digestive tract from the esophagus to the rectum, and eosinophils can invade the intestinal wall from the epithelium to the serosa with a variable depth. According to the Klein classification [1] and the predominant intestinal layer involved, eosinophilic enteritis is divided into three distinct anatomical forms including predominant mucosal disease, predominant disease of the muscle layer and serosal disease. Recently, some progress has been made in the understanding of the pathogenesis of eosinophilic enteritis involving allergy and delayed Th2 response in the development of the disease [5]. Also, recent studies investigating recruitment and activation of eosinophils have allowed the development of new therapeutic strategies in EGIDs such as monoclonal antibodies directed against IL-5 (mepolizumab) [6]. Mepolizumab is currently used for the treatment of hypereosinophilic syndrome, asthma and eosinophilic esophagitis [7–9]. Eosinophilic enteritis is still away from this new treatment because of its rarity and its benign course with good response to corticosteroids in most cases. Herein, we will review the recent findings regarding eosinophilic enteritis pathogenesis, epidemiology, clinical characteristics and treatment.

Pathogenesis of Eosinophilic Enteritis

The eosinophilic granulocyte is characterized by a lobed nucleus and the presence of specific intracytoplasmic granules having a high affinity for acid dyes such as eosin. Eosinophil granules contain acidophilic cationic proteins that are responsible for the specific eosin staining including major basic protein, eosinophil cationic protein, eosinophil peroxidase and eosinophil-derived neurotoxin [10]. These cationic proteins are able to disrupt membranes and are toxic to helminths and bacteria. They also have an RNase activity that could neutralize viruses. Moreover, cationic proteins are toxic to different cell types from numerous organs, including bronchial epithelium, keratinocytes, pneumocytes, gut epithelium and could activate numerous cells such as eosinophils themselves, basophils, neutrophils and mast cells. Under activation, the eosinophils are able to secrete these granules and act as a major inflammatory cell involved in allergic diseases and parasitic infections [11].

Eosinophils are produced in the bone marrow, where they undergo a period of maturation before reaching the bloodstream. Differentiation, proliferation and presence of eosinophils in the peripheral blood are dependent on GM-CSF, IL-3 and IL-5 signaling pathways [12]. From there, eosinophils migrate to different organs where they are normal resident, including thymus, uterus, mammary glands and gastrointestinal tract. This physiological homing of eosinophils is under the control of eotaxin-1, a major eosinophilopoietin [12]. In the gastrointestinal tract, eosinophils are located in the lamina propria of every segment of the gut except the esophagus. At baseline, eosinophils do not cause any inflammation or tissue damage and allow for effective surveillance and protection against parasitic infections [2].

Eosinophils are activated by nonspecific tissue damage, allergens or infections and are responsible for gastrointestinal lesions and symptoms observed in eosinophilic enteritis [13, 14]. Activation of eosinophils will trigger degranulation leading to the direct cytotoxicity of cationic proteins and secretion of IgE [2]. Activated eosinophils will also release numerous proinflammatory cytokines such as IL-4, IL-5, IL-13 and RANTES, amplifying the local inflammatory response and recruiting immune cells to the site of inflammation [15]. Currently, eosinophil is considered as a multifunctional leukocyte expressing a wide array of surface markers that were previously thought to be exclusively expressed by other cell types including TLRs, gamma delta TCR (innate immune receptors) and MHC class II molecules. Although eosinophils were before defined only as a terminal effector of the innate immune response, their ability to secrete cytokines and chemokines and to interact with lymphocytes clearly shows their role in the activation and action of the adaptive immune response [15].

The initial stimulus leading to eosinophilic enteritis is still unknown, and both direct IgE-mediated response and delayed Th2-adaptive response are suspected to be involved in the development of eosinophilic inflammation of the intestinal mucosa [5].

Epidemiology of Eosinophilic Enteritis

Eosinophilic enteritis is a rare condition. Since its first description by Kaiser in 1937, less than 400 cases have been reported in the literature, either in the form of clinical cases or in single-center retrospective series [1, 4, 16–21]. Its prevalence is estimated to be 1 per 100,000 population [4]. Diagnoses of eosinophilic enteritis have been reported in different countries from North America to South East Asia and Japan. Eosinophilic enteritis is probably misdiagnosed because of nonspecific gastrointestinal symptoms which do not lead systematically to endoscopy with biopsies. Also, the time between first symptoms and diagnosis may be long, with more than 2 years of delay in some case series. Eosinophilic enteritis can affect all age groups, with a peak incidence between the third and fourth decades, and presents a male predominance [4, 20].

The allergic origin of eosinophilic enteritis has long been suspected and is still debated. Patients with eosinophilic enteritis have a personal or family history of atopy and/or allergy in 25–75% of cases [22]. The elevation of IgE levels in the blood also argues in favor of an allergic origin of eosinophilic enteritis. Several patients with eosinophilic enteritis or other EGIDs present positive skin test to food allergens. Moreover, allergy survey based on dietary questionnaire may identify some products possibly implicated in the development of the eosinophilic disease.

Clinical Characteristics of Patients with Eosinophilic Enteritis

Gastrointestinal symptoms of patients with eosinophilic enteritis are nonspecific. The main inaugural symptoms are abdominal pain, nausea and/or vomiting, diarrhea and ascites [4, 20, 21]. Other gastrointestinal symptoms may be indicative such as dysphagia, rectal bleeding or jaundice. Eosinophilic enteritis may also be revealed by a complication requiring surgery (obstruction, stenosis, peritonitis) [23].

The clinical presentation of eosinophilic enteritis varies with the depth of the eosinophilic infiltration through the bowel wall. In 1970, Klein et al. [1] classified the eosinophilic enteritis into three different forms according to the predominantly involved intestinal layer: the mucosal, muscular and subserosal forms of eosinophilic enteritis. This classification of eosinophilic enteritis was established from the study of a group of patients in whom the depth of the lesion was evaluated on surgical specimens. When the eosinophilic infiltration involves predominantly the mucosa, patients have symptoms related to mucosal inflammation (diarrhea, abdominal pain, gastrointestinal bleeding) as well as signs of malabsorption and protein-losing enteropathy. When the muscular layer is predominantly involved, patients present mostly obstructive signs and symptoms. A predominant subserosal infiltration is characterized by the presence of an ascites which is rich in eosinophils associated with bloating and abdominal pain [1]. In the literature, the predominantly mucosal disease represents about 50% of patients with less muscular and subserosal disease. Talley et al. [4] reported a proportion of mucosal, muscular and subserosal disease of 57.5, 30 and 12.5%, respectively [4]. In our experience, there was a predominance of mucosal forms (44%) with a higher proportion of subserosal forms (49%) and few muscular diseases (12%) [20]. Variation in the proportion of anatomical patterns in eosinophilic enteritis may be due to limitation in the evaluation of the depth of infiltration in patients without surgical resection.

Clinical manifestations of eosinophilic enteritis also depend on the distribution of eosinophilic infiltration along the digestive tract. Esophageal involvement is systematically associated with the infiltration of one or more other intestinal segments, and its frequency is probably underestimated due to the lack of systematic esophageal biopsies in the different series of eosinophilic enteritis. Infiltration of esophagus mucosa is responsible for esophageal motility disorders leading to dysphagia [13]. The stomach and proximal small intestine are reported to be the most frequently involved intestinal segments, in about 40–80% of cases, and systematic biopsies to look for eosinophilic infiltration of the mucosa in patients with gastrointestinal symptoms are required [4, 20, 24, 25]. Eosinophilic infiltration of the proximal small intestine may be associated with protein-losing enteropathy, malabsorption and iron deficiency anemia. Colonic localization seems more rarely reported [4]. The frequency of this involvement is probably underestimated, and in a case series where colonic exams with biopsies were almost systematic, a pathologic eosinophilic infiltration of the colon was present in 60–80% of cases [20].

Biology of Eosinophilic Enteritis

The two main laboratory abnormalities present in patients with eosinophilic enteritis are increased number of eosinophils in the blood and increased serum IgE levels [20]. Peripheral blood eosinophilia (eosinophils >500/mm^3) is reported to be present in at least 70–80% of patients with eosinophilic enteritis. This increased number of blood eosinophils is often transient concomitant to flares of the disease and could reach a high level of eosinophilia especially in subserosal disease with ascites. In these particular patients, the analysis of peritoneal liquid samples showed a high level of eosinophils in ascites. The peripheral blood eosinophilia is neither sufficient nor necessary for the diagnosis of eosinophilic enteritis, missing in 1 of 5 patients. Serum IgE levels are abnormally high in over 50% of patients with eosinophilic enteritis without any specificity of the IgE identified. Biological signs of malabsorption (steatorrhea, martial or vitamin deficiency), losing enteropathy (hypoalbuminemia), and intestinal inflammation (increased CRP) may be also present in patients with eosinophilic enteritis [23].

Morphological Characteristics of Eosinophilic Enteritis

Upper gastrointestinal endoscopy and ileocolonoscopy with biopsies are necessary for the diagnosis of eosinophilic enteritis. The endoscopic appearance may be normal or present nonspecific mucosal abnormalities such as erythema, edema, erosions, ulcers, nodules and stenosis [26]. New endoscopic techniques like wireless capsule endoscopy are useful to explore the entire small intestine and reveal mucosal abnormalities not identified by conventional endoscopy [27]. However, if eosinophilic infiltration is not present in the stomach or proximal small intestine, patients with distal lesions in the small intestine will require enteroscopy in order to perform biopsies and confirm the diagnosis of eosinophilic enteritis [28]. Radiologic exams including abdominal ultrasound, CT scan and MRI are also useful for the diagnosis of eosinophilic enteritis and to characterize the depth of eosinophilic infiltration. Abdominal ultrasound is the investigation of choice to confirm the presence of ascites. Small bowel follow-through was used in the past decade to investigate the small bowel mucosa in patients with eosinophilic enteritis. In these patients, small bowel follow-through could identify wall thickening of the proximal small intestine, stenosis, dilatation of the intestinal lumen and terminal

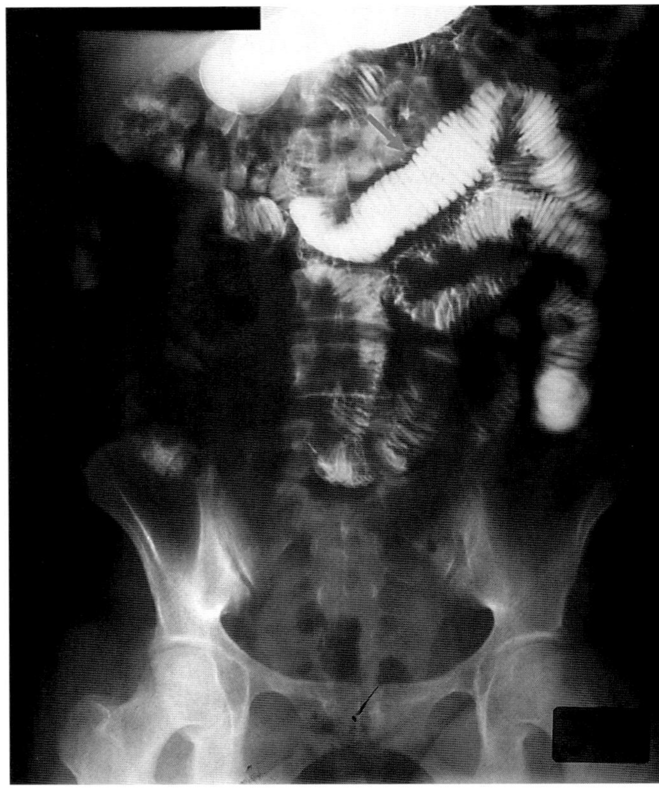
Color version available online

Fig. 1. Edema of the jejunum. Picture of a small bowel follow-through examination in a patient with a subserosal eosinophilic enteritis showing a thickening wall of the jejunum (arrow).

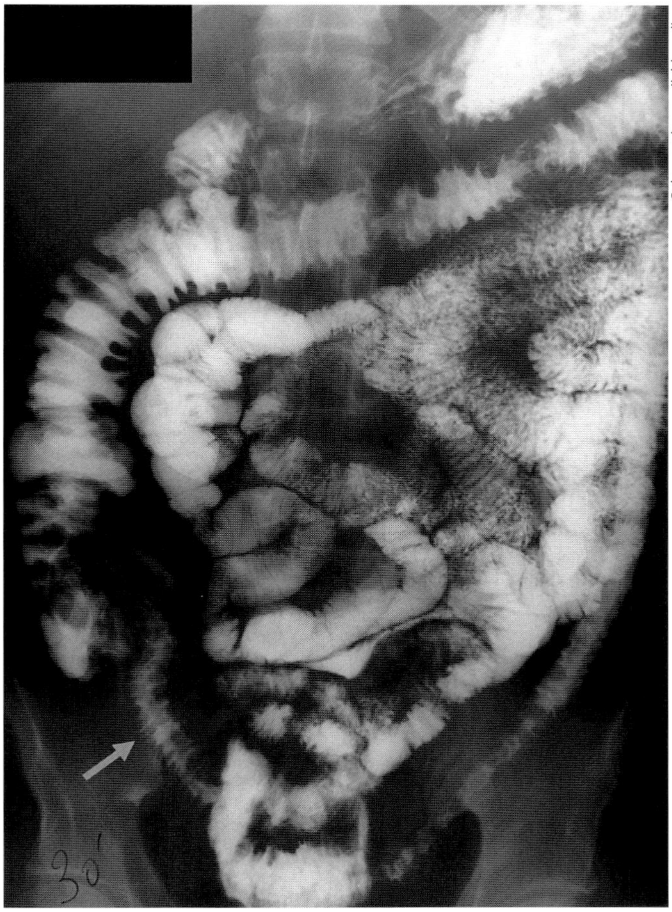

Color version available online

Fig. 2. Terminal ileitis. Picture of a small bowel follow-through examination in a patient with a mucosal eosinophilic gastroenteritis showing an inflamed and ulcerated terminal ileum (arrow).

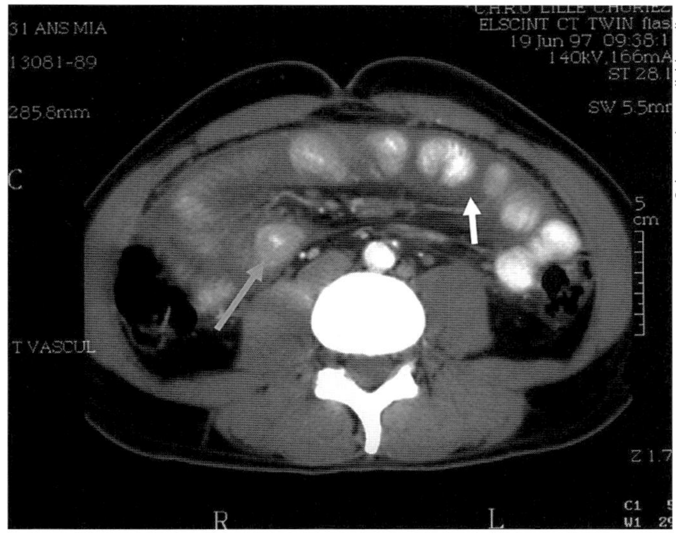

Color version available online

Fig. 3. Diffuse small bowel thickening with ascites. Picture representing a computed tomography slide in a patient with subserosal eosinophilic gastroenteritis. This patient presented diffuse thickening of the small bowel (red arrow; red color refers to the online version only) and ascites (white arrow).

ulcerated ileitis (fig. 1, 2). Abdominal CT and MRI are useful to evaluate the thickening of the intestinal wall, the extension along the intestine and the presence of ascites (fig. 3).

Diagnosis of Eosinophilic Gastroenteritis

The diagnosis of eosinophilic enteritis may be elusive and is defined as the presence of gastrointestinal symptoms associated with eosinophilic infiltration of the intestinal mucosa and exclusion of secondary causes of intestinal or blood eosinophilia [4]. Gastrointestinal symptoms observed during eosinophilic enteritis are nonspecific, and the key element of the diagnosis is the demonstration of a pathological eosinophilic infiltration of the mucosa. Eosinophils are usually present in the gut wall except in the esophagus, where they are located in the lamina propria. Their number varies along the digestive tract, and the cutoff to define a pathological infiltration is still debated. In most studies, the threshold of 20 eosinophils per high-power field (×400) is used for the diagnosis of eosinophilic enteritis [4, 16]. The presence of eosinophils in other layers of the intestinal wall should also be considered as pathologic especially if eosinophils present signs of activation (degranulation). Other findings such as crypt abscesses and architectural abnormalities could increase the likelihood of a pathologic eosinophilic infiltration of the gut. Diagnosis of eosinophilia is based on biopsies during gastrointestinal endoscopy, analysis of ascites fluid in the subserosal forms or analysis of surgical specimens when available.

Pathologic infiltration of the intestinal mucosa with eosinophils is not specific to eosinophilic enteritis, and differential diagnoses should be considered in patients with gastrointestinal symptoms and eosinophilia [29]. Intestinal parasites are one of the most common causes of digestive eosinophilia associated with peripheral blood eosinophilia and must be ruled out by direct stool examination, intestinal biopsies and serological tests. The poor sensitivity of tests used to detect parasites may justify systematic anti-parasitic treatment in patients with

Dig Dis 2015;33:183–189
DOI: 10.1159/000369540

gastrointestinal eosinophilia. Several medications could also be associated with peripheral blood and tissue eosinophilia [30]. Gastrointestinal vasculitis may be accompanied by an increase in eosinophils in the intestinal mucosa [31]. Numerous other gastrointestinal disorders may be associated with eosinophilic infiltration of the intestinal mucosa such as gastroesophageal reflux disease, *Helicobacter pylori* gastritis, celiac disease or inflammatory bowel disease. Finally, it is essential to exclude a hypereosinophilic syndrome which is defined by a peripheral blood eosinophilia >1,500 eosinophils/mm for more than 6 months associated with the involvement of at least one organ [32].

If allergy is suspected to be the cause of eosinophilic enteritis, dietary survey, skin tests and research of specific IgE should be conducted in order to discover specific food allergen. In other cases without allergic history or increased IgE, sequential exclusion of food allergens potentially incriminated is not recommended and mostly not useful to obtain sustained clinical improvement [4].

Treatment of Eosinophilic Enteritis

Treatment of eosinophilic enteritis is not clearly established as there is no randomized controlled trial available in patients with eosinophilic enteritis due to the rarity of the disease. However, it was demonstrated that spontaneous remission may occur in approximately 40% of patients [20]. The main treatment used in patients with eosinophilic enteritis is systemic corticosteroids with a good efficacy in the majority of patients at a loading dose of 20–40 mg/day of prednisone [2, 31]. Budesonide, a corticosteroid that is mostly eliminated by the liver after intestinal absorption, is a therapeutic alternative with fewer systemic side effects. After drug withdrawal, some patients may present a relapse of the disease that requires new treatment with corticosteroids. Steroid-refractory or -dependent cases of eosinophilic enteritis could be treated with immunosuppressive drugs such as azathioprine. Mepolizumab, an anti-IL-5 monoclonal antibody which was previously tested in eosinophilic esophagitis, would be an interesting alternative in patients with a complicated course of eosinophilic enteritis.

Other treatments such as antihistaminic drugs, montelukast and sodium cromoglycate have been used for the treatment of eosinophilic enteritis with conflicting results [31]. Specific diet with exclusion of food allergens previously identified can be useful in selected patients.

Natural History of Eosinophilic Enteritis

The long-term prognosis of eosinophilic enteritis remains unclear. In our case series of patients with eosinophilic enteritis, we were able to describe the natural history of the disease [20]. Indeed, after a median follow-up of 15 years (range 1–27), we identified three distinct clinical courses of eosinophilic enteritis: 18 cases (44%) of which 9 were subserosal forms had a single inaugural flare without recurrence (defined as single flare), 14 (36%) had multiple flares separated by periods of remission (defined as recurring course) and 9 (21%) a chronic form without remission (continuous course). More than 80% of the continuous courses were characterized by a mucosal predominant disease. Subserosal forms evolved in more than 50% of cases a single flare without any recurrence [20]. No myeloproliferative transformation was observed in our cohort of patients with eosinophilic enteritis [20].

Conclusions

Eosinophilic enteritis is responsible for various gastrointestinal symptoms depending on the anatomical form of the disease. The critical finding for eosinophilic enteritis diagnosis is the presence of a pathologic eosinophilic infiltration of the intestinal wall, which should be systematically sought by taking intestinal biopsies in patients with unspecific gastrointestinal symptoms and peripheral blood eosinophilia. The etiology of eosinophilic enteritis is still debated, and the implication of allergy in the pathogenesis remains controversial. Eosinophilic enteritis is often characterized by a benign course without recurrence. However, half of the patients may present a more complex natural history characterized by unpredictable relapses and a chronic course.

Disclosure Statement

The authors declare no conflicts of interest.

References

1 Klein NC, Hargrove RL, Sleisenger MH, et al: Eosinophilic gastroenteritis. Medicine (Baltimore) 1970;49:299–319.

2 Yan BM, Shaffer EA: Primary eosinophilic disorders of the gastrointestinal tract. Gut 2009;58:721–732.

3 Kaijser R: Zur Kenntnis der allergischen Affektionen des Verdauungs-Kanals vom Standpunkt des Chirurgien aus. Arch Klin Chir 1937;188:36–64.

4 Talley NJ, Shorter RG, Phillips SF, et al: Eosinophilic gastroenteritis: a clinicopathological study of patients with disease of the mucosa, muscle layer, and subserosal tissues. Gut 1990;31:54–58.

5 Ingle SB, Hinge Ingle CR: Eosinophilic gastroenteritis: an unusual type of gastroenteritis. World J Gastroenterol 2013;19:5061–5066.

6 Rothenberg ME: Eosinophilic gastrointestinal disorders (EGID). J Allergy Clin Immunol 2004;113:11–28; quiz 9.

7 Nair P, Pizzichini MM, Kjarsgaard M, et al: Mepolizumab for prednisone-dependent asthma with sputum eosinophilia. N Engl J Med 2009;360:985–993.

8 Rothenberg ME, Klion AD, Roufosse FE, et al: Treatment of patients with the hypereosinophilic syndrome with mepolizumab. N Engl J Med 2008;358:1215–1228.

9 Straumann A, Conus S, Grzonka P, et al: Anti-interleukin-5 antibody treatment (mepolizumab) in active eosinophilic oesophagitis: a randomised, placebo-controlled, double-blind trial. Gut 2010;59:21–30.

10 Hogan SP, Rosenberg HF, Moqbel R, et al: Eosinophils: biological properties and role in health and disease. Clin Exp Allergy 2008;38: 709–750.

11 Blanchard C, Rothenberg ME: Biology of the eosinophil. Adv Immunol 2009;101:81–121.

12 Mishra A, Hogan SP, Lee JJ, et al: Fundamental signals that regulate eosinophil homing to the gastrointestinal tract. J Clin Invest 1999; 103:1719–1727.

13 Desreumaux P, Seguy D, Dutoit E, et al: La gastroentérites à éosinophiles. Hépato-Gastro Oncol Dig 1996;3:279–286.

14 Torpier G, Colombel JF, Mathieu-Chandelier C, et al: Eosinophilic gastroenteritis: ultrastructural evidence for a selective release of eosinophil major basic protein. Clin Exp Immunol 1988;74:404–408.

15 Rothenberg ME, Hogan SP: The eosinophil. Annu Rev Immunol 2006;24:147–174.

16 Chen MJ, Chu CH, Lin SC, et al: Eosinophilic gastroenteritis: clinical experience with 15 patients. World J Gastroenterol 2003;9:2813–2816.

17 Kinoshita Y, Furuta K, Ishimaura N, et al: Clinical characteristics of Japanese patients with eosinophilic esophagitis and eosinophilic gastroenteritis. J Gastroenterol 2013;48: 333–339.

18 Lee CM, Changchien CS, Chen PC, et al: Eosinophilic gastroenteritis: 10 years experience. Am J Gastroenterol 1993;88:70–74.

19 Naylor AR: Eosinophilic gastroenteritis. Scott Med J 1990;35:163–165.

20 Pineton de Chambrun G, Gonzalez F, Canva JY, et al: Natural history of eosinophilic gastroenteritis. Clin Gastroenterol Hepatol 2011; 9:950–956.e1.

21 Zhang L, Duan L, Ding S, et al: Eosinophilic gastroenteritis: clinical manifestations and morphological characteristics, a retrospective study of 42 patients. Scand J Gastroenterol 2011;46:1074–1080.

22 Khan S, Orenstein SR: Eosinophilic gastroenteritis: epidemiology, diagnosis and management. Paediatr Drugs 2002;4:563–570.

23 Coton T: Gastroentérite à éosinophiles. EM Consulte DOI: 10.1016/S1155-1968(09) 27499-2.

24 Chang JY, Choung RS, Lee RM, et al: A shift in the clinical spectrum of eosinophilic gastroenteritis toward the mucosal disease type. Clin Gastroenterol 2010;8:669–675, quiz e88.

25 Katz AJ, Goldman H, Grand RJ: Gastric mucosal biopsy in eosinophilic (allergic) gastroenteritis. Gastroenterology 1977;73:705–709.

26 Navab F, Kleinman MS, Algazy K, et al: Endoscopic diagnosis of eosinophilic gastritis. Gastrointest Endosc 1972;19:67–69.

27 Endo H, Hosono K, Inamori M, et al: Capsule endoscopic evaluation of eosinophilic enteritis before and after treatment. Digestion 2011; 83:134–135.

28 Attar A, Cazals-Hatem D, Ponsot P: Videocapsule endoscopy identifies stenoses missed by other imaging techniques in a patient with eosinophilic gastroenteritis. Clin Gastroenterol Hepatol 2011;9:A28.

29 Desreumaux P, Colombel JF: Diagnostic étiologique d'une éosinophilie digestive. Rev Prat 1992;171:668–673.

30 de Weck AL: Drug allergy, immunotherapy, immune complexes and anaphylaxis. Curr Opin Immunol 1989;2:548–557.

31 Khan S: Eosinophilic gastroenteritis. Best Pract Res Clin Gastroenterol 2005;19:177–198.

32 Klion A: Hypereosinophilic syndrome: current approach to diagnosis and treatment. Annu Rev Med 2009;60:293–306.

Dig Dis 2015;33:190–199
DOI: 10.1159/000369538

Tropheryma whipplei, Immunosuppression and Whipple's Disease: From a Low-Pathogenic, Environmental Infectious Organism to a Rare, Multifaceted Inflammatory Complex

Thomas Marth

Division of Internal Medicine, Krankenhaus Maria Hilf, Daun, Germany

Key Words
Whipple's disease · *Tropheryma whipplei* · Polymerase chain reaction · Immunosuppression · Therapy

Abstract

Background: The actinobacterium *Tropheryma whipplei* was detected 20 years ago by molecular techniques, and following its culture has been characterized as the cause of a systemic infection known as Whipple's disease (WD). *T. whipplei* occurs in the environment, is prevalent only in humans, is believed to be transmitted via oral routes and to be host dependent. ***Key Messages:*** The classical form of *T. whipplei* infection, i.e. classical WD (CWD), is rare. It is well defined as slowly progressing chronic infection with arthralgia, diarrhea and weight loss, mostly in middle-aged men. However, current research revealed a much broader spectrum of clinical features associated with *T. whipplei* infection. Thus, *T. whipplei* may cause acute and transient infections (observed primarily in children) and the bacterium, which is found in soil and water, occurs in asymptomatic carriers as well as in CWD patients in clinical remission. In addition, *T. whipplei* affects isolated and localized body compartments such as heart valves or the central nervous system. Subtle immune defects and HLA associations have been described. New findings indicate that the progression of asymptomatic *T. whipplei* infection to clinical WD may be associated with medical immunosuppression and with immunomodulatory conditions. This explains that there is a discrepancy between the widespread occurrence of *T. whipplei* and the rareness of WD, and that *T. whipplei* infection triggered by immunosuppression presents with protean clinical manifestations. ***Conclusions:*** This review highlights recent findings and the clinical spectrum of infection with *T. whipplei* and WD, focusing specifically on the role of host immunity and immunosuppression. Current concepts of the pathogenesis, diagnosis and therapy are discussed.

Microbiology of *Tropheryma whipplei*

As visualized by electron microscopy, *T. whipplei* is morphologically a characteristic, rod-shaped organism (0.25 × 2 μm) with a trilaminar plasma membrane and a homogeneous cell wall with two inner layers and an outer trilaminar membrane-like structure [1]. In 1992, by polymerase chain reaction (PCR) techniques, the bacterium was phylogenetically classified to a new genus and species [2].

KARGER 125

E-Mail karger@karger.com
www.karger.com/ddi

0257–2753/15/0332–0190$39.50/0

Prof. Dr. med. Thomas Marth
Division of Internal Medicine
Krankenhaus Maria Hilf
DE–54550 Daun (Germany)
E-Mail t.marth@krankenhaus-daun.de

In 1997, the bacterium was isolated from heart valve tissue and had been propagated for a short time in peripheral blood mononuclear cells, which were deactivated by dexamethasone, interleukin (IL)-4 or IL-10 [3]. The culture of the bacillus was later stably established in human fibroblasts using specific cell culture techniques. The growth of *T. whipplei* requires several weeks due its long replication time (up to 18 days) [4]. In special mammalian cell-free ('axenic') growth media, the doubling time of the organism is shorter, and strains from cardiac valves, blood, synovial fluid, cerebrospinal fluid, duodenal biopsies, stool and saliva in cultures have been obtained [5]. The genotype of *T. whipplei* does not influence the course of the infection [6].

Sequencing of *T. whipplei* shows a small genomic size (it possesses a unique circular chromosome with 927 kbp), 800 protein-coding genes and a guanin/cytosin content of 47% [7]. Some of these characteristics are seen in intracellular bacteria. Together with 16S–23S intergenic sequence analysis, taxonomically *T. whipplei* is an actinobacteria placed between the subdivision of Gram-positive actinomycetes with B peptidoglycan and the Cellulomonadaceae. *T. whipplei* is deficient in genes that encode energy metabolism and amino acids synthesis (e.g. lack or impairment of 16 amino acids, no thioredoxine reductase homologs). Genomic analysis revealed a large chromosomal inversion and the presence of common repeats, pointing to a high genetic diversity. This results in the expression of many cell surface proteins. Thus, the genomic characteristics suggest a host-dependent lifestyle (requirement on external nutrients) and hint to mechanisms for evasion from the host's immune response ('parasitic lifestyle').

Contaminated soil as a possible route of infection with *T. whipplei* was suspected for years as farmers are at higher risk for Whipple's disease (WD) [1]. As actinobacteria are essentially environmental microorganisms from soil, freshwater, or seawater sediments, it is not surprising that *T. whipplei* has been found in a high percentage of influxes to sewage plants. *T. whipplei* can be detected in stool and saliva samples from patients with WD as well as in asymptomatic carriers. The prevalence of *T. whipplei* in stools is found to be between 1 and 11% in healthy individuals, and between 12 and 26% in sewage plant workers [8]. In saliva samples, the prevalence of *T. whipplei* is much lower. In Africa, the carrier rate of *T. whipplei* in healthy subjects has been observed to be 31% in stool samples. The prevalence of *T. whipplei* is dependent on poor living conditions of homeless people in shelters, on the absence of toilets, on close contact with *T. whipplei* carriers or on WD patients within families [9–11]. Of treated classical WD (CWD) patients, 20% excrete *T. whipplei* in their stools [unpubl. observation]. There are some reports on familial cases of WD and on local clusters of WD 'outbreaks' [12]. Environmental and animal studies (>1,000 samples, >100 animals) looking for the presence of *T. whipplei* by PCR were essentially negative [13]. These data suggest a solely human-to-human transmission of the bacterium via the fecal-oral or oral-oral route.

Immunopathogenesis

An immunologic defect in the pathogenesis of WD seems probable because of the specific features of the *T. whipplei* genome which show an immune evasion and host-adapted lifestyle. The rather loose HLA association [14] does not sufficiently explain the very low incidence of WD despite the ubiquitous presence of *T. whipplei*. However, the immunologic defect in WD is apparently subtle as it usually does not lead to susceptibility to other infections.

The histologic features of the lamina propria in WD are unique because – despite the massive influx of macrophages which persists even in remission – the intestinal tissue shows a paucity of lymphocytic infiltration and plasma cells. The replication of *T. whipplei* is mostly intracellularly, but it may be metabolically active extracellularly as well.

Active WD is characterized by a reduced CD4+/CD8+ T-cell ratio, a reduced number of *T. whipplei*-specific CD4+ cells, a shift toward mature T-cell subpopulations and increased cell activation markers on the peripheral and mucosal level. Patients exhibit diminished production of Th1 cytokines in response to *T. whipplei* and other antigens, but there is an increase in functional Th2 responses [15–18]. CWD patients show higher numbers of CD4+ T regulatory cells (Treg), elevated secretion of IL-10 and TGF-β in the lamina propria, and peripheral Treg of patients were activated [19].

The T cell pattern might contribute to an inhibition of dendritic cell maturation, to deactivation of macrophages, and to the chronic infection and systemic spread of *T. whipplei*. Some older studies showed that macrophages have decreased intracellular degradation and phagocytosis. Patients with WD have reduced numbers of cells expressing CD11b, which serves as a facilitator of microbial phagocytosis and antigen processing and mediates IFN-γ-induced intracellular bacterial killing [20]. Impaired macrophage functions in WD may be due to reduced IL-12 [15, 17, 18]. Additionally, in WD patients, IL-12-dependent signal transduction, i.e. activation (phosphorylation) of Stat4 expression, is much lower than in controls (percentage of phosphorylated Stat4 11.7% on lymphocytes of WD patients vs. 47.9% of controls, n = 7, $p < 0.05$ [unpubl. observation]). Intestinal macrophages show an alternatively activated ('M2') phenotype and produce IL-10 in a higher amount leading to a Th2 skewed immune response [21]. *T. whipplei* was propagated in mononuclear cells deactivated by IL-4 and IL-10 [3]. *T. whipplei* also replicates in monocytes and macrophages from normal individuals if deactivated with IL-16. High levels of IL-16 might promote the dissemination of *T. whipplei* via the induction of macrophage apoptosis [22, 23].

Reduced numbers of IgA-positive B cells (translating into impaired secretory IgA production), but increased numbers of surface IgM-positive cells in the lamina propria have been found. Peripheral IgM and IgG2 subclass levels are often decreased, and IgA is increased in acute stages of the disease [12, 15, 16, 24, 25]. The observation of decreased IgG2 levels deserves comment. IgG2 is the main IgG subclass induced in response to bacterial polysaccharides, and is quite specifically induced by IFN-γ. For example, IgG2 deficiency is associated with defective IFN-γ production [26]. The human Ig Fc receptor IIA (i.e. CD32) is the sole FcγR class capable of binding IgG2 complexes. Genetically determined allotypes of this receptor have different reactivities with IgG2 and are associated with recurrent bacterial infections [27]. In WD patients, we observed low ratios of IgG2 and IgM as compared to IgA (table 1). In addition, preliminary studies in a small number of WD patients showed a low expression of surface CD32 (15.4% on peripheral lymphocytes of WD patients vs. 25.4% in controls, n = 4 [unpubl. observation]). Therefore, low CD32 expression, reduced IgG2 production and decreased IFN-γ levels may be interrelated in patients with WD. It will be interesting to study whether low CD32 expression or reduced IgG2 levels are secondary to infection or genetically determined in WD patients.

Taken together, in patients with WD, the mucosal immune responses are insufficient to kill ingested *T. whipplei*. However, the weak HLA association and the data on the immunopathogenesis are lacking a discernable momentum or trigger to explain why the high prevalence of the slow-growing, low-pathogenic *T. whipplei* in humans translates so rarely in classical (systemic) WD. Thus, other additional or essential host-related cofactors, which are discussed below, have to be existent in the pathogenesis, which leads to clinical manifestations of WD.

Table 1. Studies of immunoglobulin levels in WD patients

	WD patients	Normal levels
IgG2, mg/dl	292±28	429±107
IgM, mg/dl	119±26	155±46
IgA, mg/dl	421±63	242±86
Ratio $= \frac{\text{IgG2} + \text{IgM}}{\text{IgA}}$	0.97	2.4

For WD patients n = 29 for IgG2, and n = 27 for IgM and IgA. Data adapted from Marth [12] and Kalt et al. [25].

Clinical Features of *T. whipplei* Infection

Transient and Acute T. whipplei Infection/Transient and Acute WD

A transient (i.e. self-limiting) and acute form of *T. whipplei* infection has been shown in children presenting with gastroenteritis, fever, cough or sleep disturbance (table 2). In a study including 241 young French children with diarrhea, *T. whipplei* was found as the most frequent pathogen in 15% of the cases; one third were coinfected with other diarrheal pathogens [28]. In West Africa, up to three quarters of young patients with short-term and self-limiting diarrheal disease may carry or excrete *T. whipplei* in stools; others have *T. whipplei* bacteremia or cough [29].

Asymptomatic Carriers of T. whipplei/Asymptomatic WD

Presumably, asymptomatic individuals have acquired *T. whipplei* via a subclinical or short-term acute infection and later may pass *T. whipplei* with their stools. *T. whipplei* may also be present in their saliva, or individuals have serum antibodies. The prevalence of the bacterium in fecal samples from healthy adults ranges between 1 and 11%. A high proportion (up to 26%) of asymptomatic carriers were found in workers who have close contact with sewage [8, 9]. It is not known how many individuals with asymptomatic WD will develop systemic WD later in their lives. Also, the bacterial load in the stool of these patients is lower than in untreated patients with untreated CWD.

Localized T. whipplei Infection/Localized WD

This clinical form presents only with WD manifestations in isolated organs, i.e. without systemic features of WD, and without positive duodenal biopsy. Localized WD (LWD) manifestations occur most frequently as cul-

Table 2. Clinical features and spectrum of *T. whipplei* infection

Category	Transient and acute	Asymptomatic	Localized	Classic	Associated with immunosuppression
Acronym	TWD	AWD	LWD	CWD	IS → WD
Definition	Occurs mostly in children with diarrhea and fever (in Africa)	Asymptomatic carriers More frequent e.g. in sewage workers	Localized infection, e.g. endocarditis or CNS disease without systemic symptoms	Classical form with weight loss, arthralgia, diarrhea and a broad spectrum of other (systemic) symptoms	Occurrence of diarrhea or localized disease after immunosuppression Coinfection in HIV patients IRIS
Remarks	Newly recognized Probably frequently occurring (up to 75%) Frequency in Western countries yet unknown Hints to fecal-oral route of infection	Frequency varies from 1 to 26% Development to CWD unproven, presumably rare	LWD is most frequent form of culture-negative endocarditis Severe CNS damage possible LWD is very difficult to diagnose	CWD is rare Published cases exemplify the immense spectrum of clinical symptoms	Protean clinical features hinder early diagnosis IS → WD may be explained by parasitic features of *T. whipplei* and immune defects

ture-negative bacterial endocarditis, e.g. on degenerative valve lesions leading to a slowly progressive valve damage. Clinical symptoms depend on the stage of the disease and may include cardiac murmur and valve (aortic or mitral) insufficiency, leading finally to valve replacement; however, patients often do not fulfill Duke criteria for infective endocarditis, and progress more slowly than patients with, e.g. streptococcal or staphylococcal endocarditis. LWD endocarditis is typically diagnosed by PCR (or histology) on the explanted valve. In one retrospective series with >1,100 patients, more than 6% of all infective endocarditis cases were due to *T. whipplei*, and it was thus the most frequent cause of culture-negative endocarditis [30]. In 2011, 33 cases of LWD endocarditis had been described in the literature [31].

In addition, LWD can be found localized in lymph nodes (often mesenterial lymphadenopathy), the lung, the joints (e.g. isolated synovitis), in the eye (uveitis), and in the central nervous system (CNS). Particularly CNS involvement is difficult to diagnose, and may have a progressive course; around one third of patients with isolated CNS involvement have a lethal course [32].

Classical and Systemic WD

CWD shows the leading symptoms of weight loss, diarrhea, and arthropathies. While in three quarters of cases these symptoms are found together by the time of diagnosis, the clinical presentation of patients may vary to a great extent. The rare disorder has been described most frequently in Whites, and only rare occurrences have been reported in other populations. Symptoms of CWD occur at a mean age of 50 years. Male patients without arthropathies and females exhibit symptoms 7 years later. In the mean, there is a diagnostic delay of 8 years. The medium age at diagnosis is 56 years, but 6% are under 30 years. CWD is approximately eight times more common in men than in women (some newer series find a male-to-female ratio of 3:1) [1, 33, 34]. In a European cohort, an HLA association (with DRB1*13 and DQB1*06) was observed [14].

CWD begins in two thirds insidiously with arthropathy which may precede the diagnosis for many years (in one study, mean of 8 years) [34]. Arthritis consists often of chronic migratory, nondestructive, and seronegative peripheral joint disease, and often is accompanied by myalgias. Interestingly, 29% (5 out 17) of CWD patients with arthritis reported about rheumatic disease in mothers [12].

Weight loss is found very often patients with CWD; it occurs more than 4 years before diagnosis and is clinically relevant (mean ≥20% of initial weight) [34].

Gastrointestinal symptoms, which usually begin later and ultimately lead to the diagnosis of CWD, consist of episodic and watery diarrhea or steatorrhea. They may be accompanied by colicky abdominal pain. Diarrhea may lead to the full picture of a malabsorption syndrome with severe weight loss, weakness, and cachexia. Occult blood in the stool is quite frequent and has been described in around 25% [1, 33, 35]. Despite the leading role of endoscopy in diagnosis, it is remarkable that in one series, 30% (8 out of 27) patients had a history of duodenal or stomach ulcers while they were already complaining of unspecific arthropathies, but endoscopy did not reveal WD [12]. In another analysis, in 13 of 46 (28.3%) patients, the first endoscopy done under the suspicion of WD did not reveal the diagnosis, which was established later by another endoscopy or by other organ biopsies [36].

In CWD, systemic symptoms occur frequently [1, 33]. Peripheral edema, ascites, pleuritis or polyserositis may be noted. Other frequent symptoms consist of intermittent, mostly low-grade fever, night sweats, or peripheral and abdominal lymphadenopathy. Skin hyperpigmentation, particularly affecting light-exposed skin has been observed. In addition, chronic, nonproductive cough, reversible pulmonary hypertension, chest pain and other cardiac symptoms have been described. Hepatomegaly or splenomegaly may be present in some patients with this disorder.

Involvement of the CNS is potentially serious. Patients may present with memory disorders, personality changes, and dementia. Other frequent clinical signs include ophthalmoplegia, nystagmus, or myoclonia. These may be found in combination with a disturbed sleep pattern, ataxia, seizure, or symptoms of cerebral compression (owing to hydrocephalus). Various cranial nerve symptoms, such as hearing loss and blurred vision, have been reported. In some patients, a specific, if not pathognomonic, oculomasticatory myorhythmia or myoclonus with ophthalmoplegia has been described. There seem to exist some characteristic radiologic signs of CNS WD using specific or sequences of magnetic resonance imaging. CNS symptoms have a frequency of around 15% in CWD [1, 33, 35, 36].

WD in Association with Immunosuppression

This form of WD is of importance because the WD diagnosis probably often could be established earlier. Apparently, immunomodulation or (medical) immunosuppression is able to disturb the delicate balance of homeostasis of immunity against the host-dependent, parasitic and slow-growing pathogen *T. whipplei* in some asymptomatic hosts leading to an array of clinical symptoms which are detailed below.

Immunosuppression Favors the Occurrence of Diarrhea, Leading to Diagnosis of Systemic WD

While there is no gross immune deficit in WD, i.e. patients do not exhibit the classical form of severe immunodeficiency, some data show that medical immunosuppression may trigger intestinal manifestations, particularly diarrhea which leads usually to endoscopy and to the diagnosis of WD. In one study with 27 patients, immunosuppressive therapy with corticosteroids, azathioprine, or other immunosuppressants (given for the treatment of unclear arthropathy) accelerated the progression of WD. The median time to occurrence of gastrointestinal symptoms after initiation of immunosuppressive therapy was 4 months, and another 2 months were necessary to establish the diagnosis [34]. In another retrospective study in 113 patients, it was shown that up to 50% of patients received immunosuppressive medication. Most had a rapid deterioration directly or soon after medication onset (75%), and in the rest of the patients the immunosuppressants were ineffective. Many patients with deterioration after immunosuppressive therapy developed diarrhea (57%), weight loss (40%) or fever (26%) [35].

Occurrence of LWD after Immunosuppressive Therapy

LWD is a heterogeneous clinical picture which may be a result after immunosuppressive therapy used for unclear arthritis. In recent years, LWD was quite often reported after the use of immunosuppressives, particularly after tumor necrosis factor-α inhibitor (TNFI) therapy. Medical immunosuppression therapy may be associated with isolated endocarditis, spondylitis or CNS manifestations. Thus, in one study 5 out of 16 patients with endocarditis had received immunosuppressive previously (2/16 had received TNFI) [35]. In a recent comprehensive case-control study which covers 19 publications, 41 patients were identified who were diagnosed with WD following therapy with TNFI. Ten out of 41 patients (24.4%) developed endocarditis or pericarditis. Other complications of TNFI therapy manifesting as LWD were lymphadenopathy, severe CNS or eye complications (including blindness), spondylitis or sacroiliitis. Also other, systemic WD complications such as septic fever or *T. whipplei* septicemia, colitis, and skin manifestations were observed frequently [37]. Interestingly, following immunosuppressive therapy with TFNI, in two thirds of patients PAS staining was false negative, but >90% of PCR tests were diagnostic.

There are a number of other reports which describe LWD after immunosuppressive therapy, e.g. in one case secondary vitreitis was followed by renal transplantation [38].

Association of WD with Malignancies

As peripheral and abdominal lymphadenopathy is frequent in WD (up to 50%), in some cases at first lymphomas are suspected, and sometimes lymphoma and WD are associated. There are several reports on non-Hodgkin lymphoma (NHL) at the time of WD diagnosis, or NHL occurring after treatment for WD [39, 40]. In addition, in one large prospective case series, there were 3/40 patients with Hodgkin's lymphoma (previously treated) or NHL [41]. It is unclear whether lymphoma associated with WD may be due to prior immunosuppressive therapy or chemotherapy. Other authors described clonal B cell expansions (in one case bcl-2 related) which regressed after antibiotic therapy. It is possible that the chronic inflammatory stimulus by *T. whipplei* infection triggers clonal expansion in the lymphoid system, in analogy to *Helicobacter pylori* infection and MALT lymphoma, or to small bowel immunoproliferative disease, and thereby induces lymphoma in few cases [42, 43]. In another study, 3/27 WD patients had a prior diagnosis of malignancies and were treated by chemotherapy or radiation [12]. Also, in other reports, WD clinically occurred after chemotherapy.

Association of WD with Granulomatous Diseases, Autoimmune Disorders and Infections

It was repeatedly reported that the inflammatory reaction in WD may be granulomatous, and this is described in the intestinal tract and in various organs in approximately 9% of the WD patients [1]. Most frequently, sarcoid-like epithelioid noncaseating granulomas have been described [1, 44]. They are distinct from WD macrophages (PAS negative) and are speculated to be a result of partially digested antigen, although no products of bacterial degradation have been observed. Especially when WD affects the lung, sarcoidosis may be confused with WD [1, 45]. In a recent series of 40 patients, 2 had sarcoid-like lesions [41].

Amyloidosis has been reported in a few patients with WD [1, 46], but it is unclear whether the amyloid deposits result from a chronic inflammatory response. It has to be pointed out that amyloid deposits may be faintly PAS positive and thus may be misinterpreted as WD.

There are some other histopathologic pitfalls in the diagnosis of WD. Infections with *Rhodococcus equi* and non-*Mycobacterium tuberculosis* complex in patients with AIDS (which have been named 'pseudo-WD'), infections with fungi, *Histoplasma* spp., and others may be histologically similar to WD, but may be ruled out by a Ziehl-Neelsen stain [1, 33, 47].

WD can be associated in some instances with opportunistic infections, e.g. in patients with AIDS. In 3% of bronchioalveolar lavages of ICU patients and in 13% of HIV patients, *T. whipplei* was found by PCR [48]. In addition, WD has been found in some cases to be associated in patients with *Serratia marcescens, Strongyloides stercoralis, Nocardia* or more often with *Giardia* infections [49]. The association of WD with giardiasis has been reported in many cases (in about 10% of cases) [50]. In the recent series of a mostly German group of 40 patients, 10% had had giardiasis [41]. It is speculated that an infection by one infectious mucosal agent may promote the infection with the other, and it has been assumed that *Giardia* and *T. whipplei* occupy an identical ecologic niche in the environment.

In one study, 15/27 had severe systemic infections such as hepatitis, polio, malaria, or worm diseases prior to diagnosis of WD (in addition, 3/27 WD patients had malignancies and 12/27 had received immunosuppressive therapy) [12].

It is increasingly noted in the literature, for example in one large retrospective study comprising 15 patients, that unusual presentations of WD and autoimmune comorbidities are associated with immunomodulatory conditions [51].

Association of WD with the Immune Reconstitution Inflammatory Syndrome

Many WD patients experience a complete and long-lasting remission after antibiotic therapy. However, in some cases inflammation reappears after initial improvement after antibiotics. While at first sight this may be interpreted as refractory or recurrent WD, PCR for *T. whipplei* in the tissue of these patients is frequently negative, indicating absence of vital bacteria; in addition, the reinflammation does not respond to antimicrobials, but does respond to corticosteroids. This pathological condition was first described in HIV patients with low CD4 T cells after initiation of highly active antiretroviral therapy, and later in tuberculosis or in leprosy patients, and was named immune reconstitution inflammatory syndrome (IRIS). Recent studies found IRIS in 10% of patients with WD [52]. Interestingly, IRIS in Whipple's disease is correlated with the HLA DQB1*06 allele, and HLA alleles DQB1 are also overrepresented in leprosy [53]. IRIS outcome varied from mild to fatal, and almost all WD patients who developed IRIS had previous immunosuppressive therapy (which had been given under the suspected diagnosis of rheumatic disease). IRIS has to be considered in patients with WD in whom inflammatory symptoms recur after effective treatment. Early diagnosis and treatment with steroids may be beneficial, but patients have to be followed closely.

This is because, on the other hand, the effect of corticosteroids in patients with established diagnosis WD usu-

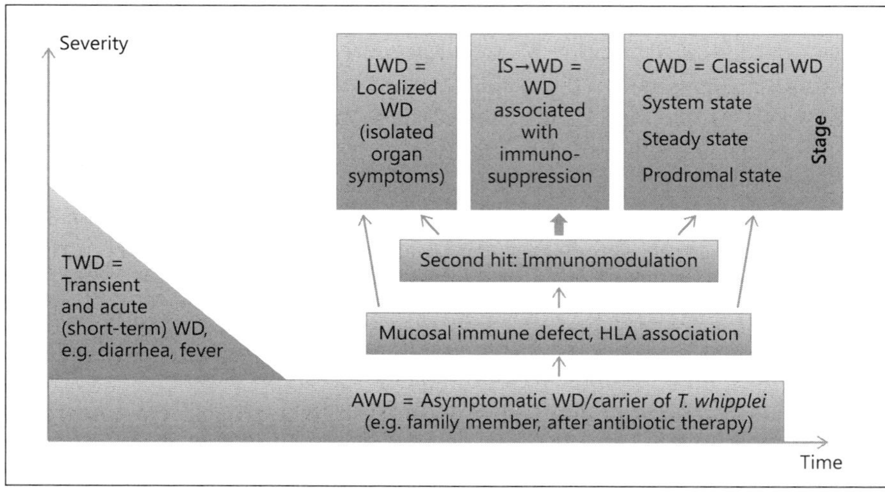

Fig. 1. Clinical features of and pathogenetic factors in *T. whipplei* infection: the 'second hit' hypothesis.

ally is not favorable, and thus is a double-edged sword. This is well known when looking back at the older literature. For example, in 1963 Davis reported 15 WD patients, 8 of whom were treated successfully with antibiotics, and the 7 that were treated with steroids relapsed, did poorly or died [54]. Still, the role of corticosteroids as adjunctive treatment for WD remained controversial for years [55], as older series had observed some positive effects of steroids [56]. Nowadays, in some cases with longstanding CNS WD, in addition to antibiotics, adjunctive therapy with corticosteroids are discussed as detailed below.

Summary for WD in Association with Immunosuppression

Taken together, because the weak HLA association or the subtle immune defects seem to be insufficient prerequisites in every WD case, the clinical form of WD in association with immunosuppression underscores the role of *T. whipplei* as an opportunistic invader and illustrates that an intact immune system in controlling an asymptomatic or subclinical *T. whipplei* infection is essential. Several factors associated with immunomodulatory effects in the host contribute to the development from asymptomatic carriage of *T. whipplei* to clinically manifested WD [56a]. It is currently unclear whether immunosuppression as a cofactor ('second hit') possesses a broader or essential role in the conversion of asymptomatic *T. whipplei* infection to various clinical manifestations of WD (fig. 1). Based on the presented data, it is possible that the pathogenetic concept of *T. whipplei* infection and WD has to be expanded.

Diagnosis

The diagnosis of CWD usually is made by upper endoscopy. Sometimes, pale yellow shaggy mucosa or whitish-yellow plaques in the duodenum or the jejunum can be seen. For diagnosis, 5 sufficiently sized and deep specimens should be taken from the distal duodenum or the jejunum as involvement can be patchy or submucosal. The diagnosis usually can be established if the characteristic PAS-positive material is present. Based on clinical manifestations, other samples may be tested [33].

Although the clinical picture together with a typical PAS-positive histology from the duodenum might be sufficient to establish the diagnosis in most cases, a specific diagnostic test, such as PCR and/or immunohistology, is recommended in every newly identified patient; it is mandatory in cases of doubt, or if the diagnosis is based on extraduodenal tissue (fig. 2). This recommendation reflects the fact that PAS staining is of limited value in extraintestinal tissue for monitoring the effect of therapy, and is unreliable in patients who have received immunosuppressive therapy (see the section above). Importantly, as 50% of the WD patients are positive for *T. whipplei* in the liquor [41], and these patients have a higher probability to develop overt CNS disease or dangerous CNS relapses, the cerebrospinal fluid (CSF) of all WD patients should be tested by PCR before initiation of therapy. PCR-based detection of *T. whipplei* DNA has become a very important diagnostic technique. Most sample specimens can be used for PCR-based diagnosis of WD. While quantitative PCR of *T. whipplei* in stool or saliva in individuals with WD often differs greatly (e.g. approx. 1–75%

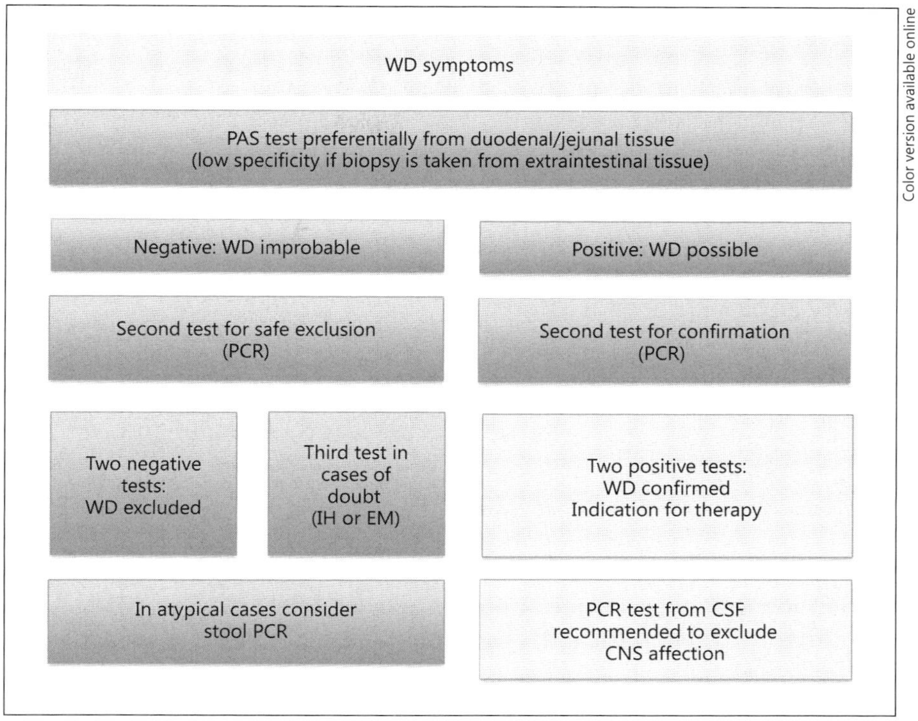

Fig. 2. Diagnostic approach to WD. EM = Electron microscopy; IH = immunohistochemistry.

in stool), these assays could be used for noninvasive screening or follow-up purposes in the future as the diagnosis of CWD is highly probable with a high bacterial load [57].

The clinical laboratory workup in WD patients often shows signs of chronic inflammation (increased acute-phase proteins), anemia, low serum albumin and decreased vitamin levels. Additionally, reduced IgG2 and IgM but increased IgA levels have been observed (table 1).

The clinician has to weigh the histopathological and laboratory findings in the context of the clinical features of the patient before antibiotic therapy is initiated, and in unclear situations specialists should be consulted.

Treatment

Antibiotic therapy often leads to a rapid improvement of the patient and to a lasting remission.

Current treatment recommendations are based on retrospective analysis and on prospective trials [41]. Recommendations include an induction treatment for 2 weeks with intravenous antibiotics that achieve high CSF levels such as ceftriaxone (2 g daily). This is followed by one year of oral trimethoprim-sulfamethoxazole (960 mg twice daily). This treatment regimen in therapy trials shows a very high rate of clinical remission. In cases of allergy to ceftriaxone, alternative induction therapies may consist of meropenem or penicillin. An alternative to long-term oral co-trimoxazole is doxycycline (2 × 100 mg/day) in combination with hydroxychloroquine (600 mg/day) [58]. Recently, a short treatment duration of only 3 months has been reported [59], an issue which is still controversial, particularly as others argue for a life-long treatment instead [60]. Further treatment trials on the issue are awaited.

WD may relapse despite an adequate and prolonged antibiotic treatment, even after many years of remission, more than once, and remarkably even with different strains of *T. whipplei* [29, 60]. Particularly relapses of CNS disease can take a detrimental course. In WD patients with CNS symptoms, neurologic defects are difficult to reverse. While some focal lesions or ophthalmoplegia respond usually to antibiotics, other structural changes such as granulomas, abscesses, or atrophic changes, may lead to persistent symptoms or even to fatal courses. Additional treatment with corticosteroids, which may reduce local inflammation, edema and endothelial damage, has been beneficial in cases of severe structural CNS manifestations [61].

WD patients should be followed lifelong, particularly closely in the first years after diagnosis, usually by duodenal biopsies and (in cases of initial cerebral involvement) with CSF analysis at 6 months and 1 year after diagnosis. Antibiotic therapy can be stopped, if PAS-positive material is absent and PCR is negative after 1 year.

Disclosure Statement

The author declares no conflict of interest.

References

1 Dobbins WO III: Whipple's Disease. Springfield, Charles C Thomas, 1987.
2 Relman DA, Schmidt TM, Macdermott RP, et al: Identification of the uncultured bacillus of Whipple's disease. N Engl J Med 1992;327: 293–301.
3 Schoedon G, Goldenberger D, Forrer R, et al: Deactivation of macrophages with interleukin-4 is the key to the isolation of *Tropheryma whipplei*. J Infect Dis 1997;176:672–677.
4 Raoult D, Birg ML, La Scola B, et al: Cultivation of the bacillus of Whipple's disease. N Engl J Med 2000;342:620–625.
5 La Scola B, Fenollar F, Perreal C, Raoult D: Epidemiologic implications of the first isolation and cultivation of *Tropheryma whipplei* from a saliva sample. Ann Intern Med 2011; 154:443–444.
6 Li W, Fenollar F, Rolain JM, et al: Genotyping reveals a wide heterogeneity of *Tropheryma whipplei*. Microbiology 2008;154:521–527.
7 Bentley S, Maiwald M, Murphy LD, et al: Sequencing and analysis of the genome of the Whipple's disease bacterium *Tropheryma whipplei*. Lancet 2003;361:637–644.
8 Schöniger-Hekele M, Petermann D, Weber B, et al: *Tropheryma whipplei* in the environment: survey of sewage plant influxes and sewage plant workers. Appl Environ Microbiol 2007;73:2033–2035.
9 Fenollar F, Trani M, Davoust B, et al: Prevalence of asymptomatic *Tropheryma whipplei* carriage among humans and nonhuman primates. J Infect Dis 2008;197:880–887.
10 Keita AK, Mediannikov O, Ratmanov P, Diatta G, Bassene H, Roucher C, Tall A, Sokhna C, Trape JF, Raoult D, Fenollar F: Looking for *Tropheryma whipplei* source and reservoir in rural Senegal. Am J Trop Med Hyg 2013;88: 339–343.
11 Fenollar F, Keita AK, Buffet S, Raoult D: Intrafamilial circulation of *Tropheryma whipplei*, France. Emerg Infect Dis 2012;18:949–955.
12 Marth T: Untersuchungen zur Klinik, Therapie und zellulären Immunität des M. Whipple; University of Bonn, 1993.
13 Dutly F, Altwegg M: Whipple's disease and *'Tropheryma whippelii'*. Clin Microbiol Rev 2001;4:561–583.
14 Martinetti M, Biagi F, Badulli C, et al: The HLA alleles DRB1*13 and DQB1*06 are associated to Whipple's disease. Gastroenterology 2009;136:2289–2294.
15 Marth T, Neurath M, Cuccherini BA, et al: Defects of monocyte interleukin 12 production and humoral immunity in Whipple's disease. Gastroenterology 1997;113:442–448.
16 Geelhaar A, Moos V, Schinnerling K, et al: Specific and nonspecific B-cell function in the small intestines of patients with Whipple's disease. Infect Immun 2010;78:4589–4592.
17 Moos V, Kunkel D, Marth T, et al: Reduced peripheral and mucosal *Tropheryma whipplei*-specific Th1 response in patients with Whipple's disease. J Immunol 2006;177: 2015–2022.
18 Marth T, Kleen N, Stallmach A, et al: Dysregulated peripheral and mucosal Th1/Th2 response in Whipple's disease. Gastroenterology 2002;123:1468–1477.
19 Schinnerling K, Moos V, Geelhaar A, et al: Regulatory T cells in patients with Whipple's disease. J Immunol 2011;187:4061–4067.
20 Marth T, Roux M, von Herbay A, Meuer SC, Feurle GE: Persistent reduction of complement receptor 3 alpha-chain expressing mononuclear blood cells and transient inhibitory serum factors in Whipple's disease. Clin Immunol Immunopathol 1994;72:217–226.
21 Moos V, Schmidt C, Geelhaar A, et al: Impaired immune functions of monocytes and macrophages in Whipple's disease. Gastroenterology 2010;138:210–220.
22 Desnues B, Lepidi H, Raoult D, et al: Whipple disease: intestinal infiltrating cells exhibit a transcriptional pattern of M2/alternatively activated macrophages. J Infect Dis 2005;192: 1642–1646.
23 Gorvel L, Al Moussawi K, Ghigo E, et al: *Tropheryma whipplei*, the Whipple's disease bacillus, induces macrophage apoptosis through the extrinsic pathway. Cell Death Dis 2010; 1:e34.
24 Dobbins WO 3rd: Is there an immune deficit in Whipple's disease? Dig Dis Sci 1981;26: 247–252.
25 Kalt A, Schneider T, Ring S, Hoffmann J, Zeitz M, Stallmach A, Persing DH, Marth T: Decreased levels of interleukin-12p40 in the serum of patients with Whipple's disease. Int J Colorectal Dis 2006;21:114–120.
26 Inoue R, Kondo N, Kobayashi Y, Fukutomi O, Orii T: IgG2 deficiency associated with defects in production of interferon-gamma; comparison with common variable immunodeficiency. Scand J Immunol 1995;41:130–134.
27 Sanders LA, van de Winkel JG, Rijkers GT, Voorhorst-Ogink MM, de Haas M, Capel PJ, Zegers BJ: Fc gamma receptor IIa (CD32) heterogeneity in patients with recurrent bacterial respiratory tract infections. J Infect Dis 1994; 170:854–861.
28 Raoult D, Fenollar F, Rolain JM, Minodier P, Bosdure E, Li W, Garnier JM, Richet H: *Tropheryma whipplei* in children with gastroenteritis. Emerg Infect Dis 2010;16:776–782.
29 Keita AK, Bassene H, Tall A, Sokhna C, Ratmanov P, Trape JF, Raoult D, Fenollar F: *Tropheryma whipplei*: a common bacterium in rural Senegal. PLoS Negl Trop Dis 2011; 5:e1403.
30 Geissdorfer W, Moos V, Moter A, Loddenkemper C, Jansen A, Tandler R, Mirguet AJ, Raoult D, Bogdan C, Schneider T: High frequency of *Tropheryma whipplei* in culture-negative endocarditis. J Clin Microbiol 2012; 50:216–222.
31 Love SM, Morrison L, Appleby C, Modi P: *Tropheryma whipplei* endocarditis without gastrointestinal involvement. Interact Cardiovasc Thorac Surg 2012;15:161–163.
32 Fenollar F, Puéchal X, Raoult D: Whipple's disease. N Engl J Med 2007;356:55–66.
33 Marth T, Raoult D: Whipple's disease. Lancet 2003;361:239–246.
34 Mahnel R, Kalt A, Ring S, Stallmach A, Strober W, Marth T: Immunosuppressive therapy in Whipple's disease patients is associated with the appearance of gastrointestinal manifestations. Am J Gastroenterol 2005;100: 1167–1173.
35 Lagier JC, Lepidi H, Raoult D, Fenollar F: Systemic *Tropheryma whipplei*: clinical presentation of 142 patients with infections diagnosed or confirmed in a reference center. Medicine (Baltimore) 2010;89:337–334.
36 Compain C, Sacre K, Puéchal X, Klein I, Vital-Durand D, Houeto JL, De Broucker T, Raoult D, Papo T: Central nervous system involvement in Whipple disease: clinical study of 18 patients and long-term follow-up. Medicine (Baltimore) 2013;92:324–330.

37 Marth T: Complicated Whipple's disease and endocarditis following tumor necrosis factor inhibitors. World J Cardiol 2014;6:1278–1284.
38 Razonable RR, Pulido JS, Deziel PJ, Dev S, Salomão DR, Walker RC: Chorioretinitis and vitreitis due to *Tropheryma whipplei* after transplantation: case report and review. Transpl Infect Dis 2008;10:413–418.
39 Gillen CD, Coddington R, Monteith PG, Taylor RH: Extraintestinal lymphoma in association with Whipple's disease. Gut 1993;11:1627–1629.
40 Gruner U, Goesch P, Donner A, Peters U: Whipple disease and non-Hodgkin lymphoma. Z Gastroenterol 2001;41:305–309.
41 Feurle GE, Junga NS, Marth T: Efficacy of ceftriaxone or meropenem as initial therapies in Whipple's disease. Gastroenterology 2010;138:478–86.
42 Wang S, Ernst LM, Smith BR, Tallini G, Howe JG, Crouch J, Cooper DL: Systemic *Tropheryma whipplei* infection associated with monoclonal B-cell proliferation: a *Helicobacter pylori*-type pathogenesis? Arch Pathol Lab Med 2003;12:1619–1622.
43 Fest T, Pron B, Lefranc MP, Pierre C, Angonin R, de Wazières B, Soua Z, Dupond JL: Detection of a clonal BCL2 gene rearrangement in tissues from a patient with Whipple disease. Ann Intern Med 1996;8:738–740.
44 Rouillon A, Menkes CJ, Gerster JC, Perez-Sawka I, Forest M: Sarcoid-like forms of Whipple's disease. Report of 2 cases. J Rheumatol 1993;20:1070–1072.
45 Dzirlo L, Hubner M, Mueller C, Blaha B, Formann E, Dellinger C, Petzelbauer P, Muellauer L, Huber K, Kneussl M, Gschwantler M: A mimic of sarcoidosis. Lancet 2007;369:1832.
46 Niemczyk S, Filipowicz E, Wozniacki L, Grochowski J, Zaleski L, Grzejszczak A, Ptasinska AP, Koperski L, Rowinska JM: Renal amyloidosis in Whipple disease: a case report. Cases J 2009;2:8444.
47 Dray X, Vahedi K, Delcey V, Lavergne-Slove A, Raskine L, Bergmann JF, Marteau P: *Mycobacterium avium* duodenal infection mimicking Whipple's disease in a patient with AIDS. Endoscopy 2007;39(suppl 1):E296–E297.
48 Lozupone C, Cota-Gomez A, Palmer BE, Linderman DJ, Charlson ES, Sodergren E, Mitreva M, Abubucker S, Martin J, Yao G, Campbell TB, Flores SC, Ackerman G, Stombaugh J, Ursell L, Beck JM, Curtis JL, Young VB, Lynch SV, Huang L, Weinstock GM, Knox KS, Twigg H, Morris A, Ghedin E, Bushman FD, Collman RG, Knight R, Fontenot AP; Lung HIV Microbiome Project: Widespread colonization of the lung by *Tropheryma whipplei* in HIV infection. Am J Respir Crit Care Med 2013;187:1110–1117.
49 Meier-Willersen HJ, Maiwald M, von Herbay A: Whipple's disease associated with opportunistic infections. Dtsch Med Wochenschr 1993;118:854–860.
50 Fenollar F, Lepidi H, Gerolami R, Drancourt H, Raoult D: Whipple disease associated with giardiasis. J Infect Dis 2003;188:828–834.
51 Arnold CA, Moreira RK, Lam-Himlin D, De Petris G, Montgomery E: Whipple disease a century after the initial description: increased recognition of unusual presentations, autoimmune comorbidities, and therapy effects. Am J Surg Pathol 2012;36:1066–1073.
52 Feurle GE, Moos V, Schinnerling K, et al: The immune reconstitution inflammatory syndrome in Whipple disease: a cohort study. Ann Intern Med 2010;153:710–717.
53 Biagi F, Trotta L, Di Stefano M, et al: Previous immunosuppressive therapy is a risk factor for immune reconstitution inflammatory syndrome in Whipple's disease. Dig Liver Dis 2012;44:880–882.
54 Davis TD, McBee JW, Borland JL, Kurtz SM, Ruffin JM: The effect of antibiotic and steroid therapy in Whipple's disease. Gastroenterology 1963;44:112–116.
55 Comer GM, Brandt LJ, Abissi CJ: Whipple's disease: a review. Am J Gastroenterol 1983;78:107–114.
56 Holt PR, Isselbacher KJ, Jones CM: The reversibility of Whipple's disease. Report of a case, with comments on the influence of corticosteroid therapy. N Engl J Med 1961;264:1335–1339.
56a Marth T: Systematic review: Whipple's disease (Tropheryma whipplei infection) and its unmasking by tumour necrosis factor inhibitors. Aliment Pharmacol Ther 2015;41:709–724.
57 Fenollar F, Lauira S, Lepidi H, Rolain JM, Raoult D: Value of *Tropheryma whipplei* quantitative polymerase chain reaction assay for the diagnosis of Whipple disease: usefulness of saliva and stool specimens for first-line screening. Clin Infect Dis 2008;47:659–667.
58 Lagier JC, Fenollar F, Lepidi H, Giorgi R, Million M, Raoult D: Treatment of classic Whipple's disease: from in vitro results to clinical outcome. J Antimicrob Chemother 2014;69:219–227.
59 Feurle GE, Moos V, Blaker H, et al: Intravenous ceftriaxone, followed by 12 or three months of oral treatment with trimethoprim-sulfamethoxazole in Whipple's disease. J Inf 66;2013:263–270.
60 Lagier JC, Fenollar F, Lepidi H, et al: Evidence of lifetime susceptibility to *Tropheryma whipplei* in patients with Whipple's disease. J Antimicrob Chemother 2011;66:1188–1189.
61 Schneider T, Moos V, Loddenkemper C, et al: Whipple's disease: new aspects of pathogenesis and treatment. Lancet Infect Dis 2008;8:179–190.

Dig Dis 2015;33:200–207
DOI: 10.1159/000371400

Motility Alterations in Celiac Disease and Non-Celiac Gluten Sensitivity

Maria Ines Pinto-Sanchez Premysl Bercik Elena F. Verdu

Farncombe Family Digestive Research Institute, Department of Medicine, McMaster University, Hamilton, Ont., Canada

Key Words
Celiac disease · Gluten sensitivity · Motility

Abstract
Regulation of gut motility is complex and involves neuromuscular, immune and environmental mechanisms. It is well established that patients with celiac disease (CD) often display gut dysmotility. Studies have shown the presence of disturbed esophageal motility, altered gastric emptying, and dysmotility of the small intestine, gallbladder and colon in untreated CD. Most of these motor abnormalities resolve after a strict gluten-free diet, suggesting that mechanisms related to the inflammatory condition and disease process are responsible for the motor dysfunction. Motility abnormalities are also a hallmark of functional bowel disorders such as irritable bowel syndrome (IBS), where it has been proposed as underlying mechanism for symptom generation (diarrhea, constipation, bloating). Non-celiac gluten sensitivity (NCGS) is a poorly defined entity, mostly self-diagnosed, that presents clinically with IBS symptoms in the absence of specific celiac markers. Patients with NCGS are believed to react symptomatically to wheat components, and some studies have proposed the presence of low-grade inflammation in these patients. There is little information regarding the functional characterization of these patients before and after a gluten-free diet. A study suggested the presence of altered gastrointestinal transit in NCGS patients who also have a high prevalence of nonspecific anti-gliadin antibodies. Results of an ongoing clinical study in NCGS patients with positive anti-gliadin antibodies before and after a gluten-free diet will be discussed. Elucidating the mechanisms for symptom generation in NCGS patients is important to find new therapeutic alternatives to the burden of imposing a strict gluten-free diet in patients who do not have CD.

Introduction

Gut motility is the result of complex interactions between multiple systems operating at the level of the gut and systemically (fig. 1). As a consequence, alterations in gut motility will be present in a variety of inflammatory disorders (fig. 2).

Gluten-related disorders involve all diseases triggered by gluten including celiac disease (CD) in its various manifestations, as well as the recently defined non-celiac gluten sensitivity (NCGS) [1–3]. CD is defined as a chronic small-intestinal immune-mediated enteropathy precipitated by exposure to dietary gluten in genetically predisposed individuals [4]. CD is one of the best well-characterized autoimmune diseases for which we have deep knowledge of the environmental, genetic, and immuno-

KARGER 125

E-Mail karger@karger.com
www.karger.com/ddi

0257–2753/15/0332–0200$39.50/0

Elena F. Verdu
Farncombe Family Digestive Research Institute
Department of Medicine, McMaster University
Hamilton, ON L8S 4K1 (Canada)
E-Mail verdue@mcmaster.ca

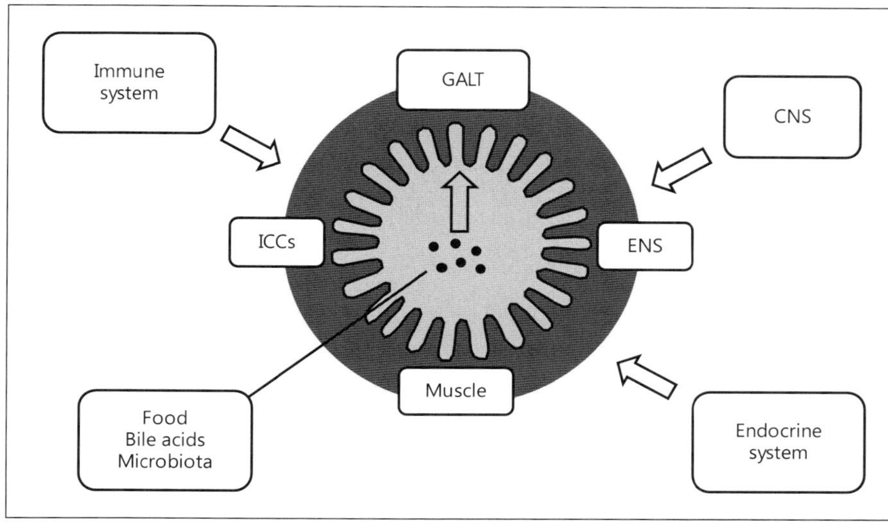

Fig. 1. Mechanisms that control gut motility. Gut motility is the result of complex interactions between the different tissues in the gut [smooth muscle, enteric nervous system (ENS), gut-associated lymphoid tissue (GALT) and pacemaker cells in the gut, and the interstitial cells of Cajal (ICCs)]. The gut generates spontaneous electrical and contractile activity that is controlled by signals from the central nervous system (CNS), and the endocrine and systemic immune systems. These interactions are bidirectional. In addition to these, luminal factors coming from the food (e.g. dietary proteins such as gluten) and intestinal microbes have an important regulatory effect on gut immune and secretomotor activity in the host.

Color version available online

logic factors involved [5]. Unlike CD, the definition of NCGS continues to be updated as new evidence arises, and there is no specific diagnostic test yet available. The latter precludes studies to accurately determine the real prevalence of NCGS, which has been estimated to be at least 6 times more frequent than CD [6]. However, this remains to be confirmed once its pathophysiology is better defined and biomarkers become available.

Intestinal dysmotility occurs in a variety of disorders in which the gut has lost its ability to coordinate muscular activity because of endogenous or exogenous causes [7–9]. Such disorders may be primary or secondary and may manifest symptomatically in a variety of ways, including abdominal distention, recurrent obstruction, abdominal colicky pain, constipation, gastroesophageal reflux disease and recurrent vomiting. In a broad sense, any alteration in the transit of foods and secretions into the digestive tract may be considered an intestinal motility disorder [10].

It is quite frequent to diagnose gastrointestinal motor abnormalities in celiac patients. Untreated celiacs can exhibit disturbed motility of the esophagus, stomach, small intestine, gallbladder, and colon. Not surprisingly, the data on motility in NCGS are just emerging. It is not the objective of this chapter to perform an in-depth review of the methods to study gut motility, which has been reviewed elsewhere in detail [11]. In the next section, we will briefly outline the main techniques used to measure gut motility in order to discuss the studies investigating this parameter in CD and, where possible, in NCGS.

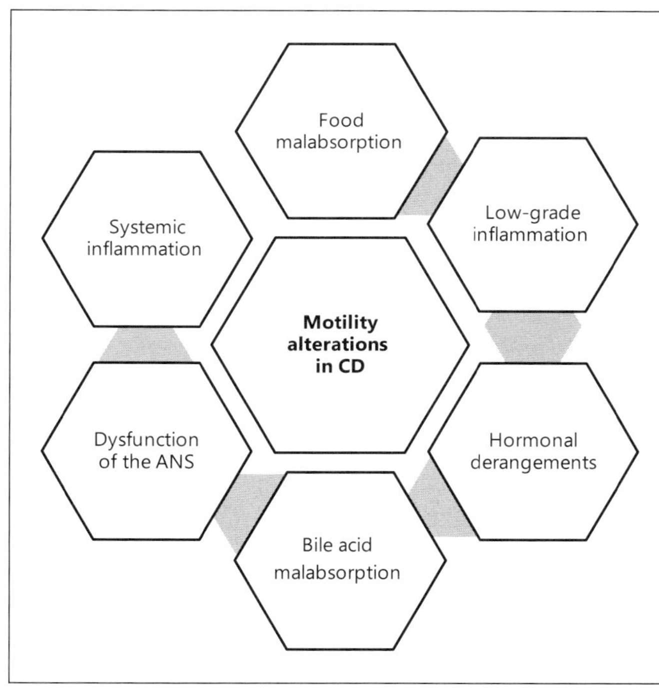

Fig. 2. Pathophysiological mechanisms involved in motility alterations in CD. ANS = Autonomic nervous system.

Brief Overview of Methods to Assess Gut Motility

Several methods are available to investigate gut motility for clinical or research purposes. The choice of method will depend on the main objective (clinical vs. research) and its availability. Overall, esophageal motility can be investigated with manometry; gastric emptying with scintigraphy, ^{13}C-octanoic breath test and ultrasound; orocecal transit time with lactulose H_2 breath test and more recently with videocapsule endoscopy (VCE). Measurement of colonic transit has been attempted with radiopaque markers, and gallbladder motility with scintigraphy.

Mouth-to-Cecum Transit Time: Lactulose H_2 Breath Test

After an overnight fast, subjects are requested to drink a lactulose-containing liquid/meal. After 30 min, breath hydrogen is measured to analyze 50-ml samples of end expiratory breath collected at 10-min intervals. A curve is drawn to show the hydrogen concentration. After a slight rise occurring in about 20 min, the breath hydrogen concentration normally falls and remains steady for a variable time, followed by a second rise steadily producing a sigmoid curve. The time to the first sustained rise (>10 parts per million above basal) in breath hydrogen concentration represents the mouth-to-cecum transit time (M-CTT). The rate of rise of the breath hydrogen is usually assessed in ppm/min from the slope of the curve lying between 10 and 50% of the maximal rise in breath hydrogen [12].

Antroduodenal Manometry

This constitutes a valuable method to assess gastroduodenal motility, and consists of the measurement of motor activity by the insertion of a manometric PVC catheter just beyond the angle of Treitz [13]. Intraluminal pressures are recorded using high-resolution solid-state transducers or water-perfused systems. The recordings are performed within fasting and postprandial periods. With this method, the three phases of interdigestive (fasting) motor activity, the migrating motor complex (MMC), can be identified. Phase I consists of motor quiescence, phase II of irregular contractile activity, and phase III (activity front) of regular contractile activity occurring at a frequency of 3 contractions per minute in the gastric antrum and contractions per minute in the duodenum-jejunum.

Ultrasound

Several approaches based on a duplex technique with serial determinations of cross-sectional areas or 3-dimensional ultrasonography with volume algorithms have been introduced to assess gastric emptying [14, 15]. Furthermore, transabdominal ultrasonography can be used to measure transpyloric flow [14, 16]. Ultrasonography is easily accessible, noninvasive and does not expose the subject to radiation. The method is operator-dependent, reliable only for liquid meals and difficult to use in obese subjects [14].

Scintigraphy

Two different isotopes can be used to measure gastric emptying by scintigraphy, a digestive solid marker and a liquid marker. ^{99}Tc sulphur colloid radiolabelled scrambled egg is often used as a digestible solid component and indium-111 diethylenetriaminepentaacetic acid in water is used as a liquid marker. The scintigraphy approach also allows for the evaluation of small-intestinal and colonic motility [14].

^{13}C-Octanoid Breath Test

The ^{13}C-octanoic acid breath test is frequently used to assess gastric emptying since it is not radioactive, it is accurate, and also safe for children [17]. Fatty acids labelled with the nonradioactive isotope ^{13}C-octanoic acid can be used to measure gastric emptying as ^{13}C is absorbed in the intestine and excreted by breath [14]. The method has the advantage that it is easy to perform and inexpensive. However, the absorption, distribution metabolism and excretion of markers require many steps that may lead to an ambiguous interpretation of results [14].

Videocapsule Endoscopy

VCE has previously been proposed as a method to assess intestinal morphology in CD [18–21]. However, its use in motility assessment has been recently evaluated. Ciaccio et al. [22] developed a method to detect and quantify differences in small-intestinal motility in celiac patients compared to controls using VCE images. Instead of investigating specific image features, as in previous studies, they used dynamic estimates of wall motility for image classification and sought to characterize motility according to frame-to-frame changes in lumen shape [22]. However, the methodology still needs to be validated before widespread implementation.

Colonic Transit Time: Radiopaque Markers

Measurement of colon transit time is the most basic and primary tool in evaluating disorders of colonic motility. Several techniques for measuring colon transit time currently exist. The standard measurement of colon transit time has been performed using radiopaque marker test. The latter is the most widely used method.

Table 1. Summary of current studies on gut motility in CD

First author, year	System	Subjects	Method	Findings
Bassotti, 1994	OCT	16 (9 adults and 7 children)	Manometry	CD adults but not children showed a greater frequency of migrating motor complexes vs. controls during fasting
Bai, 1995	OCT	55 (25 untreated, 15 treated CD and 15 controls)	Lactulose/BT SHAPE	OCT was significantly delayed and colonic transit accelerated in untreated patients
Usai, 1995	Esophagus	36 CD (14 active and 22 treated) and 144 controls	Manometry pH-metry	CD may display esophageal abnormalities in esophageal motility
Chiarioni, 1997	OCT	16 CD and 20 HV	Lactulose BT and urine D-xylose	Mouth-to-cecum transit time was increased in CD vs. controls
Spiller, 1987	OCT	27 CD and 10 controls	Lactulose BT	Delayed mouth-cecum transit in patients with steatorrhea
Perri, 1987	Gastric	20 CD before and after treatment	Gastric emptying ^{13}C-octanoic acid BT	CD patients markedly delayed gastric emptying of solids, which normalized after gluten withdrawal (6 months)
Cucchiara, 1995	Gastric	14 untreated CD 4 treated CD and 8 controls	Manometry	CD shorter duration of activity fronts and reduction in PP antral motility index vs. controls; the previous disappeared after GFD
Usai, 1997	Esophagus and gastric	30 untreated CD	Manometry Gastric emptying Scintigraphy	Esophageal abnormalities present
Fraquelli, 1999	Gallbladder	10 CD before and after GFD and 10 HV	Ultrasonography	Elevated somatostatin with increased gallbladder fasting; decreased cholecystokinin secretion reduced gallbladder emptying; GFD reversed these abnormalities
Benini, 2001	Gastric	16 CD and 24 HV	Lactulose BT	Impairment of gastric emptying in CD which is at least partially reversible after GFD
Giorgetti, 2004	Autonomic	8 CD and 8 HV	PAS	Correlation between autonomic dysfunction and CD
Bassotti, 2008	Gastric	11 CD and 33 controls	Manometry	Abnormalities >80% CD even though they were treated
Rocco, 2008	Gastric	CD controls	Gastric emptying ^{13}C-octanoic acid BT	Delayed gastric emptying in CD, not correlated with tissue ghrelin changes
Fenini, 2012	OCT	19 CD untreated, 14 CD treated and 24 controls	Mouth-to-cecum transit	M-CTT more prolonged in CD vs. controls and not reverted after GFD
Ciaccio, 2012	OCT		Videocapsule	Delayed intestinal but accelerated colonic transit?

OCT = Orocecal transit time; HV = healthy volunteers; BT = breath test.

This test is simple and inexpensive, produces minimum radiation exposure and is reliable and reproducible. However, it requires good compliance of the patient. Radiopaque markers are plastic beads or rings that are usually ingested in a capsule containing 20–50 markers. The most common capsule used is Sitzmarks® (Konsyl Pharmaceuticals, Fort Worth, Tex., USA). Several methods have been suggested including the single-capsule technique and the multiple-capsule technique. The multiple-capsule technique requires the ingestion of 1 capsule a day for 3 days, followed by abdominal X-ray on day 4 and/or day 7 [23]. Interpretation is based on the identification of markers in 3 regions, namely the right, left and rectosigmoid regions. These are defined by bony landmarks and gaseous outlines as described by Kim and Rhee [23] and Arhan et al. [24]. Colon transit times in each segment and throughout the entire colon are calculated by multiplying the number of markers by 1.2 (or by 1.0 when using a capsule containing 24 markers) [24, 25].

Esophageal Motility Alterations in CD and NCGS

Using esophageal and gastrointestinal manometry, Usai et al. [26, 27] found esophageal motor abnormalities in 50% of patients with CD and gastrointestinal motility alterations in 75% of them. In a collaborative study involving two medical centers, we evaluated esophageal motility by using manometry and pH impedance in 12 CD and 7 non-celiac controls. Preliminary results from this study demonstrated motility alterations in 83% of CD patients [28]. No studies are yet available on esophageal motility alterations in NCGS population.

Gastrointestinal Motility Alterations in CD and NCGS

Gastrointestinal motility alterations have been extensively studied in celiac patients. More than 30 years ago, Spiller et al. [12] measured for the first time M-CTT of a lactulose-labelled liquid test meal in 27 CD patients and 10 healthy controls (HC) and gastric emptying of an indium DTPA-labelled liquid test meal in 11 CD patients and 6 HC. The authors demonstrated that patients with CD and fat malabsorption tend to have a delayed mouth-cecum transit in spite of apparently normal gastric emptying and normal levels of insulin, GIP, CCC, neurotensin and PYY [12]. A delay in M-CTT in CD was also reported by Benini et al. [29].

Usai et al. [26] found gastrointestinal motility abnormalities in 75% of untreated CD patients assessed by manometry. CD patients displayed a shorter length of phase III of MMC as well as postprandial contractility in children with CD [30]. The same group performed a study in 11 untreated and 12 treated adult CD patients and demonstrated that more than 80% of untreated celiacs had discrete motor abnormalities of the upper gut, in both fasting and fed periods [31].

A recent study by Ciaccio et al. [22] evaluated motility by using VCE (Given® SB2) in 11 CD patients on a gluten-free diet (GFD) and in 10 control subjects. The authors sought to develop an automated and quantitative technique to directly characterize motility according to frame-to-frame changes in lumen shape [22]. The study revealed differences in motility in CD patients compared to controls. However, limitations related to the methodology were identified, suggesting that the results should be taken with caution [32]. Further studies are needed to validate this method and confirm its usefulness in the evaluation of celiac patients.

Gastric motility and emptying in CD have been reported to be normal [12, 33, 34] or delayed [17, 26, 29, 35]. The reason for the different findings could relate to different methods used to assess gastric emptying [17, 35]. No studies are so far available evaluating gastrointestinal motility in NCGS.

Colonic Motility Alterations in CD and NCGS

Bai et al. [36] performed a study evaluating colonic motility in 1995. The authors studied 25 patients with untreated CD, 15 treated patients and 15 HC. Transit of radiopaque makers (Metcalf method), a measure of total colonic transit, was significantly faster in untreated CD patients. The major finding was that this abnormal colonic behavior was principally due to a subpopulation of untreated patients with very fast transit times (<18 h) [36]. Using the same methodology, Benini et al. [29] measured colonic transit time in 19 CD patients and no differences in mean numbers of markers were observed. However, a limitation of the latest study is that colonic transit time was performed in only a subset of patients and healthy volunteers.

A recent study evaluated the effect of GFD on gastrointestinal motility assessed by scintigraphy in a population with diarrhea-predominant irritable bowel syndrome (IBS-D) and assessed HLA DQ2 and -8 in the population. No differences in overall GI motility after 1 month of GFD was observed in the IBS-D population, independently of HLA status [37]. We are currently conducting a study evaluating colonic motility alterations in a population with NCGS (data presented at the Falk Symposium on small-intestinal disorders in Amsterdam). Our preliminary results suggest that patients with NCGS, diagnosed by gluten-related symptoms and presence of IgG AGA, present with motility alterations that improve in the majority of cases after a GFD [38]. Further studies are needed to support these preliminary results.

Gallbladder Motility Alterations in CD and NCGS

Benini et al. [29] performed a study to assess gallbladder motility by ultrasonography, and found that gallbladder fasting volume and postprandial residual volume were significantly higher in CD patients than in controls. Fraquelli et al. [39] measured gallbladder volume and plasma levels of cholecystokinin and somatostatin by ultrasonography and radioimmunoassay in a cohort of 10 celiac patients at diagnosis, after 18 months of GFD, and 10 HC. The authors found that patients at diagnosis had significantly greater fasting gallbladder volume and higher somatostatin plasma levels than controls. No studies on gallbladder motility have been performed in NCGS. Table 1 summarizes current studies involving gut motility in CD.

Possible Mechanisms Involved in Motility Alterations in CD and NCGS

Although abnormal intestinal motility is present in CD patients, it often normalizes following a gluten-free diet [40, 41]. Similar dysmotility findings may also be present in patients with other small-intestinal conditions such as Whipple's disease, irritable bowel syndrome, food hypersensitivity, enteric neuropathies, and chronic intestinal pseudo-obstruction, suggesting that the intestine, from a motility point of view, responds in a similar manner to different pathogenic stimuli [32].

The most obvious hypothesis underlying dysmotility in active CD is related to malabsorption. Because of the reduced absorptive surface of the jejunum in CD, a longer tract of the bowel comes into contact with the products of food digestion and the previous determines the delayed gastric emptying and slower orocecal transit time [11].

Interestingly, in recent years a unifying hypothesis linking enteric dysmotility and sensation has emerged, related to the role of low-grade inflammation and disturbances of neuroimmune interactions [32]. To investigate the potential mechanisms of gut secretomotor dysfunction induced by gluten, acetylcholine release by the myenteric plexus, small-intestinal contractility, and epithelial ion transport were measured in gliadin-sensitized HLA-DQ8 mice. Although intestinal atrophy was not observed in sensitized mice, there was increased acetylcholine release from the myenteric plexus, muscle hypercontractility, and increased active ion transport that normalized after a gluten withdrawal. The study suggests a mechanism by which gluten could induce gut motor dysfunction in the context of gluten sensitivity [42]. The motor changes in the animal model described above were accompanied by low-grade inflammation in the small intestine without atrophy. It has been hypothesized that severe mucosal damage and inflammation may be more strictly related to gastrointestinal motility derangement in CD [11]. However, this is discordant with the clinical situation, where CD can present with dyspeptic symptoms without signs or symptoms of severe inflammation [13].

Another underlying mechanism for motor dysfunction in CD may relate to autonomic nervous system dysfunction [26]. It has been proposed that the severe mucosal damage observed in CD may alter the contractile upper-gut activity through perturbations of the complex hormonal and neuroimmune regulation in the intestinal mucosa [11].

Hormonal derangements as a consequence of intestinal mucosal damage in CD patients have also been proposed [11, 43–47]. For instance, a decrease in cholecystokinin and an increase in somatostatin have been implicated in gallbladder inertia, while an increase in neurotensin and plasma peptide Y levels has been suggested as a cause of delayed gastric emptying and esophageal abnormalities [11]. All these hormonal derangements could lead to an alteration in the enterohepatic circulation of bile acids, which are fundamental for intestinal absorption of lipids [11, 48]. Finally, motility alterations could also lead to bacterial overgrowth, which in turn may contribute to the development and maintenance of symptoms and inflammation in CD patients [11, 49].

The Effect of GFD on Gut Motility

Several studies have assessed the effect of a GFD on gut motility with discordant results. A positive effect of the GFD on M-CTT was reported by some groups, but not confirmed by others [29]. In a study performed by Bassotti et al. [31], motility alterations assessed by manometry persisted on those in whom CD was still active, despite the GFD. Perri et al. [17] showed that gastric motility alterations normalized after GFD. In line with this, Benini et al. [29] demonstrated that after mucosal recovery, gastric emptying of a gluten-free meal improves; however, it is still delayed compared to controls. Finally, a GFD was proven to normalize gallbladder motility in the CD population [29, 39]. Thus, it seems gut dysmotility in CD usually responds to a strict GFD, and its success may depend on resolution of inflammation.

Conclusion

Presence of dysmotility in celiacs and in NCGS patients could trigger symptoms. Motility alterations throughout the GI tract have been widely described in CD patients by using different methods. Reduced absorption of food, small-intestinal inflammation, dysfunction of the autonomic nervous system, hormonal derangements and dysbiosis are some of the mechanisms that may trigger dysmotility. Alterations in motility revert to normal after the GFD in most patients with CD. The role of low-grade inflammation and enteric nerve dysfunction and dysmotility in NCGS is beginning to emerge, and may explain some symptoms in these patients as well as improvement after the GFD. More studies are needed to elucidate the presence of and underlying mechanisms in motility alterations in NCGS.

Acknowledgements

M.I.P.-S. received a CIHR-FHP Health Professional Award Fellowship. E.F.V. holds a CRC and is funded by a CIHR grant MOP No. 8-11836.

Disclosure Statement

The authors declare that they have no conflicts of interest concerning this paper.

References

1 Ludvigsson JF, Bai JC, Biagi F, et al: Diagnosis and management of adult coeliac disease: guidelines from the British Society of Gastroenterology. Gut 2014;63:1210–1228.

2 Sapone A, Bai JC, Ciacci C, et al: Spectrum of gluten-related disorders: consensus on new nomenclature and classification. BMC Med 2012;10:13.

3 Armstrong D, Verdu EF: The spectrum of wheat sensitivity: from non-celiac gluten sensitivity to celiac disease. Clin Lab News 2014;40(8):13–19.

4 Ludvigsson JF, Leffler DA, Bai JC, et al: The Oslo definitions for coeliac disease and related terms. Gut 2013;62:43–52.

5 Alvarez-Jubete L, Arendt EK, Gallagher E: Nutritive value and chemical composition of pseudocereals as gluten-free ingredients. Int J Food Sci Nutr 2009;60(suppl 4):240–257.

6 Lundin KE: Non-celiac gluten sensitivity – why worry? BMC Med 2014;12:86.

7 Di Lorenzo C, Youssef NN: Diagnosis and management of intestinal motility disorders. Semin Pediatr Surg 2010;19:50–58.

8 Keller J, Layer P: Intestinal and anorectal motility and functional disorders. Best Pract Res Clin Gastroenterol 2009;23:407–423.

9 Venkatasubramani N, Sood MR: Motility disorders of the gastrointestinal tract. Indian J Pediatr 2006;73:927–930.

10 Ouyang A, Locke GR 3rd: Overview of neurogastroenterology-gastrointestinal motility and functional GI disorders: classification, prevalence, and epidemiology. Gastroenterol Clin North Am 2007;36:485–498, vii.

11 Tursi A: Gastrointestinal motility disturbances in celiac disease. J Clin Gastroenterol 2004; 38:642–645.

12 Spiller RC, Lee YC, Edge C, et al: Delayed mouth-caecum transit of a lactulose labelled liquid test meal in patients with steatorrhoea caused by partially treated coeliac disease. Gut 1987;28:1275–1282.

13 Patcharatrakul T, Gonlachanvit S: Technique of functional and motility test: how to perform antroduodenal manometry. Neurogastroenterol Motil 2013;19:395–404.

14 Madsen JL: Scintigraphic assessment of gastrointestinal motility: a brief review of techniques and data interpretation. Clin Physiol Funct Imaging 2014;34:243–253.

15 Bolondi L, Bortolotti M, Santi V, et al: Measurement of gastric emptying by real-time ultrasonography. Gastroenterology 1985;89: 752–759.

16 Hausken T, Gilja OH, Odegaard S, et al: Flow across the human pylorus soon after ingestion of food, studied with duplex sonography. Effect of glyceryl trinitrate. Scand J Gastroenterol 1998;33:484–490.

17 Perri F, Zicolella A, Festa VP, et al: Gastric emptying of solids is delayed in celiac disease and normalises after gluten-free diet. Gastroenterology 1998;114:A820.

18 Ciaccio EJ, Bhagat G, Naiyer AJ, et al: Quantitative assessment of the degree of villous atrophy in patients with coeliac disease. J Clin Pathol 2008;61:1089–1093.

19 Ciaccio EJ, Tennyson CA, Lewis SK, et al: Distinguishing patients with celiac disease by quantitative analysis of videocapsule endoscopy images. Comput Methods Programs Biomed 2010;100:39–48.

20 Ciaccio EJ, Tennyson CA, Bhagat G, et al: Classification of videocapsule endoscopy image patterns: comparative analysis between patients with celiac disease and normal individuals. Biomed Eng Online 2010;9:44–54.

21 Ciaccio EJ, Bhagat G, Tennyson CA, et al: Quantitative assessment of endoscopic images for degree of villous atrophy in celiac disease. Dig Dis Sci 2011;56:805–811.

22 Ciaccio EJ, Tennyson CA, Bhagat G, et al: Quantitative estimates of motility from videocapsule endoscopy are useful to discern celiac patients from controls. Dig Dis Sci 2012;57: 2936–2943.

23 Kim ER, Rhee P: How to interpret a functional or motility test – colon transit study. J Neurogastroenterol Motil 2012;18:94–99.

24 Arhan P, Devroede G, Jehannin B, et al: Segmental colonic transit time. Dis Colon Rectum 1981;24:625–629.

25 Evans RC, Kamm MA, Hinton JM, et al: The normal range and a simple diagram for recording whole gut transit time. Int J Colorectal Dis 1992;7:15–17.

26 Usai P, Usai Satta P, Lai M, et al: Autonomic dysfunction and upper digestive functional disorders in untreated adult celiac disease. Eur J Clin Invest 1997;27:1009–1015.

27 Usai P, Bassotti G, Usai Satta P, et al: Oesophageal motility in adult coeliac disease. Neurogastroenterol Mot 1995;7:239–244.

28 Nachman F, Pinto-Sanchez MI, Salím S, et al: GO-016 – disfuncion esofágica en pacientes con enfermedad celiaca (abstract). Semana Panamericana de las Enfermedades Digestivas. Buenos Aires, Octubre 2014. http://www.gastro2014.com/.

29 Benini F, Mora A, Turini D, et al: Slow gallbladder emptying reverts to normal but small intestinal transit of a physiological meal remains slow in celiac patients during gluten-free diet. Neurogastroenterol Motil 2012; 24:e100–e180.

30 Cucchiara S, Bassotti G, Castellucci G, et al: Upper gastrointestinal motor abnormalities in children with active CD. J Pediatr Gastroenterol Nutr 1995;21:435–442.

31 Bassotti G, Villanacci V, Mazzocchi A, et al: Antroduodenojejunal motor activity in untreated and treated celiac disease patients. J Gastroenterol Hepatol 2008;23:e-23–e-28.

32 Bassotti G, Villanacci V, Battaglia E: Small bowel motility from videocapsule endoscopy: beware of false prophets! Dig Dis Sci 2013;58: 1161–1162.

33 Hamlyn AN, McKenna K, Douglas AP: Gastric emptying in coeliac disease. BMJ 1977;1: 1257–1258.

34 Moberg S, Carlberger G: Gastric emptying in healthy subjects and in patients with various malabsorptive states. Scand J Gastroenterol 1974;9:17–21.

35 Rocco A, Sarnelli G, Compare D, et al: Tissue ghrelin level and gastric emptying rate in adult patients with celiac disease. Neurogastroenterol Motil 2008;20:884–890.

36 Bai JC, Mauriño E, Martínez C, et al: Abnormal colonic transit time in untreated celiac sprue. Acta Gastroenterol Latinoam 1995;25: 277–284.
37 Vazquez-Roque MI, Camilleri M, Smyrk T, et al: A controlled trial of gluten-free diet in patients with irritable bowel syndrome-diarrhea: effects on bowel frequency and intestinal function. Gastroenterology 2013;144: 903–911.
38 Pinto-Sanchez MI, Basra D, McCarville J, et al: Improvement of gastrointestinal symptoms and motility in non-celiac gluten sensitive patients after the gluten free diet (abstract FS193_0136). Celiac Disease and Other Small Bowel Disorders, Falk Symposium 193. Amsterdam, September 2014.
39 Fraquelli M, Bardella MT, Peracchi M, et al: Gallbladder emptying and somatostatin and cholecystokinin plasma levels in celiac disease. Am J Gastroenterol 1999;94:1867–1870.
40 Chiarioni G, Bassotti G, Germani U, et al: Gluten-free diet normalizes mouth-to-cecum transit of a caloric meal in adult patients with celiac disease. Dig Dis Sci 1997;42:2100–2105.
41 Sadik R, Abrahamsson H, Kilander A, et al: Gut transit in celiac disease: delay of small bowel transit and acceleration after dietary treatment. Am J Gastroenterol 2004;99:2429–2436.
42 Verdu EF, Huang X, Natividad J, et al: Gliadin-dependent neuromuscular and epithelial secretory responses in gluten-sensitive HLA-DQ8 transgenic mice. Am J Physiol Gastrointest Liver Physiol 2008;294:G217–G225.
43 Tursi A, Giorgetti GM, Brandimarte G, et al: Prevalence and clinical presentation of subclinical/silent celiac disease in adults: an analysis on a 12-year observation. Hepatogastroenterology 2001;39:462–464.
44 Besterman HS, Bloon SR, Sarson DL, et al: Gut-hormone profile in coeliac disease. Lancet 1978;1:785–788.
45 Ottaway CA: Neuroimmunomodulation in the intestinal mucosa. Gastroenterol Clin North Am 1991;20:511–529.
46 Hernanz A, Polanco I, Codocco R, et al: Gastrointestinal peptide profile in children with celiac disease. J Pediatr Gastroenterol Nutr 1987;6:341–345.
47 Fraquelli M, Bardella MT, Peracchi M, et al: Gallbladder emptying and somatostatin and cholecystokinin plasma levels in celiac disease. Am J Gastroenterol 1999;94:1866–1870.
48 Lanzini A, Lanzarotto F: Review article: the 'mechanical pumps' and the enterohepatic circulation of bile acids – defects in coeliac disease. Aliment Pharmacol Ther 2000;14: 58–61.
49 Husebye E: Gastrointestinal motility disorders and bacterial overgrowth. J Intern Med 1995;237:419–427.

Dig Dis 2015;33:208–214
DOI: 10.1159/000369517

Microscopic Colitis

Gerd Bouma[a] Andreas Münch[b]

[a]Department of Gastroenterology and Hepatology, Vrije Universiteit Medical Center, Amsterdam, The Netherlands;
[b]Division of Gastroenterology and Hepatology, Department of Clinical and Experimental Medicine, Faculty of Health Science, Linköpings University, Linköping, Sweden

Key Words
Microscopic colitis · Collagenous colitis · Lymphocytic colitis · Collagen band · Intraepithelial lymphocytes · Budesonide

Abstract
Microscopic colitis (MC) is the common denominator for lymphocytic and collagenous colitis (CC). It is now recognized as a relatively frequent cause of diarrhea that equals the prevalence of inflammatory bowel disease. Patients are typically middle-aged women, but disease may occur at every age. Patients with MC report watery, non-bloody diarrhea in the absence of endoscopic and radiologic abnormalities. Lymphocytic colitis is characterized by an increased number of intraepithelial lymphocytes, and CC by a thickened subepithelial collagen band, whereas in both an increased mononuclear infiltration of the lamina propria is found. The pathogenesis of MC is largely unknown, but may relate to autoimmunity, adverse reactions to drugs or (bacterial) toxins, and abnormal collagen metabolism in the case of CC. Budesonide is so far the only drug that has proven efficacy in randomized controlled trials both for the induction and maintenance of remission. Patients who are nonresponsive, dependent or who experience side effects on budesonide may benefit from thiopurine or anti-TNF treatment, but these options are still experimental. The long-term prognosis of MC is good; it does not appear to predispose to malignancies and can in some cases be self-limiting. Further research and randomized clinical trials are required to expand our understanding of the natural course and the pathogenesis of MC.

Introduction

In 1976, Lindström [1] described a patient with chronic watery diarrhea who had a thick, subepithelial collagen deposition in biopsy samples of endoscopically normal colonic mucosa. This disease is since then known as collagenous colitis (CC). The term lymphocytic colitis (LC) was proposed in 1989 to describe patients with pronounced lymphocytic inflammation in the absence of a thickened collagen band on histological evaluation [2]. Together, they are referred to as microscopic colitis (MC) which is now recognized as a relatively frequent cause of diarrhea, especially in elderly women. More recently, a new term has been proposed called incomplete MC to describe those patients who have similar clinical manifestations but who do not fulfil the exact histological criteria [3, 4].

KARGER 125

© 2015 S. Karger AG, Basel
0257–2753/15/0332–0208$39.50/0

E-Mail karger@karger.com
www.karger.com/ddi

Dr. Gerd Bouma, MD, PhD
Department of Gastroenterology
Vrije Universiteit Medical Center
PO Box 7057, NL–1007 MB Amsterdam (The Netherlands)
E-Mail g.bouma@vumc.nl

Epidemiology

In the past, MC was considered a rare disorder. More recently, it has become apparent that MC is a common cause of diarrhea, especially in middle-aged or elderly patients. A recent population-based study from the USA found that the incidence of MC was 21.0 cases per 100,000 person-years [5]. The incidence of LC was 12.0 per 100,000 person-years and CC 9.1 per 100,000 person-years. The prevalence in this study was 219 cases per 100,000 persons (90.4 per 100,000 persons for CC and 128.6 per 100,000 persons for LC). These findings demonstrate that MC is not a rare disorder at all, and in fact that the prevalence approaches that of the classical inflammatory bowel diseases (IBD) ulcerative colitis and Crohn's disease. It has been suggested that the incidence of MC has been rising over the last decades. Indeed, in the above-mentioned population-based study from Olmsted County, Minn., USA, the annual incidence for CC and LC increased between 1985 and 2001 from 0.3 and 0.5 to 7.1 and 12.6, respectively [6], but stabilized over the period 2002–2010 [5].

CC is a disease predominantly affecting elderly women, with a female-to-male ratio of around 7:1 [7]. The peak incidence is around 65 years, but the age at onset can range between 10 and 90 years [4, 6, 7]. The peak onset for LC is comparable to that of CC, with similar age ranges, but here the female preponderance is less pronounced according to some studies [6–9].

Etiology and Pathogenesis

The etiology of MC is unknown, and studies to unravel disease pathogenesis are still in their infancy. Similar to IBD, the current concept is that disease occurs as the consequence of a disturbed immune response to an unknown agent in a predisposed host with a disturbed mucosal barrier function. Factors suggested to be implicated in disease pathogenesis include a genetic susceptibility, exogenous or luminal factors, infections and disturbed bile acid absorption. Whether or not LC and CC are manifestations of the same disease in different stages of development is an unanswered question. The combination of increased numbers of intraepithelial lymphocytes and a thickened collagenous band is frequently observed within one patient. In addition, co-occurrence of LC and CC within one family has been described, as well as conversion from LC to CC [10–12].

Genetic Factors and Concomitant Autoimmune Diseases

A genetic susceptibility is suggested by the fact that familial cases have been described occasionally and, more importantly, the observation that co-occurrence of autoimmune diseases is frequently found in these patients [10–12]. In particular, there is a strong association between celiac disease and MC. Thus, co-occurrence of MC and celiac disease is approximately 50-fold higher than seen in the general population [13]. Prevalence of CD in patients with MC varies between 5 and >20%, although several of these studies are hampered by small data sets and potential bias [14–16]. Vice versa, the prevalence of MC in patients with CD is around 4% [17].

Co-occurrence of various other autoimmune diseases has been reported, including thyroid diseases in up to 20% of patients, diabetes in 10% and rheumatoid arthritis in 2.5% [14, 18–21]. Concomitant autoimmune disorders may be more common in CC patients than in LC patients [22].

A few studies have investigated the association between disease susceptibility and potential risk genes, in particular the genes of the human leukocyte antigen [23, 24]. The outcomes of these association studies need to be interpreted with great caution because of lack of sufficient sample size. So far, no hypothesis-free genome-wide studies have been performed.

Luminal Agents

It has been suggested that a luminal agent or an immunological reaction against an endogenous antigen might trigger MC. Indeed, diversion of the fecal stream can reduce or even normalize the histopathological changes in CC [25].

The possibility of an infectious etiology for MC is supported by the finding of a history suggesting an acute gastrointestinal infection in many patients with MC. Also the resolution of CC after antibiotic treatment for *Helicobacter pylori* and the observed improvement after treatment with bismuth may support this possibility [26, 27]. However, systematic microbiological studies in MC have so far not provided a clear explanation. *Yersinia enterocolitica* and *Clostridium difficile* have been suggested, but studies involved small numbers of patients and have not been uniform [28].

Drugs

The development of MC has been suggested to be an adverse drug effect. Best known are NSAID- and lansoprazole-associated MC [29–32]. Withdrawal of these drugs may resolve the clinical and histological abnormalities, and recurrence has been reported after rechallenge [33–35]. Similar observations have been reported for other proton pump inhibitors (PPIs), and a large number of other drugs including, among others, statins and selective serotonin reuptake inhibitors (SSRIs) have also been implicated as possible causes of MC [33, 36–43]. It should be noted that a direct cause-effect relationship has not been established for any of these drugs. Additionally, these drugs are commonly prescribed in the general population, especially in older patients, and reported associations are therefore prone to bias. Indeed, a recent large nationwide case-control study identified significant positive associations between a recorded diagnosis of MC and exposure to 4 classes of drugs (PPIs, NSAIDs, statins and SSRIs). Notably, the use of these drugs was also associated with an increased likelihood to undergo an endoscopy presumably because these drugs can cause diarrhea leading to subsequent endoscopic investigations. Adjustment for more frequent endoscopic examinations in this category of patients attenuated all of the associations, and only the association between PPIs and CC and the association between LC and SSRIs remained significant [44].

Smoking

Smoking is increasingly recognized as a risk factor for CC. Thus, in a study by Vigren et al. [45], it was found that 37% of CC patients smoked compared to 17% in the control group, whereas in the age group 16–54 years, this was as high as 50% compared to 18% in the control group. Furthermore, in this study active smokers were diagnosed with CC 10 years earlier compared to nonsmokers, results that were corroborated by Fernandez-Banares et al. [46]. Similarly, current and past cigarette smoking significantly increases the risk for LC [47].

Bile Acid Malabsorption

It has been suggested that bile acid malabsorption may be responsible for the diarrhea in CC. Indeed, one study found that increased bile acid malabsorption, as measured with ^{75}SeHCAT, was found in 44% of patients. Bile acid binding treatment was followed by a rapid, marked, or complete improvement in 78% of patients, and was not restricted to those with established bile acid malabsorption [48]. Whilst bile acid binding treatment can be clinically effective, it does not appear to change the histopathological abnormalities found in CC.

Clinical Presentation

Patients with MC present with watery, non-bloody diarrhea. Other symptoms include nocturnal diarrhea, fecal urgency and incontinence, abdominal pain, and may include weight loss. The symptoms associated with MC may closely resemble those found in diarrhea-predominated irritable bowel syndrome (IBS). Indeed, a high proportion of patients fulfil the criteria for IBS, and a substantial number is being treated as IBS before the diagnosis of MC is established. So far, no extraintestinal manifestations of the disease have been reported.

Differential Diagnosis

Gastrointestinal diseases with a similar presentation include celiac disease, which may occur concomitantly, as described above. IBD should also be considered; this can usually be excluded by characteristic endoscopic and histopathological features. The onset of MC can be sudden and mimic infectious diarrhea. Also malabsorption can be a cause of diarrhea; the clinical presentation as well as fecal analyses and cultures are useful to differentiate the latter diseases from MC. Amyloidosis can present with diarrhea, and can be differentiated from CC by Congo red staining and the absence of an inflammatory infiltrate. Collagenosis (e.g. scleroderma) presents with fibrosis of the lamina propria that extends around crypts. Tangential sectioning of the biopsy specimen can mimic a thickened collagen band, and finally a slightly increased subepithelial collagen band can be found in hyperplastic polyps.

Diagnostic Methods

The diagnosis of MC is based on classical symptoms of chronic watery diarrhea without blood, in combination with the absence of abnormalities in blood test results, microbiology, radiology and endoscopic findings, although subtle endoscopic changes, including mucosal edema, erythema or mucosal paleness may occur. Additionally, there are reports of hemorrhagic mucosal laceration and even perforation after endoscopic insufflation in CC patients, particularly in the right hemicolon [49, 50]. Biopsies obtained during endoscopy remain the cornerstone of the diagnosis of MC. The primary histological feature of MC is an intraepithelial lymphocytosis, with more than 20 lymphocytes per 100 epithelial cells, whereas healthy subjects typically have fewer than 5 lymphocytes per 100 epithelial cells. Lymphocytic infiltration of the lamina propria is more pronounced in LC but is also present in CC and is dominated by lymphocytes and plasma cells [9]. Eosinophils and mast cells can be found, but neutrophils are very rarely observed. Similar to the normal intestinal mucosa, the intraepithelial lymphocytes found in MC are predominantly CD8+ T lymphocytes [51].

A diffuse thickening of the collagen layer beneath the basement membrane in a patchy manner throughout the colon is the hallmark of CC, and is absent in LC [9]. A thickened collagen layer has also been demonstrated, although infrequently, in stomach, duodenum, terminal ileum and ileo-anal pouches [52–54]. The thickness of the subepithelial layer in normal individuals varies from 0 to 3 μm. A thickness of 10 μm or more has been accepted to establish the diagnosis of CC. There are conflicting data about the topographical distribution of the thickened collagen band leading to some uncertainty about where and how many colonic biopsies should be taken to establish the diagnosis. Based on the data from 2 prospective multicenter trials, it seems advisable to perform a complete colonoscopy as the thickened subepithelial collagenous band is mainly found in the right colon [55, 56]. Left-sided colonic biopsies alone will miss the characteristic finding of a thickened subepithelial band in 20–40% of patients [57].

Laboratory findings in patients with MC are generally uneventful. Microbiological stool analyses usually remain negative. Fecal calprotectin (FCP) is a cytosolic protein with antibacterial, antiproliferative and immunomodulating effects that is now frequently used as a biomarker for monitoring disease activity in IBD. In MC, the FCP level is generally mildly elevated in patients with active disease, with a median of 80 μg/g according to one study, and decreases to normal when disease is in remission [58]. However, robust data on FCP in MC are lacking, and therefore it can currently not be recommended for disease monitoring. Steatorrhea and increased excretion of fecal leukocytes are reported in more than 50% of patients [4].

Treatment

In the absence of a true concept of disease pathogenesis, current treatment aims include resolution of symptoms, improvement of quality of life, and prevention of symptom relapse. Whether or not improvement of histology should be a treatment goal is uncertain; so far, there are no indications that long-standing MC is associated with an increased colorectal cancer risk or otherwise unfavorable outcome.

It has been suggested that the first step in the treatment of MC is to ban NSAIDs and other colitis-inducing medication, but the effectiveness of this approach has not been systematically evaluated. Furthermore, more and more data suggest that smoking cessation should be recommended.

Several drugs have been implicated in the treatment of MC, yet most reports rely on small retrospective case series. More recently, several randomized trials have demonstrated the efficacy of budesonide in the induction of remission in CC. Budesonide 9 mg was significantly more effective in the induction of remission than placebo-treated patients [59–61]. Similar findings apply to patients with LC [62].

The majority of patients will relapse once therapy is stopped. In a randomized controlled trial with 6 mg budesonide maintenance treatment for 6 months, only 24% of CC patients were in clinical remission at follow-up 24 weeks after stopping medication. The median time to relapse was 40 days [63]. Relapse also occurs after drug withdrawal in patients with LC, but rates appeared to be somewhat lower in this group of patients (44% within 14 months) [62].

In patients with chronic active disease, long-term treatment with budesonide can be justified, and the aim should be to taper to the lowest dose achieving clinical remission in the individual patient. Two RCTs have shown that budesonide 6 mg is effective in maintaining clinical response and is well tolerated with continuation of response after 6 months of treatment in 75% of patients, compared to 25% in the placebo group [55, 63].

Prednisolone has also been evaluated for the treatment of MC. In a historical cohort study, patients treated with budesonide had a higher rate of complete response than those treated with prednisone (82.5 vs. 52.9%). Additionally, patients treated with budesonide were less likely to recur after drug withdrawal than those treated with prednisone. Taking into account that corticosteroid therapy is also more likely to induce significant side effects, the use of prednisone is not recommended as primary therapy in MC [64].

So far, there has been only one randomized controlled trial that has evaluated the effectiveness of mesalazine in CC. In this trial, mesalazine 3 g/day was compared with budesonide 9 mg/day versus placebo for 8 weeks. It was concluded that budesonide was superior to mesalazine, with remission rates in patients treated with mesalazine not exceeding those in the placebo group [56]. These findings contrast a prospective single-center study in which mesalamine 2.4 g was compared with mesalamine plus cholestyramine 4 g. After 6 months, a remission rate, confirmed by histology, of 73% in the mesalazine group was found. Addition of cholestyramine improved the remission rate to 100%. Similarly, an 85% remission rate was reported for LC, and here, no differences were detected with the addition of cholestyramine [65]. Unfortunately, no placebo group was included in this unblinded trial. In a retrospective analysis of 25 patients with MC, 85% showed improvement with an average mesalazine dose of 1,500 mg during a 6-week period [66].

Bismuth subsalicylate possesses antidiarrheal, antibacterial, and anti-inflammatory properties. This drug has only been studied in a small open-label study including 14 patients. Treatment was associated with improvement in symptoms in the large majority of patients and resolution of colitis in 70% [26]. Although based on these limited data, the use of bismuth appears to be effective and well tolerated, its use in Western Europe is limited because it is not regularly available.

Azathioprine (AZA) and 6-mercaptopurine (MP) can be considered in steroid-dependent and steroid-refractory patients. In 2 small open-label studies including a total of 15 patients, AZA or MP were clinically effective in the large majority of patients, though 3 patients were intolerant to therapy [67, 68]. In a more recent retrospective case series involving 46 patients treated with of AZA or MP, the majority (67%) of chronic, active MC patients were intolerant to AZA leading to cessation of treatment. Some of these patients were successfully switched to MP, resulting in an overall response rate of 41% [69]. Preliminary data from our hospital indicate that MP or 6-thioguanine was well tolerated. In a series of 19 patients, only 3 (16%) were intolerant to these drugs, and treatment resulted in clinical and histological improvement in the majority of patients [Bouma, unpubl. results].

A retrospective case series involving 19 patients identified 16 patients with CC who responded to 2–3 weeks of oral treatment with methotrexate (MTX) 5–25 mg/week [70]. On the other hand, an open case series of 9 patients with CC intolerant or refractory to budesonide failed to identify an effect after 12 weeks of subcutaneous MTX treatment, limiting the enthusiasm for this drug [71].

Treatment with TNF-α blockers has only been anecdotic, but long-term remission following treatment with adalimumab or infliximab has been described [72].

Finally, probiotic therapy with *Lactobacillus* and *Bifidobacterium* species did not induce histological improvement in a placebo-controlled trial [73].

The indication for surgical intervention is currently limited given the improved pharmacological treatment options. However, in a small minority of patients diarrhea can persist despite extensive medical treatment. In 9 patients with severe diarrhea due to CC, a diverting ileostomy decreased symptoms and reduced the thickness of the collagen band to normal ranges. However, recurrence of disease occurred after restoration of intestinal continuity [25].

In daily practice, the treatment of histologically confirmed MC starts with eliminating drugs suspected to induce diarrhea. Budesonide is recommended as first treatment option for inducing and maintaining clinical remission since the evidence in well-designed trials showed clear benefit with a favorable safety profile. Other treatment options are poorly investigated, but antidiarrheals (loperamide) and cholestyramine can be considered in patients with mild symptoms. In unresponsive or intolerant patients, thiopurines may be effective as maintenance therapy, and MP or 6-thioguanine may be better tolerated than AZA. However, in patients with severely deteriorated quality of life due to budesonide nonresponse, clinical remission might be achieved faster with anti-TNF agents.

Complications and Their Management

While the symptoms of MC can be debilitating, the disease generally has a benign course. It should be kept in mind that recurrence rates are high after drug withdrawal, and these patients require long-term maintenance therapy with the lowest possible dose of budesonide or thiopurines. No increased risk for colorectal cancer has been reported so far, eliminating the need for endoscopic surveillance.

Disclosure Statement

The authors declare that no financial or other conflict of interest exists in relation to the content of the article.

References

1 Lindström CG: 'Collagenous colitis' with watery diarrhoea – a new entity? Pathol Eur 1976;11:87–89.
2 Lazenby AJ, Yardley JH, Giardiello FM, Jessurun J, Bayless TM: Lymphocytic ('microscopic') colitis: a comparative histopathologic study with particular reference to collagenous colitis. Hum Pathol 1989;20:18–28.
3 Carmack SW, Lash RH, Gulizia JM, Genta RM: Lymphocytic disorders of the gastrointestinal tract: a review for the practicing pathologist. Adv Anat Pathol 2009;16:290–306.
4 Munch A, Langner C: Microscopic colitis: clinical and pathologic perspectives. Clin Gastroenterol Hepatol 2014, Epub ahead of print.
5 Gentile NM, Khanna S, Loftus EV Jr, Smyrk TC, Tremaine WJ, Harmsen WS, et al: The epidemiology of microscopic colitis in Olmsted County from 2002 to 2010: a population-based study. Clin Gastroenterol Hepatol 2014;12:838–842.
6 Pardi DS, Loftus EV Jr, Smyrk TC, Kammer PP, Tremaine WJ, Schleck CD, et al: The epidemiology of microscopic colitis: a population based study in Olmsted County, Minnesota. Gut 2007;56:504–508.
7 Wickbom A, Bohr J, Eriksson S, Udumyan R, Nyhlin N, Tysk C: Stable incidence of collagenous colitis and lymphocytic colitis in Orebro, Sweden, 1999–2008: a continuous epidemiologic study. Inflamm Bowel Dis 2013;19: 2387–2393.
8 Pardi DS, Ramnath VR, Loftus EV Jr, Tremaine WJ, Sandborn WJ: Lymphocytic colitis: clinical features, treatment, and outcomes. Am J Gastroenterol 2002;97:2829–2833.
9 Munch A, Aust D, Bohr J, Bonderup O, Fernandez BF, Hjortswang H, et al: Microscopic colitis: current status, present and future challenges: statements of the European Microscopic Colitis Group. J Crohns Colitis 2012;6: 932–945.
10 Jarnerot G, Hertervig E, Granno C, Thorhallsson E, Eriksson S, Tysk C, et al: Familial occurrence of microscopic colitis: a report on five families. Scand J Gastroenterol 2001;36: 959–962.
11 Abdo AA, Zetler PJ, Halparin LS: Familial microscopic colitis. Can J Gastroenterol 2001; 15:341–343.
12 van Tilburg AJ, Lam HG, Seldenrijk CA, Stel HV, Blok P, Dekker W, et al: Familial occurrence of collagenous colitis. A report of two families. J Clin Gastroenterol 1990;12:279–285.
13 Stewart M, Andrews CN, Urbanski S, Beck PL, Storr M: The association of coeliac disease and microscopic colitis: a large population-based study. Aliment Pharmacol Ther 2011; 33:1340–1349.
14 Vigren L, Tysk C, Strom M, Kilander AF, Hjortswang H, Bohr J, et al: Celiac disease and other autoimmune diseases in patients with collagenous colitis. Scand J Gastroenterol 2013;48:944–950.
15 Matteoni CA, Goldblum JR, Wang N, Brzezinski A, Achkar E, Soffer EE: Celiac disease is highly prevalent in lymphocytic colitis. J Clin Gastroenterol 2001;32:225–227.
16 Thorn M, Sjoberg D, Ekbom A, Holmstrom T, Larsson M, Nielsen AL, et al: Microscopic colitis in Uppsala health region, a population-based prospective study 2005–2009. Scand J Gastroenterol 2013;48:825–830.
17 Green PH, Yang J, Cheng J, Lee AR, Harper JW, Bhagat G: An association between microscopic colitis and celiac disease. Clin Gastroenterol Hepatol 2009;7:1210–1216.
18 Cindoruk M, Tuncer C, Dursun A, Yetkin I, Karakan T, Cakir N, et al: Increased colonic intraepithelial lymphocytes in patients with Hashimoto's thyroiditis. J Clin Gastroenterol 2002;34:237–239.
19 Bohr J, Tysk C, Eriksson S, Abrahamsson H, Jarnerot G: Collagenous colitis: a retrospective study of clinical presentation and treatment in 163 patients. Gut 1996;39:846–851.
20 Olesen M, Eriksson S, Bohr J, Jarnerot G, Tysk C: Lymphocytic colitis: a retrospective clinical study of 199 Swedish patients. Gut 2004;53: 536–541.
21 Holstein A, Burmeister J, Plaschke A, Rosemeier D, Widjaja A, Egberts EH: Autoantibody profiles in microscopic colitis. J Gastroenterol Hepatol 2006;21:1016–1020.
22 Madisch A, Miehlke S, Bartosch F, Bethke B, Stolte M: Microscopic colitis: clinical presentation, treatment and outcome of 494 patients. Z Gastroenterol 2014;52:1062–1065.
23 Fine KD, Do K, Schulte K, Ogunji F, Guerra R, Osowski L, et al: High prevalence of celiac sprue-like HLA-DQ genes and enteropathy in patients with the microscopic colitis syndrome. Am J Gastroenterol 2000;95:1974–1982.
24 Koskela RM, Karttunen TJ, Niemela SE, Lehtola JK, Ilonen J, Karttunen RA: Human leucocyte antigen and TNFalpha polymorphism association in microscopic colitis. Eur J Gastroenterol Hepatol 2008;20:276–282.
25 Jarnerot G, Bohr J, Tysk C, Eriksson S: Faecal stream diversion in patients with collagenous colitis. Gut 1996;38:154–155.
26 Fine KD, Lee EL: Efficacy of open-label bismuth subsalicylate for the treatment of microscopic colitis. Gastroenterology 1998;114: 29–36.
27 Narayani RI, Burton MP, Young GS: Resolution of collagenous colitis after treatment for *Helicobacter pylori*. Am J Gastroenterol 2002; 97:498–499.
28 Erim T, Alazmi WM, O'Loughlin CJ, Barkin JS: Collagenous colitis associated with *Clostridium difficile*: a cause effect? Dig Dis Sci 2003;48:1374–1375.
29 Castellano VM, Munoz MT, Colina F, Nevado M, Casis B, Solis-Herruzo JA: Collagenous gastrobulbitis and collagenous colitis. Case report and review of the literature. Scand J Gastroenterol 1999;34:632–638.
30 Yagi K, Nakamura A, Sekine A, Watanabe H: Nonsteroidal anti-inflammatory drug-associated colitis with a histology of collagenous colitis. Endoscopy 2001;33:629–632.
31 Hilmer SN, Heap TR, Eckstein RP, Lauer CS, Shenfield GM: Microscopic colitis associated with exposure to lansoprazole. Med J Aust 2006;184:185–186.
32 Chande N, Driman DK: Microscopic colitis associated with lansoprazole: report of two cases and a review of the literature. Scand J Gastroenterol 2007;42:530–533.
33 Thomson RD, Lestina LS, Bensen SP, Toor A, Maheshwari Y, Ratcliffe NR: Lansoprazole-associated microscopic colitis: a case series. Am J Gastroenterol 2002;97:2908–2913.
34 Al-Ghamdi MY, Malatjalian DA, Veldhuyzen van ZS: Causation: recurrent collagenous colitis following repeated use of NSAIDs. Can J Gastroenterol 2002;16:861–862.
35 Freston JW: Long-term acid control and proton pump inhibitors: interactions and safety issues in perspective. Am J Gastroenterol 1997;92(suppl):51S–55S.
36 Wilcox GM, Mattia A: Collagenous colitis associated with lansoprazole. J Clin Gastroenterol 2002;34:164–166.
37 Wilcox GM, Mattia AR: Microscopic colitis associated with omeprazole and esomeprazole exposure. J Clin Gastroenterol 2009;43: 551–553.
38 Berrebi D, Sautet A, Flejou JF, Dauge MC, Peuchmaur M, Potet F: Ticlopidine induced colitis: a histopathological study including apoptosis. J Clin Pathol 1998;51:280–283.
39 Duncan HD, Talbot IC, Silk DB: Collagenous colitis and cimetidine. Eur J Gastroenterol Hepatol 1997;9:819–820.
40 Beaugerie L, Patey N, Brousse N: Ranitidine, diarrhoea, and lymphocytic colitis. Gut 1995; 37:708–711.
41 Mahajan L, Wyllie R, Goldblum J: Lymphocytic colitis in a pediatric patient: a possible adverse reaction to carbamazepine. Am J Gastroenterol 1997;92:2126–2127.
42 Chagnon JP, Cerf M: Simvastatin-induced protein-losing enteropathy. Am J Gastroenterol 1992;87:257.
43 Chauveau E, Prignet JM, Carloz E, Duval JL, Gilles B: Lymphocytic colitis likely attributable to use of vinburnine (Cervoxan) (in French). Gastroenterol Clin Biol 1998;22:362.
44 Bonderup OK, Fenger-Gron M, Wigh T, Pedersen L, Nielsen GL: Drug exposure and risk of microscopic colitis: a nationwide Danish case-control study with 5,751 cases. Inflamm Bowel Dis 2014;20:1702–1707.

45 Vigren L, Sjoberg K, Benoni C, Tysk C, Bohr J, Kilander A, et al: Is smoking a risk factor for collagenous colitis? Scand J Gastroenterol 2011;46:1334–1339.

46 Fernandez-Banares F, de Sousa MR, Salas A, Beltran B, Piqueras M, Iglesias E, et al: Impact of current smoking on the clinical course of microscopic colitis. Inflamm Bowel Dis 2013; 19:1470–1476.

47 Yen EF, Pokhrel B, Du H, Nwe S, Bianchi L, Witt B, et al: Current and past cigarette smoking significantly increase risk for microscopic colitis. Inflamm Bowel Dis 2012;18:1835–1841.

48 Ung KA, Gillberg R, Kilander A, Abrahamsson H: Role of bile acids and bile acid binding agents in patients with collagenous colitis. Gut 2000;46:170–175.

49 Cruz-Correa M, Milligan F, Giardiello FM, Bayless TM, Torbenson M, Yardley JH, et al: Collagenous colitis with mucosal tears on endoscopic insufflation: a unique presentation. Gut 2002;51:600.

50 Allende DS, Taylor SL, Bronner MP: Colonic perforation as a complication of collagenous colitis in a series of 12 patients. Am J Gastroenterol 2008;103:2598–2604.

51 Goranzon C, Kumawat AK, Hultgren-Hornqvist E, Tysk C, Eriksson S, Bohr J, et al: Immunohistochemical characterization of lymphocytes in microscopic colitis. J Crohns Colitis 2013;7:e434–e442.

52 Lagorce-Pages C, Fabiani B, Bouvier R, Scoazec JY, Durand L, Flejou JF: Collagenous gastritis: a report of six cases. Am J Surg Pathol 2001;25:1174–1179.

53 Navarro-Llavat M, Domenech E, Masnou H, Ojanguren I, Manosa M, Lorenzo-Zuniga V, et al: Collagenous duodeno-ileo-colitis with transient IgG deficiency preceded by *Yersinia enterocolitica* intestinal infection: case report and review of literature. Gastroenterol Hepatol 2007;30:219–221.

54 Shen B, Bennett AE, Fazio VW, Sherman KK, Sun J, Remzi FH, et al: Collagenous pouchitis. Dig Liver Dis 2006;38:704–709.

55 Miehlke S, Madisch A, Bethke B, Morgner A, Kuhlisch E, Henker C, et al: Oral budesonide for maintenance treatment of collagenous colitis: a randomized, double-blind, placebo-controlled trial. Gastroenterology 2008;135: 1510–1516.

56 Miehlke S, Madisch A, Kupcinskas L, Petrauskas D, Bohm G, Marks HJ, et al: Budesonide is more effective than mesalamine or placebo in short-term treatment of collagenous colitis. Gastroenterology 2014;146:1222–1230.

57 Tanaka M, Mazzoleni G, Riddell RH: Distribution of collagenous colitis: utility of flexible sigmoidoscopy. Gut 1992;33:65–70.

58 Wildt S, Nordgaard-Lassen I, Bendtsen F, Rumessen JJ: Metabolic and inflammatory faecal markers in collagenous colitis. Eur J Gastroenterol Hepatol 2007;19:567–574.

59 Baert F, Schmit A, D'Haens G, Dedeurwaerdere F, Louis E, Cabooter M, et al: Budesonide in collagenous colitis: a double-blind placebo-controlled trial with histologic follow-up. Gastroenterology 2002;122:20–25.

60 Miehlke S, Heymer P, Bethke B, Bastlein E, Meier E, Bartram HP, et al: Budesonide treatment for collagenous colitis: a randomized, double-blind, placebo-controlled, multicenter trial. Gastroenterology 2002;123:978–984.

61 Bonderup OK, Hansen JB, Birket-Smith L, Vestergaard V, Teglbjaerg PS, Fallingborg J: Budesonide treatment of collagenous colitis: a randomised, double blind, placebo controlled trial with morphometric analysis. Gut 2003;52:248–251.

62 Miehlke S, Madisch A, Karimi D, Wonschik S, Kuhlisch E, Beckmann R, et al: Budesonide is effective in treating lymphocytic colitis: a randomized double-blind placebo-controlled study. Gastroenterology 2009;136:2092–2100.

63 Bonderup OK, Hansen JB, Teglbjaerg PS, Christensen LA, Fallingborg JF: Long-term budesonide treatment of collagenous colitis: a randomised, double-blind, placebo-controlled trial. Gut 2009;58:68–72.

64 Gentile NM, Abdalla AA, Khanna S, Smyrk TC, Tremaine WJ, Faubion WA, et al: Outcomes of patients with microscopic colitis treated with corticosteroids: a population-based study. Am J Gastroenterol 2013;108: 256–259.

65 Calabrese C, Fabbri A, Areni A, Zahlane D, Scialpi C, Di FG: Mesalazine with or without cholestyramine in the treatment of microscopic colitis: randomized controlled trial. J Gastroenterol Hepatol 2007;22:809–814.

66 Bonner GF, Petras RE, Cheong DM, Grewal ID, Breno S, Ruderman WB: Short- and long-term follow-up of treatment for lymphocytic and collagenous colitis. Inflamm Bowel Dis 2000;6:85–91.

67 Pardi DS, Loftus EV Jr, Tremaine WJ, Sandborn WJ: Treatment of refractory microscopic colitis with azathioprine and 6-mercaptopurine. Gastroenterology 2001;120:1483–1484.

68 Vennamaneni SR, Bonner GF: Use of azathioprine or 6-mercaptopurine for treatment of steroid-dependent lymphocytic and collagenous colitis. Am J Gastroenterol 2001;96: 2798–2799.

69 Munch A, Fernandez-Banares F, Munck LK: Azathioprine and mercaptopurine in the management of patients with chronic, active microscopic colitis. Aliment Pharmacol Ther 2013;37:795–798.

70 Riddell J, Hillman L, Chiragakis L, Clarke A: Collagenous colitis: oral low-dose methotrexate for patients with difficult symptoms: long-term outcomes. J Gastroenterol Hepatol 2007; 22:1589–1593.

71 Munch A, Bohr J, Vigren L, Tysk C, Strom M: Lack of effect of methotrexate in budesonide-refractory collagenous colitis. Clin Exp Gastroenterol 2013;6:149–152.

72 Esteve M, Mahadevan U, Sainz E, Rodriguez E, Salas A, Fernandez-Banares F: Efficacy of anti-TNF therapies in refractory severe microscopic colitis. J Crohns Colitis 2011;5:612–618.

73 Wildt S, Munck LK, Vinter-Jensen L, Hanse BF, Nordgaard-Lassen I, Christensen S, et al: Probiotic treatment of collagenous colitis: a randomized, double-blind, placebo-controlled trial with *Lactobacillus acidophilus* and *Bifidobacterium animalis* subsp. *lactis*. Inflamm Bowel Dis 2006;12:395–401.

Dig Dis 2015;33:215–220
DOI: 10.1159/000370205

Drug-Induced Enteropathy

Eric V. Marietta[a–c] Amanda Cartee[c] Abdul Rishi[c] Joseph A. Murray[a, c]

Departments of [a]Immunology and [b]Dermatology, and [c]Division of Gastroenterology and Hepatology, Mayo Clinic College of Medicine, Rochester, Minn., USA

Key Words
Olmesartan · Enteropathy · Angiotensin · Diarrhea · Drug

Abstract
Background/Aims: Many medications can cause diarrhea by increasing motility, inflammation or enteropathy. Olmesartan and mycophenolic acid (CellCept) are drugs that are capable of increasing inflammation and enteropathy in some individuals and, if not recognized, can lead to chronic diarrhea. It is this type of drug-induced diarrhea that is the focus of this review. ***Methods:*** A summary of our findings (recent and earlier published) as well as a review of published works from other centers were conducted. ***Results:*** There is increasing evidence that olmesartan use is associated with enteropathy in a small number of individuals who use angiotensin receptor II blockers, and that this enteropathy is characterized by severe diarrhea capable of inducing severe dehydration and, in some instances, failure of organs such as the kidney. Typical patient demographics are Caucasian individuals who are older (>50 years old) and obese or overweight prior to weight loss. Prolonged exposure to olmesartan use for 1–2 years is typical, although case reports of irbesartan and valsartan have been reported as well. Discontinuing olmesartan leads to improvement of symptoms; however, the period for healing is variable, with some patients requiring steroid therapy and even prolonged parental nutrition support. In addition, many histological features of olmesartan-associated enteropathy are also present in celiac disease, including villi shortening and lymphocyte infiltration. Other drug-associated enteropathies have also been reported with mycophenolate mofetil used in transplantation. ***Conclusions:*** Of the drug-associated enteropathies discussed in this review, olmesartan can generate the most severe symptoms, albeit quite rare. Therefore, with patients who present with severe diarrhea and weight loss, one should consider olmesartan-associated enteropathy. In addition, many of the features associated with olmesartan-associated enteropathy are also found in celiac disease enteropathy; as such, one should review any celiac disease diagnosis for any use of olmesartan at the time of diagnosis.

Diarrhea Induced by Drugs

Diarrhea is a common consequence of many medications. It often has an acute onset shortly after starting the medication especially if the drug increases motility, such as erythromycin or other macrolides. The diarrhea may be chronic if the drug induces inflammation or enteropathy such as that recently described with olmesartan and mycophenolic acid (CellCept) and if the association goes unrecognized. It is this latter type of drug-associated enteropathic disease that is the primary focus of this review.

KARGER 125

© 2015 S. Karger AG, Basel
0257–2753/15/0332–0215$39.50/0

E-Mail karger@karger.com
www.karger.com/ddi

Joseph A. Murray
Division of Gastroenterology and Hepatology
Mayo Foundation
Rochester, MN 55905 (USA)
E-Mail murray.joseph@mayo.edu

Pathobiology of Drug-Induced Diarrhea

Because there are many different types of drugs that can induce diarrhea, there are many mechanistic pathways associated with drug-induced diarrhea. Many antibiotics that are commonly used can induce diarrhea and typically do so by decreasing the digestive function of the colonic microbiota. Antibiotics can also directly affect motility and secretion. In contrast, chemotherapeutic agents may damage the intestine, which would then lead to substantial diarrhea. Procholinergic drugs will accelerate gastrointestinal transit and may also enhance secretion. Secretagogues can induce diarrhea through neuropharmacologic effects, and metoclopramide and domperidone, both prokinetic agents, may also induce diarrhea [1].

Diagnosis

A careful review of the patient's medications at the time of onset of diarrhea is crucial to making a diagnosis of drug-induced diarrhea; once identified, the drug should be withdrawn during a trial period, and if symptoms improve, should be completely eliminated. However, if the diarrhea was not severe and the medication is important, then a cautious re-challenge should be contemplated. Much less obvious are chronic diarrheal illnesses associated with weight loss in which there was no clear temporal association with the institution of drug therapy. Certain drug-associated syndromes have enteropathy and villous atrophy and can be identified by small intestine biopsy; these include olmesartan-associated enteropathy (OAE) and villous atrophy associated with the use of mycophenolate mofetil (abbreviated MMF, trade name CellCept) [2, 3].

Olmesartan-Associated Enteropathy

The representative case below demonstrates the typical characteristics and evaluation of what proved to be OAE.

A 65-year-old Caucasian female with hypertension treated with olmesartan for the past 2 years presented to a tertiary medical center for further evaluation of abdominal pain, 20-pound weight loss, and diarrhea for 6 months. She had been overweight until then. She described 10–12 nonbloody and malodorous bowel movements daily and had been unable to identify any alleviating or aggravating factors. The extensive evaluation at that point included CBC, complete metabolic panel, TSH, tissue transglutaminase (tTG), urinary 5-HIAA, and abdominal CT, all of which were unrevealing.

The patient's symptoms continued, and she was unable to maintain adequate hydration in the setting of profuse diarrhea. She was hospitalized several times for acute kidney injury and hypotension. During each hospitalization, her antihypertensives were held due to hypotension, and her symptoms partially abated. The symptoms recurred upon each hospital dismissal when medications were restarted. During her last hospitalization, the need for total parenteral nutrition was discussed.

Given the persistent severe symptoms, both upper and lower endoscopies were performed. Diffuse duodenal villous atrophy was apparent endoscopically and confirmed by biopsy. Microscopic colitis was found on biopsies from the macroscopically normal colon. Despite the negative tTG antibodies, a strict gluten-free diet was prescribed for 1 month without any symptomatic response. Given the pathologic evidence of celiac disease in the setting of a negative tTG and the lack of a response to a gluten-free diet, HLA testing was obtained. She was HLA-DQ2$^+$. At this point, she was referred to a tertiary medical center for evaluation and treatment of presumed refractory celiac disease [2].

Based on the patient's history of improvement when olmesartan was withheld, olmesartan was suspended, and topically active budesonide taper administered. She noted significant clinical improvement within 2 weeks with minimal residual symptoms. An antihypertensive agent from a different class was initiated without any adverse effects. She underwent repeat duodenal biopsy after 6 months of a normal gluten-containing diet without any evidence of duodenal villous atrophy.

Historical Clues to Diagnosis of OAE

The above case highlights several of the key points in a patient's history that should prompt a provider to consider OAE as a diagnosis. Typical patient demographics for OAE were Caucasian, older age (i.e. >50 years old), and obesity or overweight prior to weight loss or despite weight loss [2]. All patients had hypertension treated with olmesartan. All patients had taken olmesartan for at least 1 year prior to onset of their symptoms, where reported [4]. In a large French cohort, duration of olmesartan use for 1–2 years had an adjusted rate ratio of development of OAE of 3.20 compared to other ACE inhibitors, and longer durations had successively larger rate ratios [5].

Clinical Features (table 1)

Patients with OAE presented with sudden onset, persistent, severe abdominal pain, nausea, vomiting, nonbloody diarrhea, and weight loss. Up to 20 bowel move-

Table 1. Clinical features of OAE

1	Gastrointestinal symptoms	Diarrhea, abdominal pain, vomiting
2	Enteropathy	Mostly villous atrophy, but also intraepithelial lymphocytosis and infiltration of lamina propria
3	Negative celiac serology	Negative tTG and negative EMA
4	No improvement with a gluten-free diet	At least 1-month administration for evaluation
5	Exclusion of other (non-celiac) enteropathies	Tropical sprue, autoimmune enteropathy
6	Improvement with withdrawal of olmesartan	Improved gastrointestinal symptoms and intestinal histology

OAE features are both clinical and histological and are listed in the left column. Specific examples of each feature are listed in the right column. EMA = Anti-endomysium antibody.

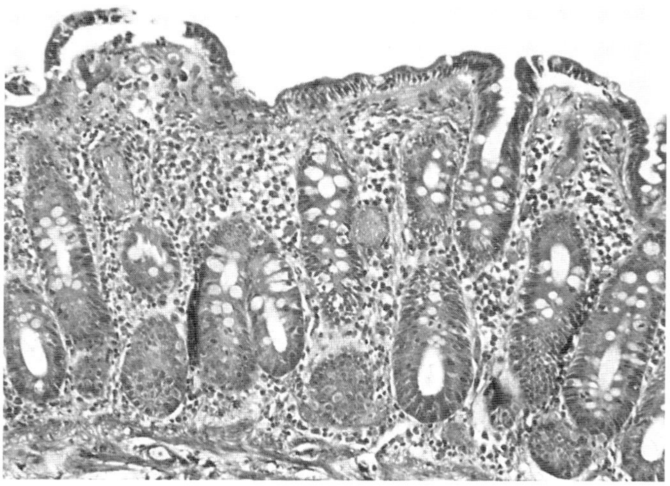

Color version available online

Fig. 1. Duodenal biopsy from a representative OAE patient while on olmesartan. Villous atrophy with variable degrees of mucosal inflammation is present in a biopsy from an OAE patient.

ments per day was not uncommon. Weight loss could be significant with one case of 59 kg reported [2]. The symptoms lasted for months despite many physician visits, tests, and various unsuccessful treatments.

With the severity and long duration of symptoms came significant morbidity. Common complications included dehydration and acute kidney injury as in the illustrated case. For others, malnutrition was obvious with extreme weight loss, and vitamin and mineral deficiencies prompted use of total parenteral nutrition. The nutritional deficiencies found in patients with OAE are further detailed in a recent review [4]. One case report describes bowel perforation thought to be secondary to OAE [6]. It is therefore not surprising that patients with OAE were admitted to the hospital, sometimes multiple times.

Diagnostic Evaluation of OAE

The diagnostic evaluations were exhaustive and extended well beyond the average workup for diarrhea. Besides elevated creatinine, hypokalemia, and evidence of micronutrient deficiencies, patients had normal laboratory findings, including tTG. Abdominal imaging was normal with one exception of bowel perforation [6]. Upper endoscopy with small bowel biopsies showed findings similar to that of celiac disease [2]. An unexpected percentage of patients seen by the senior author had gastritis and colitis, which emphasizes the importance of recognizing OAE as a disorder that affects multiple organs [2].

This then created a diagnostic dilemma: negative celiac disease screening test without other personal or family history of autoimmune conditions in the setting of a biopsy indicative of celiac disease (fig. 1). Furthermore, many had genetic predisposition for celiac disease by HLA testing but failed to improve with adequate time on a strict gluten-free diet, making the diagnosis even more unusual. Because of these findings, some patients were diagnosed with refractory sprue. Interestingly, a recent study on such a dilemma, seronegative celiac disease, found that many cases were secondary to medications, one of which was olmesartan [7].

With the unclear diagnostic evaluation, patients were often treated empirically with antidiarrheal medications, antibiotics, immunosuppressive agents, and pancreatic enzymes, without any benefit noted. The anecdotal improvement during hospitalization and recurrence of symptoms after dismissal coincided with suspension and reintroduction of olmesartan, and provided insight into the cause of the patients' symptoms. The Mini-Sentinel study on olmesartan and celiac disease by the FDA found 10 of 23 patients had a positive re-challenge.

Treatment

Removing olmesartan, the offending agent, has been the mainstay of treatment. A topically active budesonide taper has also been used, and most patients improve on this regimen (fig. 2) [2, 8]. A small number of patients do

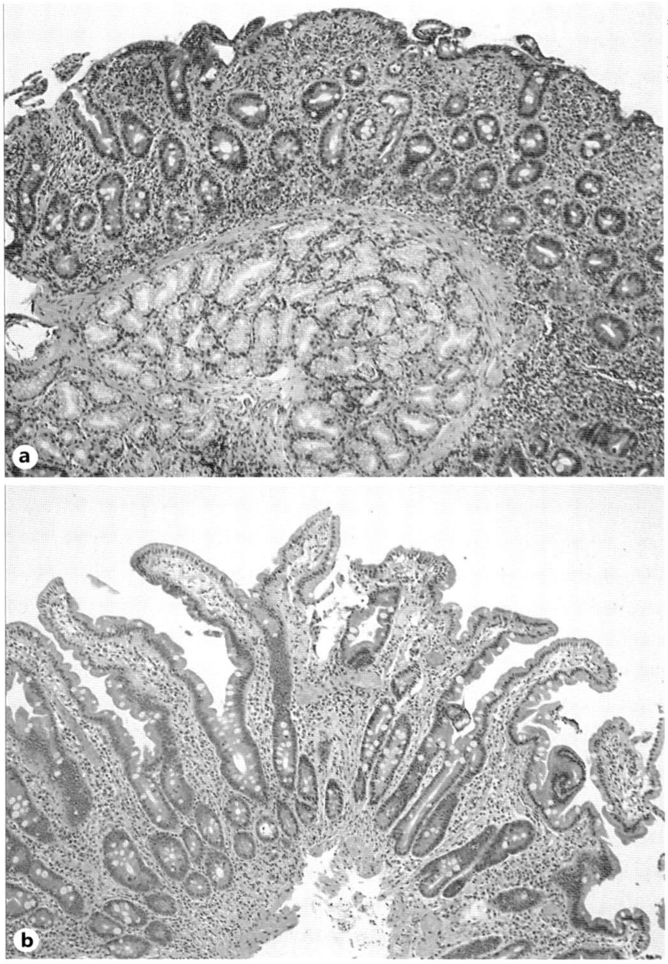

Color version available online

Fig. 2. Representative follow-up histology. **a** Flattened villi and mucosal inflammation are present in the biopsy taken whilst the OAE patient was on olmesartan. **b** Focal partial villous atrophy was observed in a follow-up duodenal biopsy obtained 54 days after suspension of olmesartan.

not improve on this regimen, and more studies are needed to determine which patients will not improve and why.

Several patients have required prolonged parenteral nutrition support due to the severity of their illness. Several patients may have received systemic steroids and even Imuran before the drug association was recognized.

Risk Factors for OAE

There is limited knowledge regarding OAE risk factors. The only identified risk factor for OAE known to date is duration of exposure. In patients seen at the Mayo Clinic, all patients had taken olmesartan for at least 1 year [4]. A recent study found a significant association between duration of exposure and risk of development of OAE [5]. Although this connection is newly recognized, it is unknown if duration of exposure itself is a risk factor or a confounding variable. In addition, duration of use was also found to be correlated with development of colitis. Finally, the percentage of patients who were HLA-$DQ2^+$ was clinically surprising. Genetic predisposition could have some role in development of OAE. Its role in development of OAE, if significant, may allow us to one day predict which patients should avoid olmesartan as an antihypertensive.

Drug-Specific or Class Effect

It is important to determine whether drugs that are similar to olmesartan in function also induce enteropathy and their relative risk. A number of case reports and a couple of previous studies demonstrated that olmesartan is associated with severe sprue and villous atrophy [9–12]. Only single case reports of enteropathy have been associated with irbesartan and valsartan [12, 13]. In a French national survey of gastroenterologists, 36 patients were identified with OAE. Only one patient was identified to have irbesartan-associated enteropathy [12]. All of these reports clearly demonstrate that administration of olmesartan to some individuals can lead to severe enteropathy. Other studies, such as the ROADMAP (Randomised Olmesartan and Diabetes Microalbuminuria Prevention) study indicated that the relative risk of developing OAE by individuals taking olmesartan is extremely low [14]. In this study, 2,232 individuals were administered olmesartan, and 2,215 individuals were administered a placebo for 3.2 years. There were 78 treatment-emergent adverse events in the olmesartan group and 94 in the placebo group. As no OAE patients were identified in the olmesartan-treated group of 2,232 individuals, the incidence must be less than 1/2,232 (less than 0.05% of olmesartan users). In another study, 10,370 individuals treated with olmesartan were followed for anywhere between 1 and 6 years. This study did not find an increased risk of GI-related hospitalization or all-cause mortality in the overall cohort as compared to the other angiotensin receptor blockers (ARBs) evaluated [15]. Both of these studies demonstrate an extremely low incidence of OAE in olmesartan-treated individuals.

Thus, there are case reports that continue to accrue demonstrating that a small number of individuals have severe adverse reactions to olmesartan and potentially irbesartan and valsartan. However, as previously noted, the number of such events for each of these drugs was found to be extremely low.

Chemical Structure of Olmesartan Medoxomil

Olmesartan medoxomil is a more recently developed ARB that differs from the previous versions of ARBs in a number of ways. One significant difference is that olmesartan is a nonpeptide ARB [16]. Two of the original versions, saralasin and sarmesin, were variants of the angiotensin II octapeptide (A-II), wherein specific amino acid residues of the A-II octapeptide were substituted [16]. Although both saralasin and sarmesin bound to the angiotensin type II receptor well and inhibited angiotensin type II from binding to the receptor, they were not efficacious as an orally administered drug due to the peptide structure and were required to be administered parenterally. To make a drug that was more suitable for oral administration, olmesartan was developed. Olmesartan was designed based on the specific forces that contribute to the binding of the A-II peptide to the receptor, but using a nonpeptide structure [17]. This structure was based on an imidazole-based core, wherein a hydroxyalkyl substituent and hydrolyzable ester group were added to the core [18]. A medoxomil unit was then added by esterification in order to make it into a prodrug that could be orally administered [19]. Esterases in the gastrointestinal mucosa would then release the active olmesartan metabolite [19].

As an active metabolite of the esterase activity, olmesartan is rapidly disseminated into the bloodstream. Peak plasma levels occur between 1 and 3 h after oral administration and the elimination half-life is 10–15 h [20]. Only 26% of olmesartan is adsorbed though, and the major route of excretion of olmesartan is in the feces with only 10–16% being excreted in the urine [20].

The second way in which olmesartan differs from previous ARBs is its selective, insurmountable inhibition of the AT1 receptor, which results in a long-lasting inhibition of the AT_1 receptor. The increased potency of olmesartan was demonstrated in studies using vasoconstriction of isolated aortas. As compared to valsartan, olmesartan is 4.2-fold more potent, and as compared to losartan, 203-fold more potent [16]. After absorption, the active olmesartan metabolite will not be further metabolized and as such may contribute to the increased potency [19].

Mycophenolate Mofetil

MMF is a commonly used drug after transplant to prevent rejection. It acts by inhibiting purine synthesis which is required for proliferation of cells. Out of the two pathways for purine synthesis, the de novo pathway depends on inosine monophosphate dehydrogenase (IMPDH), and the salvage pathway depends on hypoxanthine-guanine phosphoribosyltransferase. MMF inhibits IMPDH, thus affecting de novo synthesis of purines which is an absolute requirement for proliferation of lymphocytes. Moreover, purine synthesis in enterocytes occurs partially by the IMPDH pathway [21]. Consequently, intestinal epithelium is affected by the antiproliferative effects of MMF. Leucopenia and diarrhea are the major side effects observed in patients with renal transplant treated with MMF. The mechanism of diarrhea is unknown.

Recently, four case reports have been published showing development of villous atrophy in patients who were treated with MMF [22]. Standard stool culture, parasitological examination, and clostridium difficile investigation were negative. In each case, villous atrophy was confirmed by histopathology examination. However, pathology did not show crypt hyperplasia or increased intraepithelial lymphocytes which are features of celiac disease. In all patients, diarrhea disappeared after MMF was stopped and gluten-free diet was not required for improvement. Villous atrophy might be one of the mechanisms of diarrhea induced by MMF.

Ipilimumab

Ipilimumab is a monoclonal antibody directed against CTLA-4 (cytotoxic T-lymphocyte antigen 4) that causes upregulation of the T-cell response [23]. Although it is approved by the FDA for treatment of metastatic melanoma [23], it is also being evaluated as a potential treatment for other cancers. It is associated with gastrointestinal side effects in up to 44% of patients which include diarrhea, drug-induced enterocolitis, hepatotoxicity and pancreatitis [23]. This is likely due to an abrupt triggering of acute inflammation in the colon and small intestine. It typically occurs after the treatment and worsens with each subsequent dose. Patients are usually treated empirically with steroids and supportive care.

Recently, a case report [24] has been published showing association of ipilimumab and celiac disease. The report describes a 62-year-old man with prostatic cancer unresponsive to conventional therapy. Following inclusion in a clinical trial which involved administration of ipilimumab, the patient developed profuse diarrhea unresponsive to high-dose corticosteroids. Laboratory testing showed elevated levels of anti-tTG (IgA and IgG), antideamidated gliadin peptide IgG and HLA-DQ2 haplotype. Duodenal biopsy showed partial to near-total villous atrophy, crypt hyperplasia, chronic inflammation, decreased number of Paneth cells and intraepithelial lymphocytosis. These findings were consistent with celiac disease which started after treatment with ipilimumab. Moreover, the gastrointestinal symptoms improved and the laboratory testing revealed decreased disease activity after initiation of gluten-free diet.

Conclusions

The drug-associated enteropathy that is most common and serious is that seen with olmesartan, albeit at an extremely low rate. One should then suspect OAE in any patient who presents with severe diarrhea and weight loss. Many of the features associated with OAE are also found in the enteropathy found in celiac disease; because of this, one should review any celiac disease diagnosis for any use of olmesartan at the time of diagnosis. Features that are usually found in OAE but are not usually found in celiac disease are collagenous sprue, colitis, and gastritis. Finally, one should consider the possibility of other ARBs inducing enteropathy as there are case reports of valsartan and irbesartan associated with enteropathy.

Discosure Statement

The authors declare that no financial or other conflict of interest exists in relation to the content of the article.

References

1 Nguyen NQ, Yi Mei SL: Current issues on safety of prokinetics in critically ill patients with feed intolerance. Ther Adv Drug Saf 2011;2:197–204.
2 Rubio-Tapia A, Herman ML, Ludvigsson JF, et al: Severe spruelike enteropathy associated with olmesartan. Mayo Clin Proc 2012;87:732–738.
3 Weclawiak H, Ould-Mohamed A, Bournet B, et al: Duodenal villous atrophy: a cause of chronic diarrhea after solid-organ transplantation. Am J Transplant 2011;11:575–582.
4 Cartee A, Nadeau A, Rubio-Tapia A, Herman M, Murray JA: Characterizing olmesartan-induced enteropathy risk factors, severity, and symptom resolution, a follow-up to the 2012 case series. Gastroenterology 2014;146:S-603–S-604.
5 Basson M, Mezzarobba M, Weill A, et al: Severe malabsorption associated with olmesartan: a French nationwide cohort study. Gastroenterology 2014;146:S-114.
6 Abdelghany M, Gonzalez L 3rd, Slater J, Begley C: Olmesartan associated sprue-like enteropathy and colon perforation. Case Rep Gastrointest Med 2014;2014:494098.
7 DeGaetani M, Tennyson CA, Lebwohl B, et al: Villous atrophy and negative celiac serology: a diagnostic and therapeutic dilemma. Am J Gastroenterol 2013;108:647–653.
8 Hartranft ME, Regal RE: 'Triple phase' budesonide capsules for the treatment of olmesartan-induced enteropathy. Ann Pharmacother 2014;48:1234–1237.
9 Nielsen JA, Steephen A, Lewin M: Angiotensin-II inhibitor (olmesartan)-induced collagenous sprue with resolution following discontinuation of drug. World J Gastroenterol 2013;19:6928–6930.
10 Theophile H, David XR, Miremont-Salame G, Haramburu F: Five cases of sprue-like enteropathy in patients treated by olmesartan. Dig Liver Dis 2014;46:465–469.
11 Dreifuss SE, Tomizawa Y, Farber NJ, Davison JM, Sohnen AE: Spruelike enteropathy associated with olmesartan: an unusual case of severe diarrhea. Case Rep Gastrointest Med 2013;2013:618071.
12 Marthey L, Cadiot G, Seksik P, et al: Olmesartan-associated enteropathy: results of a national survey. Aliment Pharm Ther 2014;40:1103–1109.
13 Herman M, Rubio-Tapia A, Marietta E, Wu TT, Murray J: Severe enteropathy in a patient on valsartan. Am J Gastroenterol 2013;108:S302.
14 Menne J, Haller H: Olmesartan and intestinal adverse effects in the ROADMAP study. Mayo Clin Proc 2012;87:1230–1231; author reply 2.
15 Padwal R, Lin M, Etminan M, Eurich DT: Comparative effectiveness of olmesartan and other angiotensin receptor blockers in diabetes mellitus: retrospective cohort study. Hypertension 2014;63:977–983.
16 Mire DE, Silfani TN, Pugsley MK: A review of the structural and functional features of olmesartan medoxomil, an angiotensin receptor blocker. J Cardiovasc Pharm 2005;46:585–593.
17 Muszalska I, Sobczak A, Dolhan A, Jelinska A: Analysis of sartans: a review. J Pharm Sci 2014;103:2–28.
18 Yanagisawa H, Amemiya Y, Kanazaki T, et al: Nonpeptide angiotensin II receptor antagonists: synthesis, biological activities, and structure-activity relationships of imidazole-5-carboxylic acids bearing alkyl, alkenyl, and hydroxyalkyl substituents at the 4-position and their related compounds. J Med Chem 1996;39:323–338.
19 Scott LJ, McCormack PL: Olmesartan medoxomil: a review of its use in the management of hypertension. Drugs 2008;68:1239–1272.
20 Brunner HR: The new oral angiotensin II antagonist olmesartan medoxomil: a concise overview. J Hum Hypertens 2002;16(suppl 2):S13–S16.
21 Allison AC, Eugui EM: Immunosuppressive and other effects of mycophenolic acid and an ester prodrug, mycophenolate mofetil. Immunol Rev 1993;136:5–28.
22 Kamar N, Faure P, Dupuis E, et al: Villous atrophy induced by mycophenolate mofetil in renal-transplant patients. Transpl Int 2004;17:463–467.
23 Weber JS, Kahler KC, Hauschild A: Management of immune-related adverse events and kinetics of response with ipilimumab. J Clin Oncol 2012;30:2691–2697.
24 Gentile NM, D'Souza A, Fujii LL, Wu TT, Murray JA: Association between ipilimumab and celiac disease. Mayo Clin Proc 2013;88:414–417.

Dig Dis 2015;33:221–226
DOI: 10.1159/000369519

Refractory Celiac Disease: Epidemiology and Clinical Manifestations

Georgia Malamut[a–c] Christophe Cellier[a–c]

[a]Université Paris Descartes-Sorbonne Paris Centre, [b]Gastroenterology Department, Hôpital Européen Georges Pompidou APHP, and [c]Inserm UMR1163 Institut Imagine, Paris, France

Key Words
Refractory celiac disease · Ulcerative jejunitis · Aberrant intraepithelial lymphocytes · T-cell receptor · Clonal rearrangement

Abstract
A small subset of celiac disease (CD) patients becomes refractory to a gluten-free diet with persistent malabsorption and intestinal villous atrophy. This is a rare (probably less than 2% of adult CD patients), but serious disorder, with a high risk of progression to an overt T-cell lymphoma. Diagnosis of this condition defined as refractory CD (RCD) is made after exclusion of other small bowel diseases with villous atrophy. RCD has been subdivided into two subgroups according to the normal (RCDI) or abnormal phenotype of intraepithelial lymphocytes (RCDII). Whereas RCDI is hardly distinguishable from active noncompliant CD, RCDII has a severe clinical presentation and a very poor prognosis. We precisely describe below the different types of RCD and propose diagnostic and therapeutic guidelines for its clinical management.

Introduction

Celiac disease (CD) is an inflammatory enteropathy induced by gluten in genetically predisposed individuals. Its prevalence is 1% in Europe and USA. Treatment relies on a lifelong gluten-free diet (GFD) which prevents bone disease, autoimmune disorders and complications (nonmalignant and malignant). Resistance to a GFD is mainly due to bad compliance. Nevertheless, a small subgroup of CD patients may be primarily or secondary resistant to a GFD due to an authentic refractory CD (RCD). Diagnosis of RCD is made after exclusion of other causes of intestinal villous atrophy. RCD has been subdivided into two subgroups according to the normal [type I RCD (RCDI)] or abnormal phenotype of intraepithelial lymphocytes (IEL) [type II RCD (RCDII)]. RCDI is indistinguishable from active CD except its autonomy toward gluten exposure. RCDII is a severe enteropathy with frequent intractable ulcerative duodenojejunitis and is now considered as an intraepithelial T-cell lymphoma.

Epidemiology of RCD

The frequency of RCDI and RCDII remains unknown. Most patients show complete villous architecture recovery after a strict GFD. Nevertheless, a small percentage of patients do not respond clinically and may have a persisting villous atrophy despite a GFD. RCD is a rare disorder with prevalence estimated at 2–5% among patients diagnosed with adult CD. RCD could have been overestimated in the past because of confusion between nonresponsive CD and RCD. In fact, epidemiological studies remain very rare. The Derby cohort reports around 0.7% of RCDII patients in a series of 713 celiac patients, but the

Christophe Cellier
Hôpital Européen Georges Pompidou
20 rue Leblanc
FR–75015 Paris (France)
E-Mail christophe.cellier@egp.aphp.fr

diagnosis of RCDII patients was only based on aspects of ulcerative jejunitis [1] causing possible errors leading to the underestimation of RCDII and overestimation of RCDI. A single North American referral center study suggests a cumulative incidence of 1.5% for both RCDI and RCDII among CD patients initially diagnosed in this center [2]. A higher frequency of cases of RCDI than of RCDII was also observed in 2 other studies from the US [3] and from Germany [4]. In contrast, we and others reported a higher frequency of RCDII than RCDI [5, 6]. These discrepancies among referral centers may be due to the systematic use of FACS analysis in France and Netherlands leading to more RCDII diagnoses.

Outside RCD, persisting villous atrophy without symptoms or without aberrant IEL population is not so rare and has been observed in 5–20% among asymptomatic CD patients on GFD. The cause of this absence of 'mucosal healing' has not been assessed, but may be associated, in our experience, to a persisting iron deficiency that should probably be corrected. The long-term duration of asymptomatic CD without 'mucosal healing' is not known, but a long-term follow-up is mandatory since it may be associated with the occurrence of lymphomatous complications.

Diagnosis of RCD

Definition

RCD is defined as persisting malabsorption and villous atrophy after 1 year of strict GFD ascertained by a dietician. Indeed, bad compliance with a GFD needs to be first eliminated as less than 50% of patients are fully compliant [7]. Diagnosis of RCD also needs to exclude other causes of intestinal villous atrophy such as autoimmune enteropathy [8], tropical sprue [9] or common variable immunodeficiency (CVID) [10]. Demonstration of HLA haplotypes encoding HLA-DQ2 or DQ8 is useful as their absence excludes CD or RCD as a cause of villous atrophy [11]. Nevertheless, genotypes HLA-DQ2/DQ8 are not enough to ascertain the context of CD as they are found in 77% of CVID patients with enteropathy mimicking CD defined by intestinal intraepithelial lymphocytosis [10]. Other features such as intestinal plasmocytic rarefaction or nodular lymphoid hyperplasia allow to distinguish CVID enteropathy from CD or RCD [10]. When the diagnosis of RCD is ascertained, the next step is to define the type of RCD by analyzing the phenotype and clonality of small intestinal IEL. RCDI is defined by increased number of IEL bearing a normal phenotype with surface CD3 and CD8 expression, and RCDII is characterized by clonal expansion of abnormal IEL lacking surface markers CD3, CD8 and T-cell receptor (CD3s–, CD8s–, TCR–) and preserved expression of intracellular CD3 [12, 13].

Diagnosis

Mean age at diagnosis of RCD is around 50 years, and the diagnosis is extremely rare in children or teenagers with CD. Patients with RCDI and RCDII are primary refractory to a GFD in roughly one third and half of cases, respectively [6]. Whatever its type, RCD occurs 2–3 times more often in women than men [5–7]. RCDII has commonly a severe clinical presentation associated with endoscopic ulcerative jejunitis responsible for severe protein loss enteropathy. Symptoms are notably less severe in RCDI, and clinical features are similar to those found in active CD [6].

Diagnosis relies on endoscopic assessment of the upper gastrointestinal tract with intestinal biopsy. Double balloon enteroscopy is required in suspicion of RCDII for a better assessment of ulcers, particularly for evidence of ulcerative jejunitis found in roughly 70% of patients [6, 14]. Enteroscopy allows realization of proximal small bowel biopsy necessary for definitive diagnosis and classification of RCD. In RCDI, histological examination is similar to that found in active CD with villous atrophy and increased normal IEL. No other diagnostic criteria have yet been defined for RCDI. In contrast, the hallmark abnormal population detected by 3 combined techniques makes the diagnosis of RCDII more specific: over 25% of the CD103+ or CD45+ IEL lacking surface CD3-T-cell receptor complexes on flow cytometry or more than 50% IEL expressing intracellular CD3ε but no CD8 in formol-fixed sections and/or the presence of a detectable clonal rearrangement of the γ-chain of the TCR in duodenal biopsies [6]. Similar features allow detecting lymphocytic gastritis and colitis containing the same abnormal population in around 50 and 30% of RCDII patients, respectively. Analysis of the δ-chain rearrangement may be useful for RCDII diagnosis in patients presenting oligoclonal rearrangement of the γ-chain [6]. Others have suggested detecting the β-chain of the TCR [15]. Finally, the specificity of the PCR product needs to be attested by the formation of homoduplexes [6].

Extension of the disease is assessed by capsule endoscopy. It requires preliminary radiological imaging of the small bowel in order to rule out stricturing disease frequently observed in RCDII. In this latter condition, MRI small bowel follow-through and computed tomography scan also frequently detect enlarged mesenteric lymph nodes frequently involved by abnormal cells. Besides the diagnosis of persisting villous atrophy, capsule endoscopy allows the visualization of ulcers that may be found all along the intestinal tract in RCDII patients [16, 17]. In conclusion, upper endoscopy, capsule endoscopy and abdominal imaging are currently three complementary exams essential for the diagnosis and assessment of RCD.

Complications and Outcome

The more severe malnutrition combined with the higher risk of developing overt lymphoma explains the higher mortality in RCDII when compared to RCDI [6]. Indeed, RCDII patients have a 5-year survival rate of 44–58% [3, 5, 6]. Even if the prognosis of RCDI is much better as compared to RCDII, the rates of complications and mortality have been reported to be much higher than those of uncomplicated CD [3, 4]. Chronic inflammation could favor subepithelial accumulation of collagen and increase resistance to a GFD. In their series of 19 patients with collagenous sprue, Vakiani et al. [18] observed that 17 had CD. Nine were primary or secondary resistant to a GFD at time of diagnosis of collagenous sprue, 8 with RCDI and 1 with RCDII.

There is as yet no curative treatment for RCD, immunosuppressive treatment being poorly efficient and a possible trigger of overt lymphoma [19]. Indeed, 33–52% of RCDII patients develop enteropathy-associated T-cell lymphoma (EATL) within the 5 years after diagnosis [5, 6]. The onset of EATL in RCDI is much lower than in RCDII, with a 5-year rate of 14% in the more pessimistic studies [6]. The increased risk of transformation in RCDII probably relies on its malignant nature as it is itself a low-grade lymphoma [13]. Indeed, at this stage, clonal IEL are already engaged in malignant transformation as attested by their clonality, their abnormal phenotype, the presence of their chromosomal abnormalities, the recurrent partial trisomy 1q22–q44 and their tendency to disseminate in and outside of the intestine [6, 20]. Abnormal IEL may be found in mesenteric lymph nodes, blood, bone marrow, and in different epitheliums such as lung and skin [6]. The diagnosis of extraintestinal RCDII lesions may be made by evidence of the same clonal TCR γ/δ-chain rearrangement that presents in the duodenum but also by immunohistochemistry showing CD103+CD3i+CD8– T cells. EATL may develop into intestinal but also extraintestinal lesions of RCDII, with expression of the same IEL-specific integrin CD103. In most cases of EATL, histology reveals an infiltration of lymphoma cells of pleiomorphic appearance or large or anaplastic-like cells, with a high expression of the CD30 and KI67 mitotic index in contrast to RCDII cells, which are negative for both of these markers [21]. The clonal filiation between RCDII IEL and EATL is demonstrated by evidence of the same TCR γ-chain rearrangement [13, 21]. Regular follow-up is required for these high-risk patients; it includes control enteroscopy, computed tomography scan or MRI small bowel follow-through and positron emission tomography (PET) necessary to screen EATL as early as possible. No established interval has yet been defined. Specialized investigations can be reasonably performed every year and 6 months in RCDI and RCDII patients, respectively [6]. PET is of particular interest because high intensity is correlated with the location of proliferating overt lymphoma cells in contrast with the low intensity of nonproliferating RCDII cells [22]. It can further assist in performing radiology-guided biopsy or explorative celioscopy.

Pathogenesis

A particular genetic background differentiating RCD patients from patients with uncomplicated CD is a plausible hypothesis. The small numbers of patients are the main limitations of genetic investigations. It has been reported that the severity of CD was correlated with the number of HLA-DQ2 copies: homozygosity for HLA-DQ2 was observed in 25.5% of RCDI, 44.1% of RCDII, and 53.3% of EATL patients versus 20.7% of uncomplicated CD patients and 2.1% of controls [23]. Studies are in progress, and ongoing genome-wide association studies suggest differences in susceptibility variants between CD and RCDII [24].

Specific mechanisms underlying the pathogenesis of RCDI need to be investigated. One plausible hypothesis is that the immunological reaction initiated by gluten has evolved toward autoimmunity. Accordingly, symptoms improve under immunosuppressive treatments [5, 6]. Therefore, the hypothesis/mechanism of intestinal autoimmunity remains to be substantiated.

More progress has recently been made in the understanding of the pathogenesis of RCDII. The phenotype is now well defined with accumulation of small clonal IEL without proliferation but with apoptosis defect [25]. Ten years ago, in vitro and ex vivo experiments showed that the cytokine IL-15 could be the putative factor involved in resistance to apoptosis [25]. In active CD and RCDII, IL-15 is produced in excess by enterocytes and lamina propria mononuclear cells. On one hand, IL-15 induces the expression of cytotoxic proteins (perforin, granzymes) in RCDII IEL and stimulates their production of IFN-γ which all contribute to the prominent apoptosis observed in the flattened surface epithelium [25–27]. Moreover, IL-15 is able to activate the NKG2D-dependent cytotoxicity of IEL against enterocyte lines [28]. On the other hand, IL-15 exerts potent antiapoptotic effects that prevent the elimination of activated IEL and promote their massive accumulation despite very low in situ proliferation [25]. Indeed, IL-15 is able to activate a lymphocytic antiapoptotic signaling pathway through IL-15Rβγ by activation of Jak3, STAT5 and the anti-apoptotic factor Bcl-xL [29].

All the factors involved in the production of IL-15 represent potential triggers of RCD. Gluten exposure may increase IL-15 production. Concordantly, the risk of lymphoma was reported to be four times higher in patients noncompliant with a GFD than in compliant patients [30]. IL-15 is also induced by a variety of intracellular pathogens [31–34]. We observed B or C hepatitis at onset of refractoriness in 20 and 10% of RCDI and RCDII patients, respectively [6]. Epidemiological factors argue that viral agents such as rotavirus may increase the risk of CD in genetically predisposed individuals [35]. More than a specific virus, it is rather suspected that the components of the antiviral responses and notably type I interferons might promote the onset of chronic inflammatory disorders [reviewed in 36]. Accordingly, increased secretion of type I IFN or an IFN-stimulated gene signature is observed in a spectrum of autoimmune diseases correlating with increased disease severity [37]. Type I interferon may notably stimulate the survival and proliferation of CD8+ T cells and NK cells [37] either directly or via the induction of IL-15 [38]. A virus might also stimulate IL-15 induction via stimulation of Toll-ligand receptor 3 [39].

Treatment

It has not yet been possible to find real efficient treatment for RCDI or RCDII. Steroids transiently improved clinical symptoms in most patients with either type of RCD, with a histological response only in 30–40% of cases [6]. Steroid dependence resorted to test immunosuppressors such as azathioprine, cyclosporine or anti-TNF-α with some clinical response but rarely mucosal improvement. Indeed, in most cases of RCDI they induce clinical response but no histological effect. Finding the mechanisms underlying the pathogenesis of RCDI will probably allow investigation of new efficient treatments [6]. In RCDII, immunosuppressive drugs have no impact on the abnormal clonal IEL population and could even increase the risk of overt lymphoma as reported with azathioprine or anti-CD52 [6, 19]. The bad prognosis of RCDII has led to more aggressive treatments such as chemotherapy, but they are poorly efficient at eradicating nonproliferative RCDII cells [6]. Purine analogues such pentostatin or cladribine have been largely used in the past with slight therapeutic effect [40, 41]. Cladribine may induce clinical and even histological response but appears also to enhance the risk of transformation into EATL [6, 41]. Autologous hematopoietic stem cell transplantation constitutes another possible alternative strategy. It was shown to induce clinical and histological response but no sustained reduction of abnormal IEL in the 13 treated patients [42, 43]. The use of chemotherapy before autologous hematopoietic stem cell transplantation may probably increase hematological response, and we are currently evaluating this strategy in a prospective phase 2 trial. Setting up targeted strategy appears necessary to complete the therapeutic armory to treat RCDII. Identification of the IL-15-induced anti-apoptotic signaling pathway mechanisms underlying the onset of RCDII may help finding potential therapeutic targets [29]. Blocking IL-15 may thus help to reduce the numbers of clonal IEL and to prevent epithelial damage. The recent development of a humanized anti-IL-15 antibody which has already been used without any major side effects in a phase 1–2 trial in rheumatoid arthritis suggests the feasibility of this therapeutic approach [44]. Indeed, treatment in vivo by a human anti-IL-15 antibody of mice overexpressing human IL-15 in the small bowel suppressed the IEL hyperplasia observed in these mice [29].

Another possibility is to block the downstream molecules activated by IL-15 such as the JAK3 molecule [45]. Based on these data, JAK3 inhibitor, currently used in treating rheumatoid arthritis [46], is another interesting drug to treat RCD. Treatment of RCDII will probably combine conventional chemotherapy agents and targeted therapy by anti-IL-15 monoclonal antibody or JAK3 inhibitors in the near future. Finding an efficient treatment is necessary to prevent the onset of EATL whose prognosis is even poorer than that of RCDII [21].

Conclusion

The concept of RCD has recently emerged and refers to two distinct entities sustained by two different pathogenic mechanisms. Diagnosis requires small bowel investigations (enteroscopy, videocapsule endoscopy) and very specialized techniques of IEL analyses (immunohistochemistry, molecular biology, flow cytometry). Survival of RCDI patients has been described as worse than that of CD patients, and the onset of EATL has already been reported [3, 6]. The prognosis of RCDII is very poor due to severe malnutrition and high risk of EATL. Altogether, these rare but resistant and severe forms of CD require efficient treatments. Recent evidence of a scientific rationale for a targeted therapy for the more severe form of RCD offers some hope for an efficient treatment to cure RCD and prevent overt lymphoma.

The take-home message can be listed as follows:

- The concept of RCD has recently emerged and refers to 2 distinct entities.
- RCDI is indistinguishable from active CD except in its autonomy toward gluten exposure.
- RCDII is characterized as a low-grade intestinal lymphoma characterized by clonal expansion of abnormal intestinal IEL.
- Small bowel endoscopy such as double balloon enteroscopy with biopsy assists in diagnosis.
- Specialized analysis of intestinal IEL including immunohistochemistry, flow cytometry of isolated intestinal lymphocytes and multiplex PCR is required for diagnosis.
- Survival of patients with RCDI is slightly inferior to that of CD patients.
- The 5-year survival rate of patients with RCDII is around 50%. This poor prognosis is due to severe malnutrition and increased risk of overt lymphoma.
- Advances in the understanding of pathogenic mechanisms of RCD, RCDII in particular, offer a new therapeutic target by inhibiting IL-15 effects.

Disclosure Statement

The authors declare no competing financial interest.

References

1 West J: Celiac disease and its complications: a time traveller's perspective. Gastroenterology 2009;136:32–34.
2 Roshan B, Leffler DA, Jamma S, et al: The incidence and clinical spectrum of refractory celiac disease in a North American referral center. Am J Gastroenterol 2011;106:923–928.
3 Rubio-Tapia A, Kelly DG, Lahr BD, et al: Clinical staging and survival in refractory celiac disease: a single center experience. Gastroenterology 2009;136:99–107.
4 Daum S, Ipczynski R, Schumann M, et al: High rates of complications and substantial mortality in both types of refractory sprue. Eur J Gastroenterol Hepatol 2009;21:66–70.
5 Al-Toma A, Verbeek WH, Hadithi M, et al: Survival in refractory coeliac disease and enteropathy associated T cell lymphoma: retrospective evaluation of single centre experience. Gut 2007;56:1373–1378.
6 Malamut G, Afchain P, Verkarre V, et al: Presentation and long-term follow-up of refractory celiac disease: comparison of type I with type II. Gastroenterology 2009;136:81–90.
7 Vahedi K, Mascart F, Mary JY, et al: Reliability of antitransglutaminase antibodies as predictors of gluten-free diet compliance in adult celiac disease. Am J Gastroenterol 2003;98: 1079–1087.
8 Akram S, Murray JA, Pardi DS, et al: Adult autoimmune enteropathy: Mayo Clinic Rochester experience. Clin Gastroenterol Hepatol 2007;5:1282–1290.
9 Khokhar N, Gill ML: Tropical sprue: revisited. J Pak Med Assoc 2004;54:133–134.
10 Malamut G, Verkarre V, Suarez F, et al: The enteropathy associated with common variable immunodeficiency: the delineated frontiers with celiac disease. Am J Gastroenterol 2010;105:2262–2275.
11 Green PH, Cellier C: Celiac disease. N Engl J Med 2007;357:1731–1743.
12 Cellier C, Patey N, Mauvieux L, et al: Abnormal intestinal intraepithelial lymphocytes in refractory sprue. Gastroenterology 1998;114: 471–481.
13 Cellier C, Delabesse E, Helmer C, et al: Refractory sprue, coeliac disease, and enteropathy-associated T-cell lymphoma. French Coeliac Disease Study Group. Lancet 2000;356:203–208.
14 Daum S, Cellier C, Mulder CJ: Refractory coeliac disease. Best Pract Res 2005;19:413–424.
15 Perfetti V, Brunetti L, Biagi F, et al: TCRbeta clonality improves diagnostic yield of TCRgamma clonality in refractory celiac disease. J Clin Gastroenterol 2012;46:675–679.
16 Daum S, Wahnschaffe U, Glasenapp R, et al: Capsule endoscopy in refractory celiac disease. Endoscopy 2007;39:455–458.
17 Barret M, Malamut G, Rahmi G, et al: Diagnostic yield of capsule endoscopy in refractory celiac disease. Am J Gastroenterol 2012; 107:1546–1553.
18 Vakiani E, Arguelles-Grande C, Mansukhani MM, et al: Collagenous sprue is not always associated with dismal outcomes: a clinicopathological study of 19 patients. Mod Pathol 2010;23:12–26.
19 Goerres MS, Meijer JW, Wahab PJ, et al: Azathioprine and prednisone combination therapy in refractory coeliac disease. Aliment Pharmacol Ther 2003;18:487–494.
20 Verkarre V, Romana SP, Cellier C, et al: Recurrent partial trisomy 1q22-q44 in clonal intraepithelial lymphocytes in refractory celiac sprue. Gastroenterology 2003;125:40–46.
21 Malamut G, Chandesris O, Verkarre V, et al: Enteropathy associated T cell lymphoma in celiac disease: a large retrospective study. Dig Liver Dis 2013;45:377–384.
22 Hoffmann M, Vogelsang H, Kletter K, et al: 18F-fluoro-deoxy-glucose positron emission tomography (18F-FDG-PET) for assessment of enteropathy-type T cell lymphoma. Gut 2003;52:347–351.

23 Al-Toma A, Goerres MS, Meijer JW, et al: Human leukocyte antigen-DQ2 homozygosity and the development of refractory celiac disease and enteropathy-associated T-cell lymphoma. Clin Gastroenterol Hepatol 2006;4: 315–319.

24 Wijmenga C: Genetic and risk for associated autoimmune disorders and refractory coeliac disease. Mastering the Coeliac Condition, Florence, March 2012.

25 Mention JJ, Ben Ahmed M, Begue B, et al: Interleukin 15: a key to disrupted intraepithelial lymphocyte homeostasis and lymphomagenesis in celiac disease. Gastroenterology 2003; 125:730–745.

26 Ciccocioppo R, Di Sabatino A, Parroni R, et al: Increased enterocyte apoptosis and Fas-Fas ligand system in celiac disease. Am J Clin Pathol 2001;115:494–503.

27 Di Sabatino A, Ciccocioppo R, D'Alo S, et al: Intraepithelial and lamina propria lymphocytes show distinct patterns of apoptosis, whereas both populations are active in Fas based cytotoxicity in coeliac disease. Gut 2001;49:380–386.

28 Hue S, Mention JJ, Monteiro RC, et al: A direct role for NKG2D/MICA interaction in villous atrophy during celiac disease. Immunity 2004;21:367–377.

29 Malamut G, El Machhour R, Montcuquet N, et al: IL-15 triggers an antiapoptotic pathway in human intraepithelial lymphocytes that is a potential new target in celiac disease-associated inflammation and lymphomagenesis. J Clin Invest 2010;120:2131–2143.

30 Holmes GK, Prior P, Lane MR, et al: Malignancy in coeliac disease – effect of a gluten free diet. Gut 1989;30:333–338.

31 Doherty TM, Seder RA, Sher A: Induction and regulation of IL-15 expression in murine macrophages. J Immunol 1996;156:735–741.

32 Flamand L, Stefanescu I, Menezes J: Human herpesvirus-6 enhances natural killer cell cytotoxicity via IL-15. J Clin Invest 1996;97: 1373–1381.

33 Vazquez N, Walsh TJ, Friedman D, et al: Interleukin-15 augments superoxide production and microbicidal activity of human monocytes against *Candida albicans*. Infect Immun 1998;66:145–150.

34 Waldmann TA, Tagaya Y: The multifaceted regulation of interleukin-15 expression and the role of this cytokine in NK cell differentiation and host response to intracellular pathogens. Annu Rev Immunol 1999;17:19–49.

35 Stene LC, Honeyman MC, Hoffenberg EJ, et al: Rotavirus infection frequency and risk of celiac disease autoimmunity in early childhood: a longitudinal study. Am J Gastroenterol 2006;101:2333–2340.

36 Foxman EF, Iwasaki A: Genome-virome interactions: examining the role of common viral infections in complex disease. Nat Rev Microbiol 2011;9:254–264.

37 Gough DJ, Messina NL, Clarke CJ, et al: Constitutive type I interferon modulates homeostatic balance through tonic signaling. Immunity 2012;36:166–174.

38 Colpitts SL, Stoklasek TA, Plumlee CR, et al: Cutting edge: the role of IFN-alpha receptor and MyD88 signaling in induction of IL-15 expression in vivo. J Immunol 2012;188: 2483–2487.

39 Dafik L, Albertelli M, Stamnaes J, et al: Activation and inhibition of transglutaminase 2 in mice. PLoS One 2012;7:e30642.

40 Dray X, Joly F, Lavergne-Slove A, et al: A severe but reversible refractory sprue. Gut 2006; 55:1210–1211.

41 Al-Toma A, Goerres MS, Meijer JW, et al: Cladribine therapy in refractory celiac disease with aberrant T cells. Clin Gastroenterol Hepatol 2006;4:1322–1327.

42 Al-Toma A, Visser OJ, van Roessel HM, et al: Autologous hematopoietic stem cell transplantation in refractory celiac disease with aberrant T-cells. Blood 2007;109:2243–2249.

43 Tack GJ, Wondergem MJ, Al-Toma A, et al: Auto-SCT in refractory celiac disease type II patients unresponsive to cladribine therapy. Bone Marrow Transplant 2011;46:840–846.

44 Waldmann TA: Targeting the interleukin-15 system in rheumatoid arthritis. Arthritis Rheum 2005;52:2585–2588.

45 Yokoyama S, Perera PY, Waldmann TA, et al: Tofacitinib, a janus kinase inhibitor demonstrates efficacy in an IL-15 transgenic mouse model that recapitulates pathologic manifestations of celiac disease. J Clin Immunol 2013; 33:586–594.

46 Fleischmann R, Cutolo M, Genovese MC, et al: Phase IIb dose-ranging study of the oral JAK inhibitor tofacitinib (CP-690,550) or adalimumab monotherapy versus placebo in patients with active rheumatoid arthritis with an inadequate response to disease-modifying antirheumatic drugs. Arthritis Rheum 2012; 64:617–629.

Dig Dis 2015;33:227–230
DOI: 10.1159/000381076

Therapy in RCDII: Rationale for Combination Strategies?

Petula Nijeboer[a] Georgia Malamut[c] Gerd Bouma[a] Nadine Cerf-Bensussan[d] Frits Koning[b] Jeroen van Bergen[b] Christophe Cellier[c] Chris J.J. Mulder[a]

[a]Department of Gastroenterology, VU University Medical Centre, Amsterdam, and [b]Department of Immunohematology and Blood Transfusion, Leiden University Medical Center, Leiden, The Netherlands; [c]Department of Gastroenterology, and [d]Inserm U989, Université Paris Descartes, Hôpital Européen Georges Pompidou, Paris, France

Key Words

Refractory coeliac disease type II · Coeliac disease · Enteropathy-associated T-cell lymphoma · Tofacitinib

Abstract

Refractory coeliac disease type II (RCDII) is characterized by a continuous gluten-independent duodenal immune activation with an extremely high risk of malignant transformation. It is therefore considered as an indolent lymphoma. RCDII is characterized by the presence of villous atrophy (Marsh III A-C) in combination with an aberrant intraepithelial lymphocyte (IEL) population consisting of >20% sCD3–CD7+iCD3+ IELs. The sCD3–CD7+iCD3+ IELs are a heterogeneous lineage-negative cell population, consisting of cells that do or do not express CD127/IL7Rα. Experiments using IEL from non-RCDII patients have indicated that while the CD127– cells are IL-15 responsive, the CD127+ cells are not. Together with the observation that some patients express an aberrant (monoclonal) TCRγδ phenotype, this confirms the heterogeneity of the aberrant IEL population in RCDII and suggests that the aberrant cells are heterogeneous with respect to their response to common γ-chain cytokines. Although cladribine with or without autologous stem cell transplantation is effective in the treatment of signs and symptoms of RCDII and improves survival as compared to symptomatic topical steroid therapy, cladribine failures still bear a high risk of malignant transformation, and the rate of enteropathy-associated T-cell lymphoma (EATL) development in this subgroup is extremely high. It might be hypothesized that the heterogenous nature of aberrant IEL and the high risk of malignant transformation require a treatment strategy which is effective despite this heterogeneity. RCDII should be seen more in the light of a low-grade/no mass lymphoma or pre-EATL. We would suggest an upfront combination therapy approach integrating inhibition of downstream Jak-STAT signalling pathways with conventional therapy (2-CDA) to hopefully effectively treat signs and symptoms of RCDII and accomplish a more effective EATL prevention.

Introduction

A small subset of coeliac disease (CD) patients experiences persisting or recurring symptoms despite strict adherence to a gluten-free diet. When other causes of villous atrophy have been excluded, these patients are referred to as refractory coeliac disease (RCD). RCD can be divided

KARGER 125

E-Mail karger@karger.com
www.karger.com/ddi

0257–2753/15/0332–0227$39.50/0

Prof. Dr. Chris J.J. Mulder, MD, PhD
Department of Gastroenterology
VU University Medical Centre, PO Box 7057
NL–1007 MB Amsterdam (The Netherlands)
E-Mail cjmulder@vumc.nl

in two types based on the absence (type I) or presence (type II) of an intra-epithelial lymphocyte (IEL) population (usually clonal) with aberrant phenotype. RCDII is defined by the presence of villous atrophy (Marsh III A-C) in combination with an IEL population consisting of >20% sCD3–CD7+iCD3+ IELs determined using flow cytometry [1]. With a cumulative incidence of 0.04%, RCDII is a rare condition [unpubl. data]. RCDII is mostly diagnosed around the age of 50 years or thereafter, but younger cases may be observed [2, 3]. The most common symptoms in RCDII include persistent diarrhoea, abdominal pain and involuntary weight loss [4]. Moreover, severe malnutrition, protein-losing enteropathy and ulcerative jejunitis may be seen [5, 6]. RCDII has a high risk of malignant transformation to an enteropathy-associated T-cell lymphoma (EATL) and is therefore considered as indolent lymphoma (pre-EATL). Unfortunately, RCDII has been resistant, at least in part, to most evaluated therapies so far [2, 5, 7]. Therefore, more advanced treatment strategies aiming to treat the signs and symptoms of RCDII together with effective EATL prevention are urgently needed.

Intra- and Inter-Individual Heterogeneity in RCDII

The heterogeneous nature of RCDII IEL has been shown in various publications during the past years. Recent work from Schmitz et al. [8] has shown two major aberrant IEL populations in RCDII patients: CD56–CD127– and CD56–CD127+. Experiments evaluating the intestinal innate IEL compartment of non-CD patients as well as CD patients, revealed that the IL-2/-15 receptor B chain (CD122) is expressed by the lineage-negative CD56–CD127– population in contrast to the CD56–CD127+ population which showed lower expression of CD122. In contrast, the latter population showed co-expression of the IL-21 receptor and IL-15 receptor α-chain. What also stresses heterogeneity is the observation that the clonality of T-cell receptor rearrangements differed between RCDII cell lines [9] and within a relatively large group of RCDII patients [9, 10]. Furthermore, aberrant IELs display different stages of maturity between RCDII patients, of which only the patients harbouring the most mature aberrant IEL population developed an EATL [1]. Besides these diverse inter-individual differences, aberrant IELs in RCDII might also be characterized by intra-individual heterogeneity as RCDII cell lines show fractioned expression of different γ-chain receptors within one cell line [8]. This confirms the heterogeneity of the aberrant IEL population in RCDII and underlines the importance of extensive evaluation of CD patients refractory to a gluten-free diet using sensitive diagnostic procedures [10]. It is tempting to speculate that the heterogeneity of aberrant IEL found in RCDII might reflect the fact that proliferation and (pre-) malignant transformation of these IELs could take place at different stages of IEL development.

Cytokine Responsiveness in RCDII

It has been described that the presence of IL-15 in RCDII is likely to contribute to the expansion and survival of aberrant IEL [11]. Massive overproduction by enterocytes of IL-15 leads to continuous activation of IELs. Indeed there is evidence that this cytokine is upregulated in patients with RCD II [12]. RCDII IELs activated by enterocyte-derived IL-15 might exert cytotoxicity against epithelial cells through NKG2D and DNAM-1 ligands [8, 11], and be responsible for the severe enteropathy observed in RCDII patients. Finally, the strong anti-apoptotic effect of IL-15 might explain the accumulation and expansion of these cells despite their low in situ proliferative capacity [13]. Besides IL-15, other common γ-cytokines might play a role in the pathogenesis of RCDII as well. It can be hypothesized that the presence of different cytokine subsets in the local intestinal milieu lead to continuous IEL activation and defective apoptotic control through binding to the heterogeneous receptor subsets expressed on aberrant IELs as described above [8]. In a next step towards lymphomagenesis, a subset of IEL undergo clonal expansion and finally when chromosomal aberrations have occurred these cells transform towards a lymphoma.

Current Treatment Strategies

Unfortunately, to date there is no standardized globally accepted treatment approach for RCDII. RCDII has been resistant, at least in part, to most evaluated therapies so far. As RCDII patients often have a chronic form of malnutrition, presenting with a low BMI (<18.5) [6], the primary treatment step should be correction of nutritional deficiencies and metabolic disorders. There is no place for classic immunosuppressive drugs, such as thiopurines, in the treatment of RCDII. Although they might exert clinical effects, corticosteroids have no influence on the onset of EATL and especially do not exclude underlying EATL [14]. In a recent study, of 16 RCDII patients who developed EATL, 10 had received immunosuppressants [5]. Moreover, azathiopurine might enhance the risk or accelerate the onset of EATL [5, 15, 16]. Furthermore, combination therapy of azathioprine and prednisone in RCDII patients showed development of EATL in 7 of the 8 treated patients [16]. Based on these discouraging results, cladribine (2-CDA), a synthetic purine nucleoside homologue, has been initiated and shown to be feasible and safe for RCDII [17, 18]. 2-CDA is supposed to be especially active against low-grade CD103+ malignancies, which is one of the characteristics of the aberrant lineage-negative sCD3–CD7+iCD3+ cells. Nevertheless, 2-CDA does not prevent EATL development in all treated patients [18], and some patients died within months of RCDII diagnosis due to progressive refractory disease.

In patients with RCDII refractory to conventional 2-CDA treatment, autologous hematopoietic stem cell transplantation (auSCT) is an increasingly accepted effective treatment option. auSCT appears to be feasible and safe, and might result in clinical remission in 2-CDA failures [19, 20]. Whether the benefits from the addition of auSCT outweigh the costs and the risks of this aggressive treatment strategy needs to be substantiated in a larger cohort with longer follow-up. Furthermore, only a selected RCDII population is able to receive this aggressive treatment strategy. Recent evaluation of factors associated with EATL development in RCDII patients treated with 2-CDA revealed that histological response determines EATL development; when histological remission is achieved after 2-CDA, the frequency of EATL development is low and survival is comparable with the patients treated with 2-CDA-auSCT combination therapy. Although 2-CDA with or without autologous stem cell transplantation are both effective in the treatment of signs and symptoms of RCDII and improve survival as compared to symptomatic topical steroid therapy, 2-CDA failures who are non-eligible for auSCT still bear a high risk of malignant transformation and the rate of EATL development in this subgroup is extremely high (data from P.N.).

Future Perspectives

This underlines the need for new, advanced treatment strategies. It might be hypothesized that a small percentage, of phenotypical 'atypical' aberrant IELs might be 2-CDA resistant in some patients and that those IELs undergo continuous IEL activation resulting in persistent enteropathy and evolve into EATL over time. Therefore, we state that the heterogeneous nature of aberrant IELs as described above, and the high risk of malignant transformation, requires a treatment strategy which is effective despite this heterogeneity. As described, both lineage-negative CD127– and lineage-negative CD127+ IELs are frequently expanded in RCDII. As the IL-15 receptor B chain is expressed by the former, and the IL-7 receptor, IL-21 receptor and IL-15 receptor α-chain is expressed by the latter, treatment with anti-IL-15 is unlikely to be sufficient. Therefore, an inhibitor of common downstream signalling molecules of the different receptors expressed by aberrant IELs might be required. Considering the fact that increased Jak3 and STAT5 phosphorylation has been demonstrated in aberrant IELs [11], and these are downstream molecules of the common γ-chain receptors identified in RCDII, Jak3 or STAT5 inhibitors could serve as a potential target therapy. Tofacitinib is a Jak3 inhibitor which blocks signalling through these γ-chain receptors for several cytokines, including IL-2, -4, -7, -9, -15 and -21, and is now safely applied in rheumatoid arthritis [21, 22]. Inhibition of their signalling may thus result in modulation of the continued immune activation and the anti-apoptotic effects seen in RCDII. We expect combination therapy approaches integrating inhibition of Jak-STAT pathways with conventional therapy (2-CDA) might effectively treat signs and symptoms of RCDII and could result in a more effective EATL prevention.

In conclusion, RCDII should be seen more in the light of an indolent lymphoma (pre-EATL) and therefore upfront treatment strategies consisting of combination therapy with conventional 2-CDA and a downstream signalling blocker might be required for the initial treatment of RCDII.

Disclosure Statement

All authors state there is no actual or potential conflict of interests to disclose in relation to this article.

References

1 van Wanrooij RL, Schreurs MW, Bouma G, von Blomberg BM, Tack GJ, Verbeek WH, Mulder CJ: Accurate classification of RCD requires flow cytometry. Gut 2010;59:1732.

2 Rubio-Tapia A, Kelly DG, Lahr BD, Dogan A, Wu TT, Murray JA: Clinical staging and survival in refractory celiac disease: a single center experience. Gastroenterology 2009;136:99–107.

3 Al-Toma A, Verbeek WH, Mulder CJ: Update on the management of refractory coeliac disease. J Gastrointestin Liver Dis 2007;16:57–63.

4 Al-Toma A, Verbeek WH, Mulder CJ: The management of complicated celiac disease. Dig Dis 2007;25:230–236.
5 Malamut G, Afchain P, Verkarre V, Lecomte T, Amiot A, Damotte D, Bouhnik Y, Colombel JF, Delchier JC, Allez M, Cosnes J, Lavergne-Slove A, Meresse B, Trinquart L, Macintyre E, Radford-Weiss I, Hermine O, Brousse N, Cerf-Bensussan N, Cellier C: Presentation and long-term follow-up of refractory celiac disease: comparison of type I with type II. Gastroenterology 2009;136:81–90.
6 Wierdsma N: Refractory coeliac disease and EATL patients are characterised by malnutrition and malabsorption at presentation; a comparative study with newly diagnosed coeliac disease patients (abstract). Digestive Disease Week, Chicago, 2014.
7 Verbeek WH, Schreurs MW, Visser OJ, von Blomberg BM, Al-Toma A, Mulder CJ: Novel approaches in the management of refractory celiac disease. Expert Rev Clin Immunol 2008; 4:205–219.
8 Schmitz F, Tjon JM, Lai Y, Thompson A, Kooy-Winkelaar Y, Lemmers RJ, Verspaget HW, Mearin ML, Staal FJ, Schreurs MW, Cupedo T, Langerak AW, Mulder CJ, van Bergen J, Koning F: Identification of a potential physiological precursor of aberrant cells in refractory coeliac disease type II. Gut 2013; 62:509–519.
9 Tack GJ, van Wanrooij RL, Langerak AW, Tjon JM, von Blomberg BM, Heideman DA, van BJ, Koning F, Bouma G, Mulder CJ, Schreurs MW: Origin and immunophenotype of aberrant IEL in RCDII patients. Mol Immunol 2012;50:262–270.
10 van Wanrooij RL, Müller DM, Neefjes-Borst EA, Meijer J, Koudstaal LG, Heideman DA, Bontkes HJ, von Blomberg BM, Bouma G, Mulder CJ: Optimal strategies to identify aberrant intra-epithelial lymphocytes in refractory coeliac disease. J Clin Immunol 2014;34: 828–835.
11 Malamut G, El MR, Montcuquet N, Martin-Lanneree S, Dusanter-Fourt I, Verkarre V, Mention JJ, Rahmi G, Kiyono H, Butz EA, Brousse N, Cellier C, Cerf-Bensussan N, Meresse B: IL-15 triggers an antiapoptotic pathway in human intraepithelial lymphocytes that is a potential new target in celiac disease-associated inflammation and lymphomagenesis. J Clin Invest 2010;120:2131–2143.
12 Mention JJ, Ben AM, Begue B, Barbe U, Verkarre V, Asnafi V, Colombel JF, Cugnenc PH, Ruemmele FM, McIntyre E, Brousse N, Cellier C, Cerf-Bensussan N: Interleukin 15: a key to disrupted intraepithelial lymphocyte homeostasis and lymphomagenesis in celiac disease. Gastroenterology 2003;125:730–745.
13 Malamut G, Meresse B, Cellier C, Cerf-Bensussan N: Refractory celiac disease: from bench to bedside. Semin Immunopathol 2012;34:601–613.
14 Rubio-Tapia A, Murray JA: Classification and management of refractory coeliac disease. Gut 2010;59:547–557.
15 Malamut G, Afchain P, Verkarre V, Lecomte T, Amiot A, Damotte D, Bouhnik Y, Colombel JF, Delchier JC, Allez M, Cosnes J, Lavergne-Slove A, Meresse B, Trinquart L, Macintyre E, Radford-Weiss I, Hermine O, Brousse N, Cerf-Bensussan N, Cellier C: Presentation and long-term follow-up of refractory celiac disease: comparison of type I with type II. Gastroenterology 2009;136:81–90.
16 Goerres MS, Meijer JW, Wahab PJ, Kerckhaert JA, Groenen PJ, Van Krieken JH, Mulder CJ: Azathioprine and prednisone combination therapy in refractory coeliac disease. Aliment Pharmacol Ther 2003;18:487–494.
17 Al-Toma A, Goerres MS, Meijer JW, von Blomberg BM, Wahab PJ, Kerckhaert JA, Mulder CJ: Cladribine therapy in refractory celiac disease with aberrant T cells. Clin Gastroenterol Hepatol 2006;4:1322–1327.
18 Tack GJ, Verbeek WH, Al-Toma A, Kuik DJ, Schreurs MW, Visser O, Mulder CJ: Evaluation of cladribine treatment in refractory celiac disease type II. World J Gastroenterol 2011;17:506–513.
19 Al-Toma A, Visser OJ, van Roessel HM, von Blomberg BM, Verbeek WH, Scholten PE, Ossenkoppele GJ, Huijgens PC, Mulder CJ: Autologous hematopoietic stem cell transplantation in refractory celiac disease with aberrant T cells. Blood 2007;109:2243–2249.
20 Tack GJ, Wondergem MJ, Al-Toma A, Verbeek WH, Schmittel A, Machado MV, Perri F, Ossenkoppele GJ, Huijgens PC, Schreurs MW, Mulder CJ, Visser OJ: Auto-SCT in refractory celiac disease type II patients unresponsive to cladribine therapy. Bone Marrow Transplant 2011;46:840–846.
21 van der Heijde D, Tanaka Y, Fleischmann R, Keystone E, Kremer J, Zerbini C, Cardiel MH, Cohen S, Nash P, Song YW, Tegzova D, Wyman BT, Gruben D, Benda B, Wallenstein G, Krishnaswami S, Zwillich SH, Bradley JD, Connell CA: Tofacitinib (CP-690,550) in patients with rheumatoid arthritis receiving methotrexate: twelve-month data from a twenty-four-month phase III randomized radiographic study. Arthritis Rheum 2013;65: 559–570.
22 van Vollenhoven RF, Fleischmann R, Cohen S, Lee EB, Garcia Meijide JA, Wagner S, Forejtova S, Zwillich SH, Gruben D, Koncz T, Wallenstein GV, Krishnaswami S, Bradley JD, Wilkinson B: Tofacitinib or adalimumab versus placebo in rheumatoid arthritis. N Engl J Med 2012;367:508–519.

Dig Dis 2015;33:231–235
DOI: 10.1159/000369542

Enteropathy-Associated T-Cell Lymphoma: Improving Treatment Strategies

P. Nijeboer[a] G. Malamut[c] C.J. Mulder[a] N. Cerf-Bensussan[d] D. Sibon[e] G. Bouma[a] C. Cellier[c] O. Hermine[e] O. Visser[b]

Departments of [a]Gastroenterology and [b]Hematology, VU University Medical Centre, Amsterdam, The Netherlands; [c]Department of Gastroenterology, and [d]Inserm U989, Université Paris Descartes, Hôpital Européen Georges-Pompidou, and [e]Department of Hematology, Université Paris Descartes, Paris, France

Key Words

Enteropathy-associated T-cell lymphoma · Malignant lymphoma · Autologous stem cell transplantation · Refractory coeliac disease

Abstract

Enteropathy-associated T-cell lymphoma (EATL) is a rare and usually rapidly fatal intestinal T-cell non-Hodgkin lymphoma. It arises from intraepithelial lymphocytes and has a high association with coeliac disease. The high mortality of EATL is associated not only with the very aggressive and often chemotherapy-refractory nature of the lymphoma. The poor condition of patients due to prolonged and severe malnutrition compromises the ability to deliver chemotherapy. There are no standardized treatment protocols, and the optimal therapy for EATL remains unclear. The primary step of treatment consists of local debulking, preferably as early as possible after EATL diagnosis. Morbidity and mortality seem to rise with advanced stages of disease due to tumour size progression, worse nutritional status and a higher risk of emergency surgery due to perforation. Standard induction therapy for EATL is anthracycline-based chemotherapy, preferably resumed between 2 and 5 weeks after surgery (depending on clinical condition). Intensification of therapy using high-dose chemotherapy followed by consolidation with BEAM and autologous stem cell transplantation is associated with better outcome. Notably, this treatment strategy has only been applied in patients eligible for this aggressive regimen which might reflect selection bias. Unfortunately, prognosis of EATL remains poor; 5-year survival varies from 8 to 60% depending on the eligibility to receive additional steps of therapy. New treatment strategies are urgently needed for a better prognosis of this lethal complication of coeliac disease. Brentuximab vedotin (anti-CD30) might be promising when added to conventional chemotherapy and is suggested as upfront treatment in EATL.

Introduction

Enteropathy-associated T-cell lymphoma (EATL) is a rare intestinal lymphoma that arises from intraepithelial lymphocytes. In Western countries, this lymphoma has a high association with coeliac disease (CD). In patients with CD, EATL is identified as the main cause of increased mortality [1, 2] and develops in an estimated 0.04% of adult-onset CD patients [3]. Based on clinical presentation, EATL can be divided into two subtypes: pri-

KARGER 125

E-Mail karger@karger.com
www.karger.com/ddi

0257–2753/15/0332–0231$39.50/0

O. Visser, MD, PhD
Department of Hematology, VU University Medical Centre
De Boelelaan 1117
NL–1081 HV Amsterdam (The Netherlands)
E-Mail o.visser@vumc.nl

mary and secondary EATL. Primary EATL develops without a preceding history of CD. The first presentation could be perforation or obstruction, which leads to the diagnosis of both EATL and CD. Secondary EATL is diagnosed in patients with well-established CD or refractory CD type II (RCDII). These patients deteriorate and eventually develop EATL.

There are no validated and standardized treatment protocols for EATL due to the rarity of this disease. Treatment strategies consist of different additional steps, including surgery, chemotherapy and stem cell transplantation (SCT), each applied depending on the eligibility of the patient. EATL patients are characterized by acute malnutrition, due to both malabsorption and an alleged hypermetabolism [4]. Besides the aggressive and often chemotherapy-refractory nature of the T-cell lymphoma itself, the deprived nutritional status of most EATL patients at diagnosis seems to be an important factor which negatively affects clinical condition and therefore preventing the use of aggressive treatment strategies. This results in an extremely variable 5-year survival of EATL patients between 8 and 60% [5–11].

Since no standard therapeutic regimens are established in EATL and clinical condition is highly variable, a range of therapeutic strategies have been used. So far, treatment of EATL is only centralized in a minority of cases. This year, the European Reference Network of Coeliac Disease was started up to build a uniformly network in the field of (pre-)malignant CD. The aim of this network is to facilitate uniform standardized diagnostic and therapeutic care and to perform translational research in this field. In this paper, we summarize recently published data on different treatment strategies and present future perspectives according to the European Reference Network.

Standard Induction Therapy

Historically, patients with EATL were treated with surgery, chemotherapy or a combination of both. Unfortunately, there is a shortage of prospective observational studies, although patients with EATL have in some cases been included in trials for aggressive lymphoma. In general, chemotherapy is probably the most important factor of improved survival in lymphoma patients [12]. Due to the risk of bowel perforation during chemotherapy or symptomatic perforation or stenosis at diagnosis, the preferred first step in the treatment of EATL is surgical debulking, whether or not followed by subsequent chemotherapy. The frequency of early and late post-operative morbidity is relatively high after surgical debulking [13]. Early complications mainly include anastomotic leakage and sepsis. Stenosis at the side of the anastomosis is the most frequently reported late complication. Mortality is higher when the resection is performed in the acute setting. Resection of the tumour mass, preferably as early as possible after diagnosis, improves survival and improves the ability to receive chemotherapy after resection [8, 13]. Standard induction chemotherapy regimens applied in EATL are usually anthracycline based consisting of CHOP (cyclophosphamide, doxorubicin, vincristine, prednisolone) in most cases [8, 10, 12]. Five-year survival percentages following surgical debulking and standard induction chemotherapy vary from 8 to 28% [7–9, 14]. The most common reason for withholding chemotherapy after surgical debulking is a poor condition of the patient after surgery. Furthermore, a considerable proportion of EATL patients are unable to complete chemotherapy due to poor nutritional status, rapid progression of disease during treatment, and local or systemic complications [11].

As shown in different independent studies, patients with secondary EATL have a less favourable outcome than EATL patients without a prior diagnosis of CD [8, 9, 15]. Within the group of secondary EATL, patients who suffer from refractoriness to the gluten-free diet (RCDII) even have a worse prognosis. A potential explanation relates to the fact that these patients generally suffer from severe and long-standing malnutrition [4, 8].

Overall, patients treated with combination therapy consisting of surgical debulking and subsequent standard induction chemotherapy show a significantly better outcome than those treated with standard induction chemotherapy or surgery alone [7–9, 14]. This stresses the importance of early diagnosis of EATL and extensive nutritional assessment to optimize nutritional status at diagnosis and during therapy.

Treatment Intensification

As the role of standard induction chemotherapy (CHOP) combined with surgical debulking obtained persisting dismal survival percentages, several novel strategies are being assessed in EATL treatment. In the last decades, treatment intensification using high-dose chemotherapy and consolidation with hematopoietic SCT as upfront therapeutic option has become an increasingly accepted treatment option for aggressive T-cell non-

Hodgkin lymphomas (NHL). Two recent studies showed significant improvement of prognosis in patients treated with intensified chemotherapy (CHOP combined with etoposide [5, 6] or methotrexate [5, 7]) followed by auSCT. The specific effect of new drug combinations and intensified chemotherapy is somewhat difficult to evaluate due to a combination with SCT in most studies and the selected patient category. These studies showed a lower amount of patients failing the high-dose chemotherapy due to disease progression as compared to anthracycline-based chemotherapy. Moreover, patients treated with high-dose chemotherapy and autologous SCT (auSCT) had higher remission rates than those treated with standard induction therapy including CHOP and additional auSCT [9–11]. However, as expected, there was a higher incidence of neutropenic fever and sepsis compared with standard induction chemotherapy. This supports the notion that intensification of induction therapy might increase eligibility in EATL patients to ultimately achieve SCT.

Consolidation Therapy

As mentioned, consolidation with BEAM (carmustine, etoposide, cytarabine, melphalan) and autologous haematopoietic SCT (auSCT) has become increasingly accepted for EATL treatment. The rationale for using this strategy is tumour and immunoablation using high-dose chemotherapy, with subsequent regeneration of naïve T-lymphocytes derived from reinfused haematopoietic progenitor cells. During induction chemotherapy, stem cells are harvested by leukapheresis and are re-infused after high-dose, myeloablative BEAM chemotherapy. Various independent studies have demonstrated that auSCT combined with intensified chemotherapy and resection is feasible, also in patients with CD, and shows the most favourable outcome. Outcome for those treated with intensified chemotherapy followed by auSCT improved to a 5-year overall survival of 50–60% [6, 7]. It should be noted that these studies included a variable EATL population consisting of only primary EATL [7], various types of peripheral T-cell NHL [6] or EATL patients in whom various chemotherapy schemes preceded the auSCT [5]. In series evaluating the complete EATL population, consolidation therapy using SCT also appeared to increase survival [8, 9], although this was non-significant due to the limited amount of patients in these studies eligible for auSCT and a limited time of follow-up.

These results clearly support the idea that patients tolerating more intensive approaches may benefit. Since SCT has only been applied in patients eligible for this aggressive regimen, it remains to be seen whether adding SCT can make a significant impact on survival in all EATL patients, and international trials to evaluate this are therefore urgently needed.

Experimental Treatment Strategy

Based on the theory that allogeneic SCT (alloSCT) might be more effective than auSCT in EATL treatment due to a graft-versus-lymphoma effect, the effect of alloSCT in EATL has been assessed. However, results are conflicting. In some centres, patients who underwent alloSCT died within 2 months after transplantation due to EATL relapse [9]. Others showed alloSCT to be successful in 2 out of 3 patients treated with this regimen [8]. We hypothesize that a dismal outcome in alloSCT in some cases might be due to insufficient conditioning or a delay in the graft-versus-lymphoma effect due to the immunosuppressive medication used. Whether alloSCT has a role in treatment of EATL remains to be evaluated in future experimental prospective trials.

Future Perspectives

Due to the fact that only a limited percentage of EATL patients ultimately achieve the most aggressive consolidation step, recent studies assessed intensification strategies consisting of new chemotherapy combinations and a higher dose as described above [6, 7]. Besides high-dose chemotherapy, the evidence for the effectiveness of target therapy with monoclonal antibodies (mAbs) is increasing. Owing to their excellent potential for specific detection, delineation and selective treatment of systemic diseases, mAbs are broadly used as a treatment strategy in malignancies as B- and T-cell NHL. The rationale for using this strategy is based on the utilization of the antigens expressed by tumour cells and to deliver cytotoxic agents inside the malignant cell based on this antigen expression using antibody-drug conjugates.

EATL type I is a large-cell lymphoma and is highly associated with CD30 [16]. This type of T-cell NHL is characterized by the expression of CD30 in the majority of cases [17]. CD30 is an ideal target for mAb therapy due to its limited expression on normal tissues. Brentuximab vedotin is an anti-CD30 antibody which is conjugated to

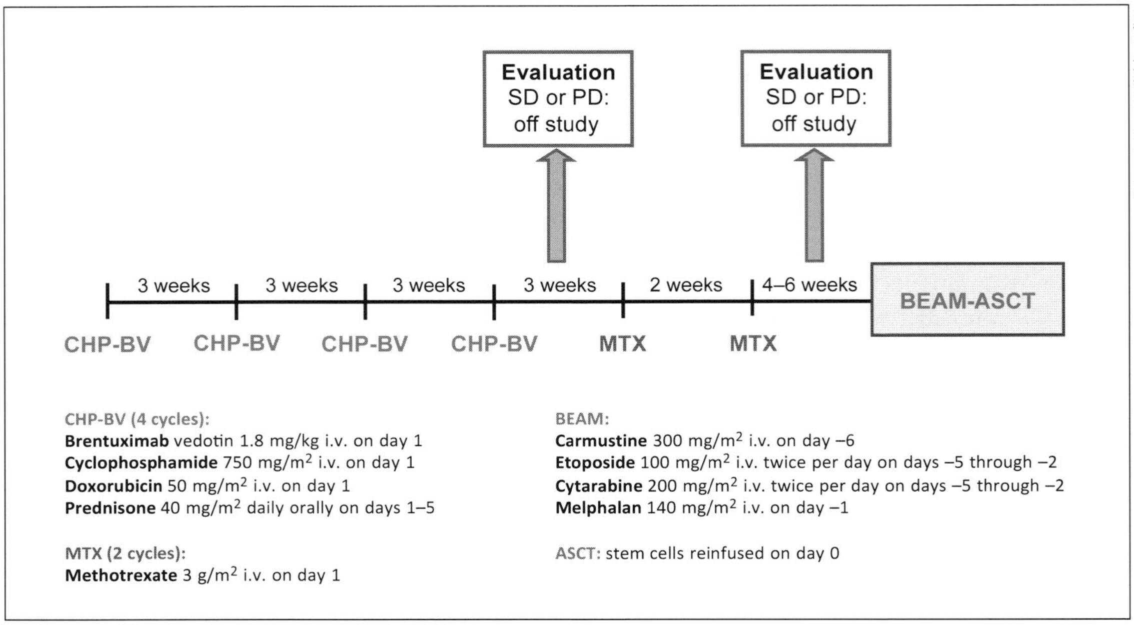

Fig. 1. Phase 2 study of brentuximab vedotin and CHP followed by auSCT as frontline treatment of EATL. SD = Stable disease; PD = progressive disease. Study coordinators: Prof. Hermine, Prof. Cellier, Dr. Sibon (Paris).

the anti-microtubule agent monomethyl auristatin E [18]. Following binding to CD30, brentuximab vedotin leads to cell cycle arrest and apoptosis of the tumour cell. Several studies showed this agent to be well tolerated and highly active in patients with relapsed Hodgkin's lymphoma [19], systemic anaplastic lymphoma or primary cutaneous T-cell NHL [18]. The most frequently reported adverse event is peripheral neuropathy [20].

This impressive response might be very promising for the relatively chemotherapy-refractory nature of EATL, and has been described to be effective for EATL in a case description [21]. Preliminary data in a limited number of EATL patients described by Malamut et al. [8] show multi-agent therapy consisting of intensive chemotherapy combined with anti-CD30 followed by consolidation with BEAM and auSCT to be safe and effective, although longer follow-up will be required. The European Reference Network of Coeliac Disease suggests implementing a uniform treatment strategy in Europe including brentuximab vedotin. This network was started up this year and consists of haematologists, gastroenterologists, researchers from the major (R)CD-referral centres in Europe (including Paris, Amsterdam; more centres are expected). The suggested treatment protocol is outlined in figure 1 and combines high-dose chemotherapeutic drugs, which are proven to be effective (CHP/MTX), with anti-CD30 targeted therapy (brentuximab vedotin) with the aim to improve the number of patients able to proceed to BEAM and auSCT.

Ultimately, the best way to treat EATL would be to prevent it. Therefore, stringent strategies for early EATL diagnosis in patients with uncomplicated CD or RCDII should be implemented. One of the options suggested by the European Reference network would be to perform radioactive labelling of mAbs with brentuximab vedotin. Since patients with RCDII show no CD30 expression on the intra-epithelial lymphocytes and EATL is characterized by CD30 expression, organ and whole-body distribution of the labelled product can be assessed using PET imaging, and early EATL development could be made more or less likely using this strategy. Besides imaging strategies for early diagnosis, brentuximab vedotin might be used for in vivo research to understand the biological process and the pathogenesis of EATL development in CD and RCDII patients. Furthermore, early diagnosis and effective treatment of RCDII is of utmost importance for secondary prevention of EATL.

Conclusion

In conclusion, prognosis for EATL patients remains extremely poor. Most studies indicate that optimising nutritional status and combination therapy including both surgical debulking and standard induction chemotherapy should be the standard of care for these patients. In addition, some studies suggest that intensification with upfront high-dose chemotherapy and consolidation using auSCT may further improve disease control and survival, although this aggressive treatment strategy is only available for a limited amount of patients. Considering the need for a uniform treatment strategy in order to combine highly specialized care and translational research in this field, we would highly suggest adding brentuximab vedotin and methotrexate to the standard induction chemotherapy in EATL patients and to perform easy accessible consolidation with BEAM and auSCT in patients aged <70 years.

Disclosure Statement

All authors state there is no actual or potential conflict of interest to disclose in relation to this article.

References

1 Mearin ML, Catassi C, Brousse N, Brand R, Collin P, Fabiani E, Schweizer JJ, Abuzakouk M, Szajewska H, Hallert C, Farre MC, Holmes GK: European multi-centre study on coeliac disease and non-Hodgkin lymphoma. Eur J Gastroenterol Hepatol 2006;18:187–194.

2 Corrao G, Corazza GR, Bagnardi V, Brusco G, Ciacci C, Cottone M, Sategna GC, Usai P, Cesari P, Pelli MA, Loperfido S, Volta U, Calabro A, Certo M: Mortality in patients with coeliac disease and their relatives: a cohort study. Lancet 2001;358:356–361.

3 Biagi F, Gobbi P, Marchese A, Borsotti E, Zingone F, Ciacci C, Volta U, Caio G, Carroccio A, Ambrosiano G, Mansueto P, Corazza GR: Low incidence but poor prognosis of complicated coeliac disease: a retrospective multicentre study. Dig Liver Dis 2014;46:227–230.

4 Wierdsma NJP, Nijeboer MAE, de van der Schueren M, Berkenpas AA, van Bodegraven AA, Mulder CJ: Refractory coeliac disease and EATL patients are characterised by malnutrition and malabsorption at presentation; a comparative study with newly diagnosed Coeliac Disease patients (abstract). Digestive Disease Week, Chicago, May 2014.

5 Jantunen E, Boumendil A, Finel H, Luan JJ, Johnson P, Rambaldi A, Haynes A, Duchosal MA, Bethge W, Biron P, Carlson K, Craddock C, Rudin C, Finke J, Salles G, Kroschinsky F, Sureda A, Dreger P: Autologous stem cell transplantation for enteropathy-associated T-cell lymphoma: a retrospective study by the EBMT. Blood 2013;121:2529–2532.

6 d'Amore F, Relander T, Lauritzsen GF, Jantunen E, Hagberg H, Anderson H, Holte H, Osterborg A, Merup M, Brown P, Kuittinen O, Erlanson M, Ostenstad B, Fagerli UM, Gadeberg OV, Sundstrom C, Delabie J, Ralfkiaer E, Vornanen M, Toldbod HE: Upfront autologous stem-cell transplantation in peripheral T-cell lymphoma: NLG-T-01. J Clin Oncol 2012;30:3093–3099.

7 Sieniawski M, Angamuthu N, Boyd K, Chasty R, Davies J, Forsyth P, Jack F, Lyons S, Mounter P, Revell P, Proctor SJ, Lennard AL: Evaluation of enteropathy-associated T-cell lymphoma comparing standard therapies with a novel regimen including autologous stem cell transplantation. Blood 2010;115:3664–3670.

8 Malamut G, Chandesris O, Verkarre V, Meresse B, Callens C, Macintyre E, Bouhnik Y, Gornet JM, Allez M, Jian R, Berger A, Chatellier G, Brousse N, Hermine O, Cerf-Bensussan N, Cellier C: Enteropathy associated T cell lymphoma in celiac disease: a large retrospective study. Dig Liver Dis 2013;45:377–384.

9 Nijeboer P, Baaij LR, Visser O, Witte BI, Cillessen SA, Mulder CJ, Bouma G: Treatment response in enteropathy associated T-cell lymphoma; survival in a large multicentre cohort (abstract). Digestive Disease Week, Chicago, May 2014.

10 Gale J, Simmonds PD, Mead GM, Sweetenham JW, Wright DH: Enteropathy-type intestinal T-cell lymphoma: clinical features and treatment of 31 patients in a single center. J Clin Oncol 2000;18:795–803.

11 Daum S, Ullrich R, Heise W, Dederke B, Foss HD, Stein H, Thiel E, Zeitz M, Riecken EO: Intestinal non-Hodgkin's lymphoma: a multicenter prospective clinical study from the German Study Group on Intestinal non-Hodgkin's Lymphoma. J Clin Oncol 2003;21: 2740–2746.

12 Sieniawski MK, Lennard AL: Enteropathy-associated T-cell lymphoma: epidemiology, clinical features, and current treatment strategies. Curr Hematol Malig Rep 2011;6:231–240.

13 van de Water JMW, Nijeboer P, de Baaij LR, Zegers J, Bouma G, Visser OJ, van de Peet DL, Mulder CJJ, Meijerink WJHJ: Surgery in (pre-)malignant coeliac disease (abstract). Digestive Disease Week, Chicago, May 2014.

14 Delabie J, Holte H, Vose JM, Ullrich F, Jaffe ES, Savage KJ, Connors JM, Rimsza L, Harris NL, Muller-Hermelink K, Rudiger T, Coiffier B, Gascoyne RD, Berger F, Tobinai K, Au WY, Liang R, Montserrat E, Hochberg EP, Pileri S, Federico M, Nathwani B, Armitage JO, Weisenburger DD: Enteropathy-associated T-cell lymphoma: clinical and histological findings from the international peripheral T-cell lymphoma project. Blood 2011;118:148–155.

15 Rubio-Tapia A, Kelly DG, Lahr BD, Dogan A, Wu TT, Murray JA: Clinical staging and survival in refractory celiac disease: a single center experience. Gastroenterology 2009;136: 99–107.

16 van de Water JM, Cillessen SA, Visser OJ, Verbeek WH, Meijer CJ, Mulder CJ: Enteropathy associated T-cell lymphoma and its precursor lesions. Best Pract Res Clin Gastroenterol 2010;24:43–56.

17 World Health Organization: Classification of Tumour of Hematopoietic and Lymphoid Tissues. Geneva, World Health Organization, 2008.

18 van de Donk NW, Dhimolea E: Brentuximab vedotin. MAbs 2012;4:458–465.

19 Pro B, Perini GF: Brentuximab vedotin in Hodgkin's lymphoma. Expert Opin Biol Ther 2012;12:1415–1421.

20 Foyil KV, Bartlett NL: Brentuximab vedotin for the treatment of CD30+ lymphomas. Immunotherapy 2011;3:475–485.

21 Khalaf WF, Caldwell ME, Reddy N: Brentuximab in the treatment of CD30-positive enteropathy-associated T-cell lymphoma. J Natl Compr Canc Netw 2013;11:137–140.

Dig Dis 2015;33:236–243
DOI: 10.1159/000371405

Serum Markers in the Clinical Management of Celiac Disease

Marlou Adriaanse Daniel A. Leffler

Division of Gastroenterology, Beth Israel Deaconess Medical Center, Boston, Mass., USA

Key Words
Celiac disease · Serology · Tissue transglutaminase · Deamidated gliadin peptide · Endomysial antibody · Biomarker · Intestinal fatty acid-binding protein

Abstract
The advent of highly reliable noninvasive celiac diagnostic tests has transformed the field of celiac disease, from diagnosis, to evaluation of epidemiology, to clinical and translational research. Serologic tests in their modern forms are highly sensitive and specific for diagnosis, allowing for consideration of avoidance of diagnostic intestinal biopsy in some settings. On the other hand, as predictors of intestinal damage and for use in monitoring disease activity, currently available noninvasive tests have been disappointing. Serologic tests, while a measure of disease activity, do not correlate well with histology or symptomatology, and it is unclear if they predict long-term risk. Additionally, while the many clinically available tests have improved accessibility, they can have widely different cutoff levels and overall performance, making the comparison of levels in individual patients over time and across populations quite difficult. In the future, we can expect to see improvement in the currently available serologic tests including tissue transglutaminase and deamidated gliadin peptide with expansion of the dynamic range of the tests, and the celiac care community should push for a standardization of assays that would simplify research and patient care. Additionally, current serologic tests are measures of the adaptive immune response in celiac disease but do not directly measure intestinal inflammation. Promising work on intestinal fatty acid-binding protein and other assays which directly measure intestinal damage may complement traditional serologic tests and further improve our ability to noninvasively diagnose and monitor celiac disease. The coming years hold promise for the continuing evolution of serum-based tests in celiac disease with the possibility of substantial improvement of patient care and clinical research.

Introduction

Celiac disease (CD) is a common immune-mediated enteropathy triggered by the intake of dietary gluten in wheat, barley and rye, in genetically susceptible individuals [1]. Gluten peptides in the intestine trigger T-helper 1-mediated immune responses resulting in epithelial inflammation, an increased number of intraepithelial lymphocytes, intestinal villous atrophy, autoantibody production, and malabsorptive symptoms. Traditionally, the diagnosis of CD relies on visualizing the typical lesion via small intestinal biopsy. Early diagnosis and treatment of CD can prevent severe complications. A gluten-free diet (GFD) generally leads to improvement in intestinal mucosal damage, clinical symptoms and CD autoantibody titers.

KARGER 125
E-Mail karger@karger.com
www.karger.com/ddi

0257–2753/15/0332–0236$39.50/0

Daniel A. Leffler
Division of Gastroenterology, Beth Israel Deaconess Medical Center
East/Dana 501, 330 Brookline Avenue
Boston, MA 02215-5400 (USA)
E-Mail dleffler@bidmc.harvard.edu

The widespread availability of highly accurate serologic testing for CD has been a fundamental driver of advances in clinical care and research in this field [2]. The serologic tests for CD are more accurate than most other antibody-based tests for immune-based disorders. In the early 1960s, the gliadin component of wheat was found to be the pathologic trigger for CD. Autoantibodies (AGA) against this protein were subsequently the first to be used as a screening tool for the disease [3]. Since that time, serologic testing advanced from an adjunctive aid in diagnosis to an integral component of diagnosis, management and clinical research. Highly sensitive and specific tests including tissue transglutaminase (tTG), endomysial (EMA) and deamidated gliadin peptide (DGP) autoantibodies have been identified optimizing diagnostics and screening studies. Indeed, for all individuals in whom CD is being considered, serologic blood testing should be the initial step in evaluation [4–6]. With improvement of serologic antibody tests and highly accurate assays, we are potentially reaching the time where a diagnosis of CD can be made without intestinal biopsies, at least in select well-defined situations [5].

Despite these advances and the overall laudable test performance of EMA, tTG and DGP for CD diagnosis, current testing still is subject to a number of important limitations that are important for both clinicians and researchers to recognize. First, one of the most practical issues currently faced by clinicians is the diversity of available testing platforms, many of which have different cutoff levels, dynamic ranges and overall test performance. This issue, which has gone largely unaddressed, can be a major impediment to both patient care and research when values are not comparable between providers or between studies. In addition, it has been noted that the excellent test performance shown in validation studies of various serologic tests may not accurately reflect test performance in clinical practice and more diverse populations.

Furthermore, monitoring disease activity in treated CD patients remains a challenge. Although the CD antibody tests show a high accuracy for selecting patients needing a diagnostic biopsy, these tests do not seem to be reliable after diagnosis as the autoantibody titers do not correlate well with histological findings or symptoms in CD patients on a GFD. To optimize the noninvasive diagnostic algorithm and improve monitoring of disease activity, different tests for CD activity have been studied. Two promising markers are intestinal fatty acid-binding protein (I-FABP), a marker reflecting enterocyte damage, and citrulline (CIT), a marker for functional enterocyte mass, and will be discussed in this review.

Also, unlike histology, there are virtually no data on the impact of serologic test results of long-term prognosis. Fortunately, work is ongoing to address these limitations, and the coming years hold promise for the continuing evolution of serum-based tests in CD with the possibility of substantial improvement of patient care and clinical research. The aim of this review is to evaluate the currently available serum markers and their accuracy in clinical practice in patients with a suspicion of CD, and their use for monitoring disease activity in CD patients on a GFD. Next to the traditional (gliadin, reticulin, actin) and modern tests (tTG, EMA and DGP), two novel promising markers for disease activity (I-FABP and CIT) will be discussed.

Traditional Autoantibody Tests: Anti-Gliadin, Anti-Reticulin and Anti-Actin

Anti-Reticulin and Anti-Actin

Anti-reticulin antibodies (ARA) were first described as a possible predictive test for CD in the early 1970s [7]. While IgA antibodies to reticulin connective tissue did see some use, primarily in pediatric CD evaluation and appeared to have test performance equal to or better than AGA [8], ARA was largely supplanted first by AGA for technical reasons and later on by EMA and tTG which had markedly better test performance, as described below.

Around the same time as ARA were described, anti-actin antibodies (AAA) were found to be present in a number of autoimmune and neoplastic conditions [9]. AAA has been evaluated on multiple occasions as a supplemental serologic test in CD. While AAA may have a higher predictive value for severe intestinal damage than other serologic tests, the relatively low sensitivity has made the clinical value of this test uncertain and AAA have never gained widespread use in CD [10, 11].

Anti-Gliadin

About one decade later, in the 1980s, the native anti-gliadin antibody (AGA) test was developed for CD [12]. This test for both IgA and IgG antibodies was relatively easy to manufacture and perform (enzyme-linked immunosorbent assay, ELISA). It was a major step forward as they were the first tests to allow some degree of noninvasive risk stratification, especially important in what was, at that time, a primarily pediatric disease, and quickly became the standard serologic test.

There is marked heterogeneity in results of studies evaluating the sensitivity and specificity of AGA tests, as a results of assay variants and cutoffs provided, a common problem for all CD diagnostic tests [13–15]. The average sensitivity and specificity of the best tests for both IgA and IgG AGA is between 80 and 90%, with lower specificities generally seen in adults compared with children [2, 13]. In recent years, AGA-IgA tests have been replaced by more accurate serological assays, such as tTG, EMA and DGP.

One historic advantage of AGA had been the availability of a moderately accurate IgG-based test. While IgA is the major component of the gluten-autoantibody interaction in the small intestinal lumen, IgG represents a longer-term immune response. As selective IgA deficiency occurs in up to 2% of patients with CD, the need for a non-IgA-based test is apparent [16, 17]. IgG AGA testing remained the standard diagnostic test for CD in individuals with selective IgA deficiency through the early 2000s. However, in the past few years, IgG-tTG and particularly IgG-DGP assays have been developed that are superior to IgG-AGA for this population [18–21].

Recently, AGA has been suggested as a marker of nonceliac gluten sensitivity (i.e. those with negative antibodies to tTG and/or EMA and normal intestinal histology) [22]. However, at this point, there are no clear data that support the use of AGA testing in any clinical setting where more modern tests are available.

Newer Tests: EMA, tTG and DGP

Endomysium

Introduction of the EMA test in the mid-1980s was a significant step forward from AGA testing. Although heterogenic, the sensitivity of EMA-IgA is generally reported to be above 90% with a specificity up to 100% [13, 23, 24]. Because of the close to 100% specific association with CD, EMA testing has generally been used as a confirmatory test for tTG. However, approximately 10% of CD patients remain negative for EMA. The test has been suggested to be less sensitive in patients with milder small intestinal lesions (Marsh 3A) [25, 26] and among CD children under 2 years of age [27]. Nevertheless, different studies suggest that EMA appears in the serum before development of villous atrophy, making it a marker of early or 'potential' CD [28, 29]. EMA is detected by an indirect immunofluorescence method (monkey esophagus or human umbilical cord tissue as antigen). A consequent disadvantage of this method is that the results are labor-intensive and operator-dependent, increasing the costs and diminishing the objectivity of the test [2].

Tissue Transglutaminase

The identification of tTG as autoantigen in the late 1990s enabled the development of an easy to perform ELISA-based test with recombinant tTG. tTG is responsible for the deamidation of gluten-derived gliadin peptides, resulting in DGP with greatly enhanced immunoreactivity [30, 31]. Gluten in this altered confirmation binds with high affinity to HLA DQ2 or HLA DQ8 molecules on antigen-presenting cells which present the deamidated gluten and bound tTG to helper T cells triggering production of antibodies to tTG and DGP [32–35]. Enteropathy is caused by cell-mediated cytotoxicity triggered also by the binding of deamidated gluten to HLA molecules on antigen-presenting cells but resulting in CD8-mediated inflammation with infiltration of lymphocytes into the mucosa along with villous destruction. (The pathogenic significance of the autoantibody response in CD patients remains unclear; however, celiac antibodies have been postulated to increase intestinal permeability, activate monocytes, disturb angiogenesis, inhibit epithelial cell differentiation or induce cell proliferation.) Since they were described, tTG quickly became the standard test used in CD diagnosis, as this method is more reproducible and objective compared with EMA. The best tests for tTG IgA have shown both sensitivity and specificity of 95% and above [2, 13, 14, 36]. The performance of commercial ELISA assays for tTG however may vary depending on the quality of the antigen, and discrepancies between different kits are also present in the cutoff values. The concordance rate of tTG and EMA test is very high, but based on its high sensitivity, lower costs and ease of interpretation, tTG is suggested as the first screening test [37, 38]. Nevertheless, in most studies, the specificity of EMA tests is higher, suggesting that this test can be performed as confirmatory in tTG-positive individuals [38, 39]. Furthermore, as discussed above, the accuracy of all serologic tests depends on disease prevalence and may be lower in clinical settings compared with highly enriched validation cohorts.

Deamidated Gliadin Peptides

Most recently, drawing off the known pathophysiology of CD, antibodies directed to DGP have been introduced into the spectrum of serologic tests for CD. DGP reflects the CD B-cell epitopes more specific than the native nonamidated peptides targeted by the traditional AGA [20], and consequently has a higher sensitivity and specificity. Although DGP-IgA was shown to be nearly as sensitive and specific as tTG-IgA [40, 41], recent studies revealed that tTG performs significantly better [36, 42]. The sensitivity and specificity for DGP-IgA have generally been shown to be around 85 and 95%, respectively [2, 36, 43]. Nevertheless, while IgG-based tTG tests in IgA-deficient patients have disappointing sensitivity, DGP-IgG tests display high specificity for CD (99%, similar to EMA) [20, 40, 42–44]. DGP-IgG allows for the identification of all CD cases in IgA-deficient patients with a high sensitivity in young children, proposing a new protocol for CD that uses only two tests.

The revolution in antibody tests has substantially improved the diagnostic algorithm for CD. Further improvement can be expected by rapid point of care tests that can be performed at the outpatient clinic, instead of requiring trained personnel and centralized laboratories. Point of care tTG-IgA tests have been developed, but reports on their accuracy are contradictory, and these tests need further exploration before clinical implementation [39, 45].

Despite the major improvements in serologic testing, no antibody test shows an absolute sensitivity and specificity for CD. In the majority of patients, the diagnosis of CD still relies on the demonstration of the characteristic small intestinal changes by duodenal biopsy. The best serologic approach for case finding might be the combined detection of a panel of antibodies. Recently, the European Society for Pediatric Gastroenterology Hepatology and Nutrition introduced a revised guideline for CD in children based on the optimization of antibody assays. According to this guideline, children can be diagnosed with CD without a duodenal biopsy when presenting with symptoms, a strongly elevated tTG-IgA (>10 cutoff value), confirmed by a positive EMA-IgA test on a separate occasion, and positive genetic testing (HLA-DQ2 and/or HLA-DQ8) [5]. Such a strategy seems premature for CD in adults, and a substantial proportion of children with suspicion of CD do not fulfill all four diagnostic criteria. Thus, currently a diagnostic biopsy remains necessary for most patients.

Other serum markers are warranted to prevent the diagnostic biopsies in all children and in adult patients. Research has been underway for many years for a noninvasive test that cannot only screen individuals at risk for CD, but also correlate with the severity of the intestinal lesions and monitor the histological response to a GFD. Potential markers are discussed below.

Experimental Tests: I-FABP and CIT

Citrulline

CIT is a nonprotein amino acid, and is a metabolic intermediate in the urea cycle. CIT is almost exclusively present in the enterocytes of the small intestine [46–48]. Consequently, circulating CIT levels have been proposed to be a potential marker of small intestinal function and mass. Recently, CIT levels have been shown to be a reliable marker of small intestinal damage in other disease associated with villous atrophy and enterocyte alterations, including HIV and tropical enteropathy [49, 50].

Publications on the value of CIT testing in CD are conflicting. A few studies showed that CIT levels are reduced in children and adults with untreated CD compared with healthy controls [51–53]. Most of these studies showed an inverse correlation between fasting plasma CIT level and the extent of villous atrophy [51, 52]. However, significant overlap was present between CD patients and controls [52, 53]. Furthermore, others found that fasting plasma CIT levels were unable to reflect a decreased intestinal energy absorption capacity in patients with enterocyte damage [54]. This may be due to a milder degree of intestinal disease [54], suggesting that significant intestinal damage must be present for CIT levels to decrease.

Initiation of a GFD in studies with decreased CIT levels at diagnosis led to an increase in CIT levels [51–53], depending on the histological responsiveness [51], and has been shown to normalize CIT levels to the levels of controls after more than 2 years of GFD [52].

As an alternative to fasting CIT levels, a CIT generation test (CGT) has been provided to assess enterocyte function [55]. Loading the enterocyte with orally administered glutamine, the natural precursor of CIT, may increase CIT output, reflecting the functional capacity of the enterocyte. This study revealed that the generation of CIT was delayed in patients with CD. This test might offer a new possibility to assess the functional capacity of enterocytes in CD. For now however, the clinical utility of CIT measurement is questionable in CD and needs further evaluation.

Intestinal Fatty Acid-Binding Protein

Measurement of circulating endogenous enterocyte proteins has been shown to be useful to estimate enterocyte damage. Fatty acid-binding protein comprises a class of low-molecular-weight (14–15 kDa) cytosolic proteins found in high concentrations in tissues involved in the uptake and consumption of fatty acids [56]. Three types of FABP are present in the gut: intestinal FABP (I-FABP), liver FABP (L-FABP) and ileal bile acid-binding protein (I-BABP). I-FABP is executively present in the gut, as is I-BABP which is exclusively present in the ileum, while L-FABP is also present in the liver and kidneys. I-FABP is primarily limited to mature enterocytes of the small intestine, with a maximal expression in the jejunum, while the expression in the colon is low [57]. Since I-FABPs are small water-soluble proteins, they are easily released into the circulation upon enterocyte damage and rapidly cleared though the kidneys (half-life of 11 min). I-FABP levels can be measured sensitively using an ELISA. It circulates in low amounts in the bloodstream of healthy individuals, likely reflecting the physiological turnover rate of enterocytes. Outside of CD, elevated circulating FABP levels have been reported in patients with intestinal ischemia, necrotizing enterocolitis and the early phase of sepsis [58–60].

Recent studies have revealed that serum I-FABP may be a sensitive marker for enterocyte damage in CD. These studies showed that I-FABP levels are significantly elevated in untreated CD adults and children at diagnosis as compared with control subjects [57, 61, 62]. Interestingly, serum I-FABP levels correlated with the severity of the histological lesions. These studies showed a sensitivity of 80 and 82%, and a specificity of 87 and 90% in adults and children, respectively, for CD, suggesting that serum I-FABP might be a useful additional marker in the diagnostic algorithm of CD [61, 62]. Patients with positive CD-specific markers and an elevated serum I-FABP level seem to suffer from CD, suggesting that a diagnostic biopsy can be omitted in these patients. Nevertheless, in patients with elevated CD, autoantibody titers and a normal serum I-FABP level, a duodenal biopsy would remain necessary.

Serum I-FABP levels may also be useful for monitoring disease activity after diagnosis. After introduction of the GFD, serum I-FABP levels decrease relatively fast. This is especially useful to confirm a diagnosis made without duodenal biopsy. In children, serum I-FABP levels have been shown to generally decrease and normalize within 6 months after initiation of gluten elimination [61]. This is faster than the decrease in tTG levels. However, in adult patients, levels appeared elevated compared with controls, even after up to 3–4 years of apparent compliance with the GFD [62]. This is in line with studies on histological healing in patients on a GFD, generally showing slow and incomplete mucosal healing in adult CD patients, while recovery in children seems to be faster and more complete [63, 64]. As postulated, a correlation has been found between serum I-FABP levels and the severity of the histological lesions in CD patients on a GFD [62]. Furthermore, a pilot study showed that I-FABP may be used as an early responsive marker during a gluten challenge procedure [unpubl. data]. Large international studies are underway to validate this marker for use in diagnosis, monitoring and research trials.

Limitations and Areas for Future Study

CD is a significant disorder with limited treatment adherence [65, 66] and adverse effects on quality of life [65, 67, 68] and nutritional [69] and metabolic indices [70, 71]. It is also associated with increased risk of malignancy and mortality [72–74]. For this reason, all major societies recommend routine follow-up of patients with CD [4–6, 75]. The goal of routine monitoring is to identify and treat coexisting disorders and manage active CD.

Thus, reliable but also easily applicable markers are needed. The modalities commonly used for CD monitoring are serologic tests and less often intestinal biopsy. While both tests are clearly supported as part of CD diagnosis, their use in monitoring is much less clear. Both small intestinal mucosal inflammation and serologic tests are reflections of different aspects of the adaptive immune response triggered by gluten in CD. When CD is highly active, as at diagnosis before the GFD is initiated, highly elevated serologic titers are correlated with intestinal damage, as both arms of adaptive immunity are fully activated [2, 76]. With initiation of the GFD however, this relationship becomes unstable. Data show that EMA, tTG and DGP titers should fall significantly in the first months after initiation of GFD and be normal or close to normal one year after diagnosis [77–79]. It is clear from gluten challenge studies that increases in antibody titers reflect increased disease activity and increased intestinal inflammation. However, elevation of CD-specific serology is delayed significantly from episodes of gluten exposure [80], and CD antibodies are poor predictors of dietary adherence with low levels of cross contamination or inadvertent gluten [81, 82]. CD serology lacks both sensitivity and specificity for ongoing enteropathy on a long-term GFD [83]. Furthermore, there are no studies that evaluate the relationship between normalization of serologic tests and risk of long-term complications. Although more research is necessary, promising experimental markers for enterocyte damage, such as I-FABP and CIT, may be more accurate for monitoring disease activity in CD patients on a GFD.

Conclusion

Serum markers for CD play an important role in CD management. In recent decades, the evolvement from detection of the disease trigger to several antibody tests has greatly improved the diagnostic algorithm, epidemiology and research, and will continue to do so.

In the upcoming years, further improvement and expansion of existing and new serological tests can be expected, with wider dynamic ranges, improved responsiveness and possibly higher sensitivity and specificity. Combination of different noninvasive markers may lead to diagnostic algorithms with greatly reduced need for diagnostic duodenal biopsies. Novel markers measuring direct mucosal damage, like I-FABP and CIT, instead of reflecting the immune response, may complement traditional serologic tests. These markers may also be more accurate predictors for monitoring disease activity after diagnosis, as the currently used antibody tests do not correlate well with histology or symptomatology. Once these novel tests are validated and clinically available, guidelines for CD diagnosis and monitoring may look very different from those available today.

At the same time, use of different antibody tests and cutoffs make comparison in individual patients over time and across populations difficult in both clinical and research situations. The range of competing tests is likely only to grow in the coming years. A centralized effort to perform an open and robust comparison across testing platforms paired with detailed clinical and histologic data is feasible and could be completed with modest resources. These data would also be essential to the next major question of whether serologic titers, either at diagnosis or in follow-up, are of any prognostic significance in diagnosed patients. A number of studies have provided important data on the relationship between histology and long-term outcomes in CD. Clearly, the fact that we have only had serologic tests for a few decades has limited the conduct of these studies. However, sufficient time has elapsed to begin to make these studies possible.

Disclosure Statement

Daniel Leffler has been a consultant for and/or received research support from the following: NIH, Shire Pharmaceuticals, Inova Diagnostics, Coranado Biosciences, Alba Therapeutics, Alvine Pharmaceuticals, Glenwood Pharmaceuticals and Ironwood Pharmaceuticals.

References

1 Green PH, Cellier C: Celiac disease. N Engl J Med 2007;357:1731–1743.
2 Leffler DA, Schuppan D: Update on serologic testing in celiac disease. Am J Gastroenterol 2010;105:2520–2524.
3 Berger E, Buergin-Wolff A, Freudenberg E: Diagnostic value of the demonstration of gliadin antibodies in celiac disease (in German). Klin Wochenschr 1964;42:788–790.
4 Rubio-Tapia A, Hill ID, Kelly CP, et al: ACG clinical guidelines: diagnosis and management of celiac disease. Am J Gastroenterol 2013;108:656–676; quiz 677.
5 Husby S, Koletzko S, Korponay-Szabo IR, et al: European Society for Pediatric Gastroenterology, Hepatology, and Nutrition guidelines for the diagnosis of coeliac disease. J Pediatr Gastroenterol Nutr 2012;54:136–160.
6 Bai JC, Fried M, Corazza GR, et al: World Gastroenterology Organisation global guidelines on celiac disease. J Clin Gastroenterol 2013;47:121–126.
7 Seah PP, Fry L, Rossiter MA, et al: Anti-reticulin antibodies in childhood coeliac disease. Lancet 1971;2:681–682.
8 Lerner A, Kumar V, Iancu TC: Immunological diagnosis of childhood coeliac disease: comparison between antigliadin, antireticulin and antiendomysial antibodies. Clin Exp Immunol 1994;95:78–82.
9 Trenchev P, Holborow EJ: The specificity of anti-actin serum. Immunology 1976;31:509–517.
10 Fabbro E, Rubert L, Quaglia S, et al: Uselessness of anti-actin antibody in celiac disease screening. Clin Chim Acta 2008;390:134–137.
11 Granito A, Muratori P, Cassani F, et al: Anti-actin IgA antibodies in severe coeliac disease. Clin Exp Immunol 2004;137:386–392.
12 O'Farrelly C, Kelly J, Hekkens W, et al: Alpha gliadin antibody levels: a serological test for coeliac disease. BMJ (Clin Res Ed) 1983;286: 2007–2010.
13 Hill ID: What are the sensitivity and specificity of serologic tests for celiac disease? Do sensitivity and specificity vary in different populations? Gastroenterology 2005;128:S25–S32.
14 Rostom A, Dube C, Cranney A, et al: The diagnostic accuracy of serologic tests for celiac disease: a systematic review. Gastroenterology 2005;128:S38–S46.
15 Naiyer AJ, Hernandez L, Ciaccio EJ, et al: Comparison of commercially available serologic kits for the detection of celiac disease. J Clin Gastroenterol 2009;43:225–232.
16 Cataldo F, Marino V, Bottaro G, et al: Celiac disease and selective immunoglobulin A deficiency. J Pediatr 1997;131:306–308.
17 Chow MA, Lebwohl B, Reilly NR, et al: Immunoglobulin A deficiency in celiac disease. J Clin Gastroenterol 2012;46:850–854.
18 Dahlbom I, Olsson M, Forooz NK, et al: Immunoglobulin G (IgG) anti-tissue transglutaminase antibodies used as markers for IgA-deficient celiac disease patients. Clin Diagn Lab Immunol 2005;12:254–258.
19 Cataldo F, Lio D, Marino V, et al: IgG(1) antiendomysium and IgG antitissue transglutaminase (anti-tTG) antibodies in coeliac patients with selective IgA deficiency. Working Groups on Celiac Disease of SIGEP and Club del Tenue. Gut 2000;47:366–369.
20 Prince HE: Evaluation of the INOVA diagnostics enzyme-linked immunosorbent assay kits for measuring serum immunoglobulin G (IgG) and IgA to deamidated gliadin peptides. Clin Vaccine Immunol 2006;13:150–151.
21 Lenhardt A, Plebani A, Marchetti F, et al: Role of human-tissue transglutaminase IgG and anti-gliadin IgG antibodies in the diagnosis of coeliac disease in patients with selective immunoglobulin A deficiency. Dig Liver Dis 2004;36:730–734.
22 Verdu EF, Armstrong D, Murray JA: Between celiac disease and irritable bowel syndrome: the 'no man's land' of gluten sensitivity. Am J Gastroenterol 2009;104:1587–1594.
23 Collin P, Kaukinen K, Vogelsang H, et al: Antiendomysial and antihuman recombinant tissue transglutaminase antibodies in the diagnosis of coeliac disease: a biopsy-proven European multicentre study. Eur J Gastroenterol Hepatol 2005;17:85–91.
24 Volta U, Fabbri A, Parisi C, et al: Old and new serological tests for celiac disease screening. Expert Rev Gastroenterol Hepatol 2010;4: 31–35.

25 Rostami K, Kerckhaert J, Tiemessen R, et al: Sensitivity of antiendomysium and antigliadin antibodies in untreated celiac disease: disappointing in clinical practice. Am J Gastroenterol 1999;94:888–894.
26 Abrams JA, Diamond B, Rotterdam H, et al: Seronegative celiac disease: increased prevalence with lesser degrees of villous atrophy. Dig Dis Sci 2004;49:546–550.
27 Maglio M, Tosco A, Paparo F, et al: Serum and intestinal celiac disease-associated antibodies in children with celiac disease younger than 2 years of age. J Pediatr Gastroenterol Nutr 2010;50:43–48.
28 Maki M, Holm K, Lipsanen V, et al: Serological markers and HLA genes among healthy first-degree relatives of patients with coeliac disease. Lancet 1991;338:1350–1353.
29 Kurppa K, Collin P, Viljamaa M, et al: Diagnosing mild enteropathy celiac disease: a randomized, controlled clinical study. Gastroenterology 2009;136:816–823.
30 Molberg O, McAdam SN, Korner R, et al: Tissue transglutaminase selectively modifies gliadin peptides that are recognized by gut-derived T cells in celiac disease. Nat Med 1998; 4:713–717.
31 Dieterich W, Ehnis T, Bauer M, et al: Identification of tissue transglutaminase as the autoantigen of celiac disease. Nat Med 1997;3: 797–801.
32 Abadie V, Sollid LM, Barreiro LB, et al: Integration of genetic and immunological insights into a model of celiac disease pathogenesis. Annu Rev Immunol 2011;29:493–525.
33 Jabri B, Sollid LM: Mechanisms of disease: immunopathogenesis of celiac disease. Nat Clin Pract Gastroenterol Hepatol 2006;3: 516–525.
34 Schuppan D, Junker Y, Barisani D: Celiac disease: from pathogenesis to novel therapies. Gastroenterology 2009;137:1912–1933.
35 Sollid LM, Jabri B: Celiac disease and transglutaminase 2: a model for posttranslational modification of antigens and HLA association in the pathogenesis of autoimmune disorders. Curr Opin Immunol 2011;23:732–738.
36 Lewis NR, Scott BB: Meta-analysis: deamidated gliadin peptide antibody and tissue transglutaminase antibody compared as screening tests for coeliac disease. Aliment Pharmacol Ther 2010;31:73–81.
37 Sardy M, Karpati S, Peterfy F, et al: Comparison of a tissue transglutaminase ELISA with the endomysium antibody test in the diagnosis of gluten-sensitive enteropathy. Z Gastroenterol 2000;38:357–364.
38 Tonutti E, Visentini D, Bizzaro N, et al: The role of antitissue transglutaminase assay for the diagnosis and monitoring of coeliac disease: a French-Italian multicentre study. J Clin Pathol 2003;56:389–393.
39 Raivio T, Korponay-Szabo IR, Paajanen T, et al: Comparison of a novel whole blood transglutaminase-based ELISA with a whole blood rapid antibody test and established conventional serological celiac disease assays. J Pediatr Gastroenterol Nutr 2008;47:562–567.
40 Sugai E, Vazquez H, Nachman F, et al: Accuracy of testing for antibodies to synthetic gliadin-related peptides in celiac disease. Clin Gastroenterol Hepatol 2006;4:1112–1117.
41 Volta U, Granito A, Fiorini E, et al: Usefulness of antibodies to deamidated gliadin peptides in celiac disease diagnosis and follow-up. Dig Dis Sci 2008;53:1582–1588.
42 Volta U, Granito A, Parisi C, et al: Deamidated gliadin peptide antibodies as a routine test for celiac disease: a prospective analysis. J Clin Gastroenterol 2010;44:186–190.
43 Volta U, Villanacci V: Celiac disease: diagnostic criteria in progress. Cell Mol Immunol 2011;8:96–102.
44 Villalta D, Tonutti E, Prause C, et al: IgG antibodies against deamidated gliadin peptides for diagnosis of celiac disease in patients with IgA deficiency. Clin Chem 2010;56:464–468.
45 Korponay-Szabo IR, Szabados K, Pusztai J, et al: Population screening for coeliac disease in primary care by district nurses using a rapid antibody test: diagnostic accuracy and feasibility study. BMJ 2007;335:1244–1247.
46 Windmueller HG, Spaeth AE: Source and fate of circulating citrulline. Am J Physiol 1981; 241:E473–E480.
47 Wakabayashi Y, Henslee JG, Jones ME: Pyrroline-5-carboxylate synthesis from glutamate by rat intestinal mucosa. Subcellular localization and temperature stability. J Biol Chem 1983;258:3873–3882.
48 Wakabayashi Y, Yamada E, Hasegawa T, et al: Enzymological evidence for the indispensability of small intestine in the synthesis of arginine from glutamate. I. Pyrroline-5-carboxylate synthase. Arch Biochem Biophys 1991; 291:1–8.
49 Crenn P, De Truchis P, Neveux N, et al: Plasma citrulline is a biomarker of enterocyte mass and an indicator of parenteral nutrition in HIV-infected patients. Am J Clin Nutr 2009;90:587–594.
50 Papadia C, Kelly P, Caini S, et al: Plasma citrulline as a quantitative biomarker of HIV-associated villous atrophy in a tropical enteropathy population. Clin Nutr 2010;29:795–800.
51 Crenn P, Vahedi K, Lavergne-Slove A, et al: Plasma citrulline: a marker of enterocyte mass in villous atrophy-associated small bowel disease. Gastroenterology 2003;124:1210–1219.
52 Ioannou HP, Fotoulaki M, Pavlitou A, et al: Plasma citrulline levels in paediatric patients with celiac disease and the effect of a gluten-free diet. Eur J Gastroenterol Hepatol 2011; 23:245–249.
53 Miceli E, Poggi N, Missanelli A, et al: Is serum citrulline measurement clinically useful in coeliac disease? Intern Emerg Med 2008;3: 233–236.
54 Peters JH, Wierdsma NJ, Teerlink T, et al: Poor diagnostic accuracy of a single fasting plasma citrulline concentration to assess intestinal energy absorption capacity. Am J Gastroenterol 2007;102:2814–2819.
55 Peters JH, Wierdsma NJ, Teerlink T, et al: The citrulline generation test: proposal for a new enterocyte function test. Aliment Pharmacol Ther 2008;27:1300–1310.
56 Pelsers MM, Hermens WT, Glatz JF: Fatty acid-binding proteins as plasma markers of tissue injury. Clin Chim Acta 2005;352:15–35.
57 Derikx JP, Vreugdenhil AC, Van den Neucker AM, et al: A pilot study on the noninvasive evaluation of intestinal damage in celiac disease using I-FABP and L-FABP. J Clin Gastroenterol 2009;43:727–733.
58 Derikx JP, Poeze M, van Bijnen AA, et al: Evidence for intestinal and liver epithelial cell injury in the early phase of sepsis. Shock 2007; 28:544–548.
59 Derikx JP, Evennett NJ, Degraeuwe PL, et al: Urine based detection of intestinal mucosal cell damage in neonates with suspected necrotising enterocolitis. Gut 2007;56:1473–1475.
60 Schellekens DH, Grootjans J, Dello SA, et al: Plasma intestinal fatty acid-binding protein levels correlate with morphologic epithelial intestinal damage in a human translational ischemia-reperfusion model. J Clin Gastroenterol 2014;48:253–260.
61 Vreugdenhil AC, Wolters VM, Adriaanse MP, et al: Additional value of serum I-FABP levels for evaluating celiac disease activity in children. Scand J Gastroenterol 2011;46: 1435–1441.
62 Adriaanse MP, Tack GJ, Passos VL, et al: Serum I-FABP as marker for enterocyte damage in coeliac disease and its relation to villous atrophy and circulating autoantibodies. Aliment Pharmacol Ther 2013;37:482–490.
63 Wahab PJ, Meijer JW, Mulder CJ: Histologic follow-up of people with celiac disease on a gluten-free diet: slow and incomplete recovery. Am J Clin Pathol 2002;118:459–463.
64 Bardella MT, Velio P, Cesana BM, et al: Coeliac disease: a histological follow-up study. Histopathology 2007;50:465–471.
65 Lee AR, Ng DL, Diamond B, et al: Living with coeliac disease: survey results from the USA. J Hum Nutr Diet 2012;25:233–238.
66 Leffler DA, Edwards-George J, Dennis M, et al: Factors that influence adherence to a gluten-free diet in adults with celiac disease. Dig Dis Sci 2008;53:1573–1581.
67 Mahadev S, Simpson S, Lebwohl B, et al: Is dietitian use associated with celiac disease outcomes? Nutrients 2013;5:1585–1594.
68 Barratt SM, Leeds JS, Sanders DS: Quality of life in coeliac disease is determined by perceived degree of difficulty adhering to a gluten-free diet, not the level of dietary adherence ultimately achieved. J Gastrointest Liver Dis 2011;20:241–245.

69 Theethira TG, Dennis M, Leffler DA: Nutritional consequences of celiac disease and the gluten-free diet. Expert Rev Gastroenterol Hepatol 2014;8:123–129.
70 Kabbani TA, Goldberg A, Kelly CP, et al: Body mass index and the risk of obesity in coeliac disease treated with the gluten-free diet. Aliment Pharmacol Ther 2012;35:723–729.
71 Abid N, McGlone O, Cardwell C, et al: Clinical and metabolic effects of gluten free diet in children with type 1 diabetes and coeliac disease. Pediatr Diabetes 2011;12:322–325.
72 Lebwohl B, Granath F, Ekbom A, et al: Mucosal healing and mortality in coeliac disease. Aliment Pharmacol Ther 2013;37:332–339.
73 Biagi F, Corazza GR: Mortality in celiac disease. Nat Rev Gastroenterol Hepatol 2010;7:158–162.
74 Rubio-Tapia A, Rahim MW, See JA, et al: Mucosal recovery and mortality in adults with celiac disease after treatment with a gluten-free diet. Am J Gastroenterol 2010;105:1412–1420.
75 AGA Institute: AGA Institute medical position statement on the diagnosis and management of celiac disease. Gastroenterology 2006;131:1977–1980.
76 Tursi A, Brandimarte G, Giorgetti GM: Prevalence of antitissue transglutaminase antibodies in different degrees of intestinal damage in celiac disease. J Clin Gastroenterol 2003;36:219–221.
77 Midhagen G, Aberg AK, Olcen P, et al: Antibody levels in adult patients with coeliac disease during gluten-free diet: a rapid initial decrease of clinical importance. J Intern Med 2004;256:519–524.
78 Dickey W, Hughes DF, McMillan SA: Disappearance of endomysial antibodies in treated celiac disease does not indicate histological recovery. Am J Gastroenterol 2000;95:712–714.
79 Dipper CR, Maitra S, Thomas R, et al: Anti-tissue transglutaminase antibodies in the follow-up of adult coeliac disease. Aliment Pharmacol Ther 2009;30:236–244.
80 Leffler D, Schuppan D, Pallav K, et al: Kinetics of the histological, serological and symptomatic responses to gluten challenge in adults with coeliac disease. Gut 2013;62:996–1004.
81 Leffler DA, Edwards George JB, Dennis M, et al: A prospective comparative study of five measures of gluten-free diet adherence in adults with coeliac disease. Aliment Pharmacol Ther 2007;26:1227–1235.
82 Vahedi K, Mascart F, Mary JY, et al: Reliability of antitransglutaminase antibodies as predictors of gluten-free diet compliance in adult celiac disease. Am J Gastroenterol 2003;98:1079–1087.
83 Tursi A, Brandimarte G, Giorgetti GM: Lack of usefulness of anti-transglutaminase antibodies in assessing histologic recovery after gluten-free diet in celiac disease. J Clin Gastroenterol 2003;37:387–391.

Dig Dis 2015;33:244–251
DOI: 10.1159/000369510

Videocapsule Endoscopy in Celiac Disease: Indications and Timing

Emanuele Rondonotti Silvia Paggi

Gastroenterology Unit, Ospedale Valduce, Como, Italy

Key Words

Celiac disease · Enteropathy-associated T-cell lymphoma · Refractory celiac disease · Ulcerative jejunitis · Videocapsule endoscopy

Abstract

Background: Because of its technical characteristics (i.e. 8-fold magnification, capability to inspect the entire small bowel) and minimal invasiveness, videocapsule endoscopy (VCE) has been proposed as a useful tool for managing patients with celiac disease (CD). ***Key Messages:*** Although VCE has been found to be highly sensitive and specific in identifying CD endoscopic markers, it is still inadequate to replace esophagogastroduodenoscopy (EGD) with biopsies in the diagnosis of CD. Nevertheless, it represents a reliable alternative in patients unable or unwilling to undergo EGD. Up to now, available studies have failed to identify any correlation between the length of small bowel involvement and the severity of symptoms. The available evidence on the use of VCE in diagnosing CD in equivocal cases (patients with positive serology and negative or nonspecific histology or those with negative serology and histologically proven villous atrophy) is limited, and its role is still under discussion. In CD patients not improving on gluten-free diet, a complete workup is necessary. In patients with nonresponsive (NRCD) or refractory CD (RCD), VCE has been shown to be able not only to detect significant findings, driving further management, but also to rule out major complications. Nevertheless, in this setting, the inability of VCE to take tissue samples and the risk of capsule retention can represent major limitations. ***Conclusions:*** At the present time, for diagnostic purposes, VCE can be proposed only in patients unable or unwilling to undergo EGD, whereas it could be useful in some equivocal cases. Conversely, there is no room for VCE either to estimate the length of the small bowel affected by villous atrophy or to follow up patients improving on gluten-free diet. In patients with NRCD or RCD, VCE can play a role, but it should be combined with other diagnostic techniques.

Introduction

Until the introduction of videocapsule endoscopy (VCE) into clinical practice, the small bowel was very difficult to explore by the available techniques. As compared with other diagnostic techniques, VCE provides a reliable noninvasive and well-tolerated method to inspect the entire small bowel, allowing a closer look at the intestinal mucosa. In fact, VCE is equipped with a wide-angle camera with an 8-fold magnification capability, and it is potentially able to assess not only obvious mucosal changes (i.e. vascular lesions, ulcers, erosions, masses, etc.) but

KARGER 125

E-Mail karger@karger.com
www.karger.com/ddi

0257–2753/15/0332–0244$39.50/0

Emanuele Rondonotti, MD, PhD
Gastroenterology Unit, Ospedale Valduce
Via Dante 10
IT–22100 Como (Italy)
E-Mail ema.rondo@gmail.com

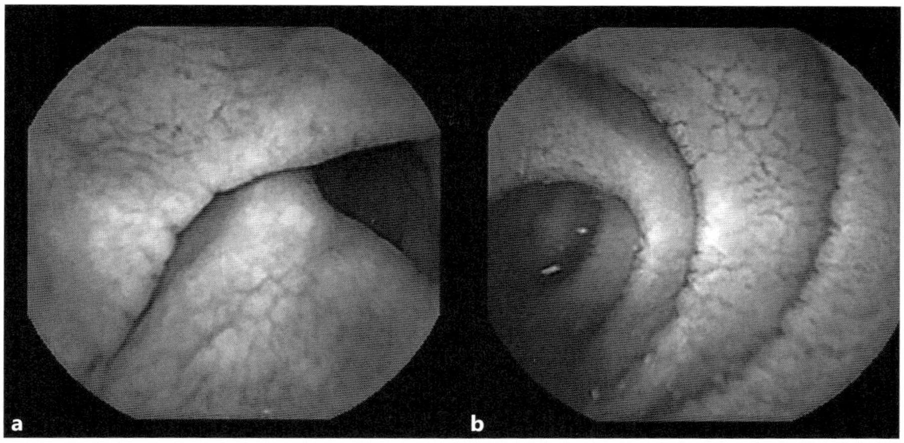

Fig. 1. Endoscopic markers identified by VCE in a patient with suspected CD: mucosal fissures (**a**) and scalloping of folds (**b**).

also villous structure. Because of its technical peculiarities and thanks to the excellent safety and diagnostic profile observed in other clinical settings (i.e. obscure gastrointestinal bleeding, Crohn's disease, etc.) VCE represents an attractive tool for the management of patients with celiac disease (CD), which primarily affects the small bowel mucosa. On the other hand, VCE has some limitations, such as the inability to collect tissue samples and the risk of device retention, which could prevent its use in the setting of CD.

Taking into account potential advantages and disadvantages of VCE, in the next few paragraphs we will review its possible role in the diagnostic workup of patients suspected to have CD (those with symptoms and positive CD serology but also in the more challenging patients in which duodenal histology and CD serology show conflicting results) and in the management of those with known CD to evaluate the response to gluten-free diet (GFD) or in case of nonresponsive or complicated CD.

Diagnosis of Suspected CD

When CD is suspected, the first diagnostic step is testing for specific antibodies. In everyday clinical practice, the IgA antiendomysial (EMA) and the IgA anti-tissue transglutaminase (TTG) tests, which are both highly sensitive and specific (values exceeding 95% in most studies), are primarily used to screen either symptomatic or asymptomatic at-risk individuals [1, 2]. Patients testing positive, together with those with high clinical suspicion despite negative antibody test, are required to undergo esophagogastroduodenoscopy (EGD) with small bowel biopsies, which is the current gold standard test for CD diagnosis [1].

Nevertheless, EGD is perceived by patients as an invasive procedure; it is unable to evaluate the small bowel mucosa beyond the duodenum and, more importantly, small bowel biopsies taken during the procedure can be affected by some pitfalls hampering the final diagnosis. Indeed, small bowel mucosal changes in CD are often patchy [3–5], and duodenal biopsy sampling may be affected by specimen orientation and fixation artifacts [6]. Therefore, several efforts have been made to find new tools to improve the sampling methods (e.g. jumbo forceps) [7], to target biopsies (e.g. immersion and/or magnification techniques) or to completely avoid small bowel biopsies (e.g. by optical coherence tomography, VCE) [8].

Noteworthy, VCE cannot take biopsies, so that the VCE diagnosis of CD is based on the recognition of the so-called 'CD endoscopic markers'. These are characteristic, although not absolute disease-specific, endoscopic findings which have been described in the duodenum and jejunum in patients with CD [9]. They include reduction in the number or scalloping of duodenal folds, mucosal fissures, mosaic pattern, visible mucosal vessels or nodularity (fig. 1). Although these endoscopic markers, when identified during conventional EGD, have shown good specificity (about 95–100%) for the diagnosis of CD, they are lacking in sensitivity (50–80%) [9–11]. However, these figures refer to endoscopic markers identified by conventional EGD. As aforementioned, VCE differs from EGD in several technical aspects (wider angle of view, 8-fold magnification, absence of insufflation, underwater navigation), which can increase its capability to recognize these endoscopic markers. Moreover, in 2008, Murray et al. [12] evaluating 35 biopsy-proven CD patients, confirmed that VCE had better overall sensitivity for the detection of endoscopic markers as compared with upper endoscopy (92 vs. 55%, $p < 0.05$). In addition, the VCE, providing an extensive view of the small bowel beyond the duodenum, can potentially overcome the issue of patchiness of mucosal lesions.

Interestingly, even when VCE is compared with duodenal histology, the diagnostic performance is high. In the meta-analysis by Rokkas and Niv [13], which included 6 studies, collecting overall 166 patients with suspected CD (the majority of them with elevated EMA or TTG antibodies titles), the pooled sensitivity of VCE for the detection of mucosal changes in the small bowel was 89% (95% CI: 82–94%), while the specificity was 95% (95% CI: 89–98%). Accordingly, the pooled positive and negative likelihood ratios were 12.90 (95% CI: 2.89–57.58) and 0.16 (95% CI: 0.1–0.25), respectively. These figures suggest that when such intestinal mucosal changes are observed during VCE, patients have a high probability of having CD, whereas, on the other hand a normal capsule endoscopy pattern cannot definitively exclude CD.

Nevertheless, these interesting data deserve a critical appraisal. Although they accurately reflect real life, when patients are selected for VCE on the basis of positive serology, the high pre-test probability of CD in this population can potentially bias the observed results, overestimating its confirmatory power. Furthermore, in the majority of studies, the VCE videos have been reviewed by endoscopists with extensive experience in capsule endoscopy. Even in this setting, the interobserver agreement is often poor or fair (K values between 0.26 and 0.5) [12, 14, 15], and it further decreases when videos are evaluated by reviewers with limited experience [14]. In addition, the described mucosal changes are not strictly disease-specific and can be observed in a variety of other conditions such as infective enteritis (i.e. giardiasis, cytomegalovirus infection, HIV enteropathy, tuberculosis, etc.), immune disorders (i.e. agammaglobulinemia), Crohn's disease, amyloidosis, etc. [16]. Last but not least, EGD with biopsies is readily available worldwide and it is cheaper in comparison with VCE, although no specific cost-effectiveness studies have been performed yet.

Taking into account all these issues, EGD with biopsies remains the gold standard for the diagnosis of CD, whereas VCE can be considered as a reliable alternative in patients unable or unwilling to undergo EGD with biopsies [1, 16–18]. In line with this, Chang et al. [19] published a case series of 4 patients, with positive CD serology, in which EGD was declined or not performed because of coagulative disorders (von Willebrand disease). In all these patients, CD diagnosis was reached by means of VCE, and all of them showed a clinical/serological improvement with GFD.

Equivocal Cases

As reported above, highly sensitive and specific serological tests for CD (namely EMA or TTG) together with the villous atrophy observed in duodenal biopsies represent 'the cornerstones' for the diagnosis of CD. Therefore, when a positive serological test is accompanied by a histologically confirmed villous atrophy, the GFD is warranted; conversely, the negative results of both these tests rule out the diagnosis of CD in the large majority of cases. However, when the two tests yield conflicting results, a clinical diagnostic challenge rises. VCE has been advocated as a helpful diagnostic tool to evaluate these equivocal cases.

Patients with Positive Serology and Negative or Nonspecific Duodenal Histology

Several studies demonstrated that histological abnormalities associated with CD can be patchy [20–22]. Therefore, multiple biopsies of the duodenum should be performed if the diagnosis of CD is considered; a recent study performed in the US collecting 132,352 patients who underwent duodenal biopsy showed that the probability of CD diagnosis was significantly increased when four specimens or more were collected [23]. Nevertheless, even with an adequate number of specimens, duodenal biopsies can be affected by a sampling error. Conversely VCE, being equipped with a wide angle and allowing to evaluate the entire organ, may overcome these limitations related to the patchiness of mucosal changes. This has been clearly shown in a patient with biopsy-proven dermatitis herpetiformis, with a positive EMA test and negative duodenal histology, in which typical patchy mucosal changes were identified by VCE [24].

Unfortunately, the studies evaluating patients with positive serology and negative or nonspecific duodenal histology are few, collect a small number of patients and yield inconsistent evidence.

In 2006, Adler et al. [25] evaluated by VCE 22 patients with symptoms (fulfilling the Rome criteria for the diagnosis of irritable bowel syndrome), positive celiac serology and normal duodenal histology. Interestingly, although VCE detected abnormalities within the small bowel in 55% of cases, the findings were mostly minor and subtle (i.e. blunted villi, erythema, fissures), which have also been described in about 10–15% of healthy controls undergoing VCE. In addition, these findings were found either in patients with and without human leukocyte antigen (HLA) genotype predisposing to CD. Last but not least, only 3 patients (13%) were EMA or TTG positive. Therefore, the authors concluded that, in this setting, VCE has a limited role, being potentially helpful in a subset of patients (those with positive HLA and small bowel mucosal changes) which is probably worth a close follow-up.

In 2011, Lidums et al. [26] focused their attention on patients with positive serological tests (EMA or TTG) and negative duodenal histology. They found that VCE did not reveal any endoscopic features of CD in all the 8 enrolled patients. More recently, Kurien et al. [27] evaluated 30 patients with nonspecific duodenal histology (namely Marsh I or Marsh II). Of them, only 6 (20%) had positive serology (EMA or TTG), and only one was finally diagnosed with CD and another one with Crohn's disease.

Given this limited evidence, at the present time, the repetition of EGD with biopsies (or push enteroscopy) [28] together with HLA testing, which may help to exclude CD, given its high negative predictive value [1, 29], remains the most viable option. Nevertheless, VCE seems to have a potential role in excluding other diseases, and further studies are warranted, mostly to better identify the subset of patients suitable to receive VCE.

Patients with Negative Serology and Histologically Proven Villous Atrophy

Although in patients with symptoms suggesting CD the positive predictive value of TTG and EMA is extremely high, TTG may be negative in 5–16% of patients with villous atrophy [1, 30, 31]. On the other hand, villous atrophy can be detected in several diseases other than CD, and it always deserves further investigation.

In the study on equivocal CD cases by Kurien et al. [27], the authors included 32 patients with antibody-negative VA. These patients were extensively investigated for CD including HLA testing, by monitoring response to GFD and in some cases by repeating duodenal biopsies. On the basis of VCE findings and other ancillary tests, 7 patients could be diagnosed with extensive villous atrophy and 2 further patients were diagnosed with small bowel Crohn's disease (9/32; 28%). Again, this is a single small study, and further work is needed to clarify the role of VCE in antibody-negative villous atrophy cases. This is particularly important as VCE alone is probably insufficient to confirm a diagnosis of CD as endoscopic markers are not specific to CD; they rather represent predictors of mucosal disease [16].

CD Extent Assessment and Follow-Up of Responsive CD Patients

Previous studies, in which extensive endoscopic evaluation of the small bowel was performed by means of push enteroscopy or ileocolonoscopy in untreated CD patients, showed that mucosal changes extend beyond the duodenum, and villous atrophy, detected in the proximal intestine, gradually decreases towards the distal intestine [32, 33]. A potential correlation between the severity of symptoms and the extent of mucosal damage has also been postulated. In addition, the complications of untreated CD tend to be located in the distal small bowel. For all these reasons, VCE, owing to the lack of invasiveness and the ability to explore the entire small bowel, appeared as an attractive diagnostic tool to estimate the extent of mucosal damage at the time of diagnosis and to monitor the mucosal changes in the deep small bowel over time.

All the studies where VCE was performed at the time of diagnosis confirmed that mucosal changes extend distally, involving the jejunum in two thirds of patients, reaching the terminal ileum in 10% of cases. Nevertheless, available studies failed in demonstrating any correlation between the extent of enteropathy and the severity of clinical manifestations at the time of diagnosis, while they reported a significant correlation with EMA titles.

So far, 2 studies have been performed to evaluate the possible role of VCE in monitoring patients over time [12, 34]. By repeating VCE after 12 months in patients on strict GFD with substantial improvement of symptoms, Lidums et al. [34] observed a significant reduction of the mucosal changes. Similarly, Murray et al. [12] confirmed that with GFD, the healing process is more evident in the distal than in the proximal small bowel.

Noteworthy, at present, a reliable method to estimate the length of the small bowel affected by CD mucosal changes is lacking. In 2 recent studies mentioned above [12, 34], the authors based the estimation of the length of the small bowel with typical mucosal changes on the percentage of the small bowel transit time. Nevertheless, in about 20% of patients VCE does not allow a complete inspection of the entire small bowel, thus preventing the calculation of small bowel transit time. Moreover, it is well documented that the capsule transit differs in different small bowel segments. In addition, recent data seem to suggest that the intestinal motility differs between CD patients and controls [35].

On the grounds of these data, the systematic assessment by VCE of the length of small bowel showing typical mucosal changes at time of diagnosis as well as the monitoring of small bowel involvement in patients improving on GFD do not seem to be justified [16, 18].

Nonresponsive and Refractory CD

In about 30% of patients diagnosed with CD, symptoms persist despite a GFD or relapse after an initial response [1, 36]. Nonresponsive CD (NRCD) is usually defined as persistent symptoms, signs or laboratory abnormalities typical of CD despite 6–12 months of dietary gluten avoidance [1, 36, 37]. The major cause of failure is a continuing ingestion of gluten. In fact, a minimal but continuous intake of gluten can prevent mucosal recovery. However, when the dietary compliance is established by a dietician and the patient still does not respond, the initial diagnosis of CD must be reassessed and other reasons for persisting symptoms (i.e. pancreatic insufficiency, irritable bowel syndrome, bacterial overgrowth, inflammatory bowel disease, microscopic colitis, tropical sprue, non-CD-related small bowel neoplasm; fig. 2) must be ruled out. When clinical symptoms and histological abnormalities persist or recur despite a strict adherence to the diet for more than 12 months, patients are defined as suffering from refractory CD (RCD) [1, 36, 37]. These cases represent a small minority of CD patients (about 1–2%) but are more prone to developing ulcerative jejunitis and enteropathy-associated T-cell lymphoma (EATL) [1, 38, 39].

Unfortunately, the papers evaluating the role of VCE in NRCD or RCD patients are few (table 1) and mostly retrospective. Moreover, a wide heterogeneity of patients included either in different studies or within the same study has to be mentioned. Some studies include mostly patients with NRCD, while other include patients with RCD or patients at increased risk of developing small bowel neoplasm [27, 40–46]. These papers often lack a control group, and the majority of them test VCE as the only diagnostic procedure. This has led to the overestimation of the possible contribution of VCE in this subset of patients. Of note, some findings identified at VCE were evaluated by reviewers as non-CD specific, and standardized criteria for classifying the clinical relevance of the VCE are lacking. In the most recently published papers [42, 45], the criteria for classifying the severity of inflammatory findings (ulcers and erosions) was the size or the

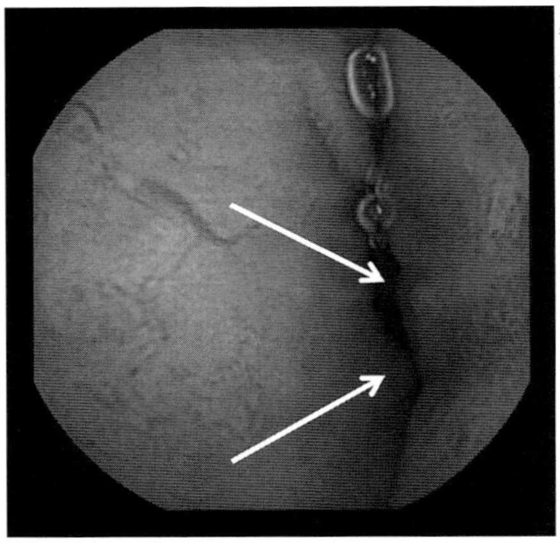

Fig. 2. Ulcerated gastrointestinal stromal tumor (arrows) diagnosed in a CD patient with long-lasting iron deficiency anemia.

number of lesions (diameter ≥1 cm or number ≥5 were considered index of severity); however, this classification is completely arbitrary and needs to be validated.

In spite of all these limitations, papers that focused on NRCD or RCD patients confirm that there are some subgroups at higher risk of developing complications (RCD type II patients or patients with a history of small bowel neoplasms) suitable to receive VCE. In this setting, VCE plays a key role: when positive, it drives further examinations (i.e. device-assisted enteroscopy) and when negative it spares other invasive diagnostic procedures. Barret at al. [45] observed that stopping investigations when VCE was normal would have led to several upper enteroscopies being spared.

In light of these studies (summarized in table 1) [27, 40–46], the use of VCE in NRCD or RCD patients may therefore be justified, keeping in mind that data coming from this procedure have to be part of a complex diagnostic workup including EGD with biopsies, flow cytometry, radiology and device-assisted enteroscopy [1, 16, 18, 47]. In line with this, the most recently published studies [42, 45] focused their attention on the contribution of VCE not only to the diagnostic process but also as a possible predictor of poor prognosis.

Barret et al. [45] compared the endoscopic findings of 38 CD patients (9 symptomatic CD patients, 11 RCDI and 18 RCDII patients) with those from 45 non-CD patients. They observed that villous atrophy, numerous or distally located small bowel ulcers are more frequent in CD patients than in controls. Among RCD patients, the mucosal damage was more extensive in RCDII than in RCDI patients and, interestingly, VCE had a major clinical im-

Table 1. VCE in NRCD and RCD: summary of available studies

Study	Year	Study design	Control group	Patients	Patient type	Patients with negative VCE, %	Patients with relevant findings at VCE[1], %	Capsule retention
Culliford et al. [46]	2005	prospective	no	47	CCD	13	59	0/47
Daum et al. [43]	2006	retrospective	no	14	RCD	7	7	0/14
Maiden et al. [40]	2007	prospective	no	19	NRCD	53	10	0/19
Collin et al. [44]	2011	retrospective	yes	33	RCD	27	49	0/16
Atlas et al. [41]	2011	retrospective	yes	42	NRCD	n.r.	5	n.r.
Barett et al. [45]	2012	retrospective	yes	38	RCD, SCD	n.r.	19	0/38
Van Weyenberg et al. [42]	2013	retrospective	no	48	NRCD	n.r.	23	0/48
Kurien et al. [27]	2013	prospective	no	69	NRCD	43	13	0/69

CCD = Complicated celiac disease; n.r. = not reported; SCD = symptomatic celiac disease.
[1] Relevant findings include EATL, diffuse inflammatory changes, small bowel masses and small bowel strictures.

pact by revealing ulcerated jejunal strictures, which turned out to be lymphomas in 2 cases, and ulcerative jejunitis warranting a specific treatment.

More recently, Van Weyenberg et al. [42] published a series of 48 NRCD patients undergoing a complete diagnostic workup (including flow cytometry and radiological or device-assisted enteroscopy, when appropriate). The authors, comparing patients with an increased risk of poor prognosis (RCDII or secondary EATL) with those without increased risk of complications (uncomplicated CD or RCDI), performed a multivariate analysis which showed that the absence of capsule progression and presence of focal erythema were independently associated with a poor prognosis. In this study, none of the 28 patients without these endoscopic features, 2/15 patients with one feature and 4/5 with both of them died during the follow-up, respectively.

Interestingly, although patients with ulcerative jejunitis and EATL carry a significant risk of small bowel strictures, none of the papers published so far reported a case of capsule retention. This can be due to the strict selection of patients included in the published studies. Therefore, in clinical practice in patients with NRCD or RCD, VCE should be preceded by other examinations aimed at excluding small bowel strictures.

Future Directions

The first video capsule endoscope was designed in 2001 by G. Iddan as a new tool for the investigation of the small bowel. It was initially manufactured and marketed by only one company (Given Imaging, Yokneam, Israel), whereas, to date, multiple VCE systems for the study of the small bowel are available. Since its introduction into clinical practice, many efforts have been made in order to overcome the limitations of VCE. Both the hardware (i.e. angle of view, battery life, automatic light control) and the software (i.e. introduction of the blue mode) improved significantly. Moreover, techniques for the active control of the capsule movement, such as a magnetic steering mechanism by external manipulation and a locomotive mechanism by internal manipulation are under evaluation as well as new technologies allowing a more accurate localization of VCE findings.

One of the main limitations of VCE in CD concerns the interobserver agreement in recognizing endoscopic markers, which is often poor or fair and strictly depends on the reviewer expertise. Various automatic image analysis algorithms (based on the shape-from-shadow 3-D image reconstruction, or image texture analysis) have been tested [48] in order to allow a quantitative evaluation of villous atrophy. Interestingly, they found that using these algorithms, celiacs were often quantitatively distinguishable from controls.

The same authors have also developed a system for analyzing images that allows estimating the motility of the VCE [35]. Although previous clinical studies had not shown significant differences in transit time through the small intestine in CD patients [49], they found a good sensitivity of the motility analysis which allowed discriminating CD patients from healthy controls.

More recently, these authors published a study in which the images obtained in celiac patients and controls were analyzed by combining motility estimation with different other image analysis techniques (such as texture analysis, volumetric reconstruction and image transformation) [50]. The aim of the study was to test the capability of the automatic system to predict villous atrophy. They found that automata-based polling may be useful to set out the presence of mucosal atrophy. Since the method is quantitative and automated, it can potentially eliminate observer bias and enable the detection of subtle abnormalities in patients lacking a clear diagnosis. This system could also be helpful in estimating the length of the small bowel affected by villous atrophy.

Unfortunately, these studies included a limited number of patients, and these image analysis systems are not readily available; therefore, further studies are needed to evaluate the impact of these new tools in clinical practice.

Disclosure Statement

All the authors declare no conflict of interest.

References

1 Rubio-Tapia A, Hill ID, Kelly CP, Calderwood AH, Murray JA; American College of Gastroenterology: ACG clinical guidelines: diagnosis and management of celiac disease. Am J Gastroenterol 2013;108:656–676.

2 Lewis NR, Scott BB: Meta-analysis: deamidated gliadin peptide antibody and tissue transglutaminase antibody compared as screening tests for coeliac disease. Aliment Pharmacol Ther 2010;31:73–81.

3 Hopper AD, Cross SS, Sanders DS: Patchy villous atrophy in adult patients with suspected gluten-sensitive enteropathy: is a multiple duodenal biopsy strategy appropriate? Endoscopy 2007;39:219–224.

4 Green PHR: Celiac disease: how many biopsies for diagnosis? Gastrointest Endosc 2008;67:1088–1090.

5 Pais WP, Duerksen DR, Pettigrew NM, Bernstein CN: How many duodenal biopsy specimens are required to make a diagnosis of celiac disease? Gastrointest Endosc 2008;67:1082–1087.

6 Ravelli A, Villanacci V: Tricks of the trade: how to avoid histological pitfalls in celiac disease. Pathol Res Pract 2012;208:197–202.

7 Dandalides SM, Carey WD, Petras R, Achkar E: Endoscopic small bowel mucosal biopsy: a controlled trial evaluating forceps size and biopsy location in the diagnosis of normal and abnormal mucosal architecture. Gastrointest Endosc 1989;35:197–200.

8 Ianiro G, Gasbarrini A, Cammarota G: Endoscopic tools for the diagnosis and evaluation of celiac disease. World J Gastroenterol 2013;19:8562–8570.

9 Lee SK, Green PH: Endoscopy in celiac disease. Curr Opin Gastroenterol 2005;21:589–594.

10 Dickey W, Hughes D: Prevalence of celiac disease and its endoscopic markers among patients having routine upper gastrointestinal endoscopy. Am J Gastroenterol 1999;94:2182–2186.

11 Barada K, Habib RH, Malli A, Hashash JG, Halawi H, Maasri K, Tawil A, Mourad F, Sharara AI, Soweid A, Sukkarieh I, Chakhachiro Z, Jabbour M, Fasano A, Santora D, Arguelles C, Murray JA, Green PH: Prediction of celiac disease at endoscopy. Endoscopy 2014;46:110–119.

12 Murray JA, Rubio-Tapia A, Van Dyke CT, Brogan DL, Knipschield MA, Lahr B, Rumalla A, Zinsmeister AR, Gostout CJ: Mucosal atrophy in celiac disease: extent of involvement, correlation with clinical presentation, and response to treatment. Clin Gastroenterol Hepatol 2008;6:186–193.

13 Rokkas T, Niv Y: The role of video capsule endoscopy in the diagnosis of celiac disease: a meta-analysis. Eur J Gastroenterol Hepatol 2012;24:303–308.

14 Petroniene R, Dubcenco E, Baker JP, Ottaway CA, Tang SJ, Zanati SA, Streutker CJ, Gardiner GW, Warren RE, Jeejeebhoy KN: Given® Capsule Endocopy in celiac disease: evaluation of diagnostic accuracy and interobserver agreement. Am J Gastroenterol 2005;100:685–694.

15 Biagi F, Rondonotti E, Campanella J, Villa F, Bianchi PI, Klersy C, De Franchis R, Corazza GR: Video capsule endoscopy and histology for small bowel mucosa evaluation: a comparison performed by blinded observers. Clin Gastroenterol Hepatol 2006;4:998–1003.

16 Rahman I, Patel P, Rondonotti E, Koulaouzidis A, Pennazio M, Kalla R, Sidhu R, Mooney P, Sanders D, Despott EJ, Fraser C, Kurniawan N, Baltes P, Keuchel M, Davison C, Beejay N, Parke C, Panter S: Small bowel capsule endoscopy; in Li Z, Mc Alindon M, et al (eds): Handbook of Capsule Endoscopy. Dordrecht, Springer Science and Business Media, 2014, pp 47–118.

17 Rondonotti E, Villa F, Saladino V, de Franchis R: Enteroscopy in the diagnosis and management of celiac disease. Gastrointest Endosc Clin N Am 2009;19:445–460.

18 Ladas SD, Triantafyllou K, Spada C, Riccioni ME, Rey JF, Niv Y, Delvaux M, de Franchis R, Costamagna G, ESGE Clinical Guidelines Committee: European Society Gastrointestinal Endoscopy (ESGE) recommendations (2009) on clinical use of video capsule endoscopy to investigate small-bowel, esophageal and colonic diseases. Endoscopy 2010;42:220–227.

19 Chang MS, Rubin M, Lewis SK, Green PH: Diagnosing celiac disease by video capsule endoscopy (VCE) when esophagogastroduodenoscopy (EGD) and biopsy is unable to provide a diagnosis: a case series. BMC Gastroenterol 2012;12:90.

20 Ravelli A, Bolognini S, Gambarotti M, Villanacci V: Variability of histologic lesions in relation to biopsy site in gluten-sensitive enteropathy. Am J Gastroenterol 2005;100:177–185.

21 Ravelli A, Villanacci V, Monfredini C, Martinazzi S, Grassi V, Manenti S: How patchy is patchy villous atrophy? Distribution pattern of histological lesions in the duodenum of children with celiac disease. Am J Gastroenterol 2010;105:2103–2110.

22 Bonamico M, Mariani P, Thanasi E, Ferri M, Nenna R, Tiberti C, Mora B, Mazzilli MC, Magliocca FM: Patchy villous atrophy of the duodenum in childhood celiac disease. J Pediatr Gastroenterol Nutr 2004;38:204–207.

23 Lebwohl B, Kapel RC, Neugut AI, Green PH, Genta RM: Adherence to biopsy guidelines increases celiac disease diagnosis. Gastrointest Endosc 2011;74:103–109.

24 Rondonotti E, Spada C, Cave D, Pennazio M, Riccioni ME, De Vitis I, Schneider D, Sprujevnik T, Villa F, Langelier J, Arrigoni A, Costamagna G, de Franchis R: Video capsule enteroscopy in the diagnosis of celiac disease: a multicenter study. Am J Gastroenterol 2007;102:1624–1631.

25 Adler SN, Jacob H, Lijovetzky G, Mulder CJ, Zwiers A: Positive coeliac serology in irritable bowel syndrome patients with normal duodenal biopsies: video capsule endoscopy findings and HLA-DQ typing may affect clinical management. J Gastrointest Liver Dis 2006;15:221–225.

26 Lidums I, Cummins AG, Teo E: The role of capsule endoscopy in suspected celiac disease patients with positive celiac serology. Dig Dis Sci 2011;56:499–505.
27 Kurien M, Evans KE, Aziz I, Sidhu R, Drew K, Rogers TL, McAlindon ME, Sanders DS: Capsule endoscopy in adult celiac disease: a potential role in equivocal cases of celiac disease? Gastrointest Endosc 2013;77:227–232.
28 Höroldt BS, McAlindon ME, Stephenson TJ, Hadjivassiliou M, Sanders DS: Making the diagnosis of coeliac disease: is there a role for push enteroscopy? Eur J Gastroenterol Hepatol 2004;16:1143–1146.
29 Cassinotti A, Birindelli S, Clerici M, Trabattoni D, Lazzaroni M, Ardizzone S, Colombo R, Rossi E, Porro GB: HLA and autoimmune digestive disease: a clinically oriented review for gastroenterologists. Am J Gastroenterol 2009;104:195–217.
30 Li M, Yu L, Tiberti C, Bonamico M, Taki I, Miao D, Murray JA, Rewers MJ, Hoffenberg EJ, Agardh D, Mueller P, Stern M, Bonifacio E, Liu E: A report on the International Transglutaminase Autoantibody Workshop for Celiac Disease. Am J Gastroenterol 2009;104: 154–163.
31 Rashtak S, Ettore MW, Homburger HA, Murray JA: Comparative usefulness of deamidated gliadin antibodies in the diagnosis of celiac disease. Clin Gastroenterol Hepatol 2008;6: 426–432.
32 Cellier C, Cuillerier E, Patey-Mariaud de Serre N, Marteau P, Verkarre V, Brière J, Brousse N, Barbier JP, Schmitz J, Landi B: Push enteroscopy in celiac sprue and refractory sprue. Gastrointest Endosc 1999;50:613–617.
33 Hopper AD, Hurlstone DP, Leeds JS, McAlindon ME, Dube AK, Stephenson TJ, Sanders DS: The occurrence of terminal ileal histological abnormalities in patients with coeliac disease. Dig Liver Dis 2006;38:815–819.
34 Lidums I, Teo E, Field J, Cummins AG: Capsule endoscopy: a valuable tool in the follow-up of people with celiac disease on a gluten-free diet. Clin Transl Gastroenterol 2011;18:2.
35 Ciaccio EJ, Tennyson CA, Bhagat G, Lewis SK, Green PH: Quantitative estimates of motility from videocapsule endoscopy are useful to discern celiac patient from controls. Dig Dis Sci 2012;57:2936–2943.
36 Leffler DA, Dennis M, Hyett B, Kelly E, Schuppan D, Kelly CP: Etiologies and predictors of diagnosis in nonresponsive celiac disease. Clin Gastroenterol Hepatol 2007;5:445–450.
37 Ludvigsson JF, Leffler DA, Bai JC, Biagi F, Fasano A, Green PH, Hadjivassiliou M, Kaukinen K, Kelly CP, Leonard JN, Lundin KE, Murray JA, Sanders DS, Walker MM, Zingone F, Ciacci C: The Oslo definitions for coeliac disease and related terms. Gut 2013; 62:43–52.
38 Malamut G, Afchain P, Verkarre V, Lecomte T, Amiot A, Damotte D, Bouhnik Y, Colombel JF, Delchier JC, Allez M, Cosnes J, Lavergne-Slove A, Meresse B, Trinquart L, Macintyre E, Radford-Weiss I, Hermine O, Brousse N, Cerf-Bensussan N, Cellier C: Presentation and long-term follow-up of refractory celiac disease: comparison of type I with type II. Gastroenterology 2009;136:81–90.
39 Roshan B, Leffler DA, Jamma S, Dennis M, Sheth S, Falchuk K, Najarian R, Goldsmith J, Tariq S, Schuppan D, Kelly CP: The incidence and clinical spectrum of refractory celiac disease in a North American referral center. Am J Gastroenterol 2011;106:923–928.
40 Maiden L, Elliott T, McLaughlin SD, Ciclitira P: A blinded pilot comparison of capsule endoscopy and small bowel histology in unresponsive celiac disease. Dig Dis Sci 2009;54: 1280–1283.
41 Atlas DS, Rubio-Tapia A, Van Dyke CT, Lahr BD, Murray JA: Capsule endoscopy in nonresponsive celiac disease. Gastrointest Endosc 2011;74:1315–1322.
42 Van Weyenberg SJ, Smits F, Jacobs MA, Van Turenhout ST, Mulder CJ: Video capsule endoscopy in patients with nonresponsive celiac disease. J Clin Gastroenterol 2013;47:393–399.
43 Daum S, Wahnschaffe U, Glasenapp R, Borchert M, Ullrich R, Zeitz M, Faiss S: Capsule endoscopy in refractory celiac disease. Endoscopy 2007;39:455–458.
44 Collin P, Rondonotti E, Lundin KE, Spada C, Keuchel M, Kaukinen K, DE Franchis R, Jacobs MA, Villa F, Mulder CJ: Video capsule endoscopy in celiac disease: current clinical practice. J Dig Dis 2012;13:94–99.
45 Barret M, Malamut G, Rahmi G, Samaha E, Edery J, Verkarre V, Macintyre E, Lenain E, Chatellier G, Cerf-Bensussan N, Cellier C: Diagnostic yield of capsule endoscopy in refractory celiac disease. Am J Gastroenterol 2012; 107:1546–1553.
46 Culliford A, Daly J, Diamond B, Rubin M, Green PH: The value of wireless capsule endoscopy in patients with complicated celiac disease. Gastrointest Endosc 2005;62:55–61.
47 Tomba C, Elli L, Bardella MT, Soncini M, Contiero P, Roncoroni L, Locatelli M, Conte D: Enteroscopy for the early detection of small bowel tumours in at-risk celiac patients. Dig Liver Dis 2014;46:400–404.
48 Ciaccio EJ, Tennyson CA, Lewis SK, Krishnareddy S, Bhagat G, Green PH: Distinguishing patients with celiac disease by quantitative analysis of videocapsule endoscopy images. Comput Methods Programs Biomed 2010; 100:39–48.
49 Urgesi R, Cianci R, Bizzotto A, Costamagna G, Riccioni ME: Evaluation of gastric and small bowel transit times in coeliac disease with the small bowel PillCam®: a single centre study in a non gluten-free diet adult Italian population with coeliac disease. Eur Rev Med Pharmacol Sci 2013;17:1167–1173.
50 Ciaccio EJ, Tennyson CA, Bhagat G, Lewis SK, Green PH: Implementation of a polling protocol for predicting celiac disease in videocapsule analysis. World J Gastrointest Endosc 2013;5:313–322.

Dig Dis 2015;33:252–259
DOI: 10.1159/000369516

Small Bowel Imaging in Celiac Disease

Stijn J.B. Van Weyenberg[a] Chris J.J. Mulder[b] Jan Hein T.M. Van Waesberghe[c]

[a]Department of Gastroenterology and Hepatology, Leiden University Medical Center, Leiden, Departments of [b]Gastroenterology and Hepatology and [c]Radiology, VU University Medical Center, Amsterdam, The Netherlands

Key Words
Celiac disease · Radiology · Enteroclysis · Magnetic resonance imaging · Small intestine

Abstract
Background: Modern small bowel imaging techniques allow detailed depiction of small-intestinal abnormalities. The role of these techniques in the investigation of celiac disease is increasing, especially in patients with suspected complicated celiac disease. ***Key Messages:*** In general, there is no need for radiological small bowel imaging in uncomplicated celiac disease. It is however important that clinicians and radiologists are aware of certain specific radiological findings that may suggest celiac disease, especially since celiac disease is often not considered in adult patients, and small bowel radiology may be performed before specific tests for celiac disease. Radiological abnormalities can be observed with both conventional small bowel radiology studies, like small bowel follow-through or double-contrast small bowel enteroclysis, and newer modalities, like computed tomography or magnetic resonance enterography or enteroclysis. These signs include a decreased number of jejunal folds, an increased number of ileal folds, small bowel dilatation, wall thickening and intussusception. Extraintestinal abnormalities include mesenteric lymphadenopathy, vascular changes and splenic atrophy. Abnormalities congruent with refractory celiac disease type II include a severe decrease in jejunal folds, infiltration of the mesenteric fat and thickening of the small bowel wall. Additionally, a severely decreased splenic volume may indicate complicated celiac disease. Malignant complications of celiac disease, such as enteropathy-associated T-cell lymphoma and small-intestinal adenocarcinoma, can be reliably investigated with cross-sectional enteroclysis techniques. ***Conclusions:*** Small bowel imaging and especially cross-sectional enteroclysis techniques are important extensions to the diagnostic workup of clinicians involved in the care of patients with celiac disease, especially those with suspected complicated disease.

Introduction

With the current possibilities of serology and histology, radiology plays no important role in the diagnosis of celiac disease (CD). However, it is important that radiological features associated with CD are recognized, especially since in patients with nonspecific symptoms abdominal imaging may be performed before the diagnosis

KARGER 125
E-Mail karger@karger.com
www.karger.com/ddi

0257–2753/15/0332–0252$39.50/0

Stijn J.B. Van Weyenberg
Department of Gastroenterology and Hepatology
Leiden University Medical Center
Albinusdreef 2, NL–2333 ZA Leiden (The Netherlands)
E-Mail s.j.b.van_weyenberg@lumc.nl

Table 1. Diagnostic modalities in small bowel radiology

Modality	Invasiveness	Enteral contrast	Radiation exposure	Luminal detail	Wall detail	Extraintestinal detail	Availability	Costs
Plain abdominal X-ray	–	None	+	+	–	–	++++	+
SBFT	+	Oral	+++	++	+	–	+++	++
Conventional enteroclysis	+++	Nasojejunal tube	+++	+++	+	–	++	++
Double-contrast enteroclysis	+++	Nasojejunal tube	+++	++++	++	–	+	++
Abdominal ultrasound	–	None	–	+	+	++	++++	+
CT enterography	++	Oral	+++	+++	+++	+++	+++	++
CT enteroclysis	+++	Nasojejunal tube	+++	++++	++++	+++	++	++
MR enterography	++	Oral	–	+++	+++	+++	++	+++
MR enteroclysis	+++	Nasojejunal tube	+ (tube placement)	++++	++++	+++	+	+++

of CD is considered and specific testing has been performed. In patients with nonresponsive CD, the possibility of refractory CD (RCD), small bowel adenocarcinoma or lymphoma has to be considered. In these circumstances, small bowel imaging may provide important information.

This review aims to provide clinicians involved with the care for patients with CD with some basic knowledge on the strengths and limitations of modern small bowel radiology. Additionally, it aims to inform on the diagnostic accuracy of radiological findings associated with CD, as well as its complications, including RCD and small bowel malignancies.

Modalities in Small Bowel Radiology

In order to be able to appreciate the findings of small bowel radiology, or to efficiently order small bowel radiology, some knowledge on the possibilities and limitations of the different modalities and ways of contrast delivery is important (table 1). The ideal small bowel imaging method is noninvasive, does not require potentially toxic (intravenous) contrast agents, does not use ionizing radiation, and is able to depict the complete small-intestinal lumen, bowel wall, as well as extraluminal structures. In addition, the ideal modality needs to be widely available, result in easy to interpret images and be cost-effective [1]. Small bowel radiological modalities can be classified by the way the image is acquired: fluoroscopy, ultrasound (US), computed tomography (CT) or magnetic resonance (MR) imaging. Except for the modality used, another important factor is whether or not luminal contrast agents are being used, and if so, how these are administered: orally (enterography) or by means of a nasojejunal catheter (enteroclysis). The latter is considered to be more invasive, but allows periprocedural increasing of luminal contrast dose when suboptimal bowel distention is seen, which seems to be particularly important when information on the jejunum is needed [2].

Up to 10 years ago, most small bowel radiology was performed using fluoroscopic techniques. The most prevalent technique was small bowel follow-through (SBFT), which requires the ingestion of at least 0.5 liters of barium suspension. Fluoroscopy is performed when the barium progresses through the intestine. Manual palpation is usually needed to separate individual small bowel loops. Although easy to perform, the poor distention of the small bowel as well as the poor separation of segments limit its accuracy [1]. These problems can be overcome when the barium is administered directly into the small intestine using a fluoroscopically placed nasojejunal catheter, a technique that is called enteroclysis. Even better distention can be achieved when this is followed by administration of methylcellulose suspension or air to enable optimal distension of individual small bowel loops [3]. Limitations of fluoroscopic techniques include the limited information they provide on mural and extraintestinal abnormalities as well as the need for ionizing radiation.

CT is a widely available cross-sectional imaging method, often used in the evaluation of abdominal symptoms. In routine settings, too little luminal contrast agent is administered to prevent collapse of the small-intestinal lumen, and therefore information on the small intestine in limited. Bowel distention can be achieved either by increasing the dose of orally ingested contrast medium (enterography) or by administering methylcellulose (neutral enteral contrast) or barium (positive enteral contrast) directly into the small bowel by means of a nasojejunal catheter (enteroclysis) [1].

1

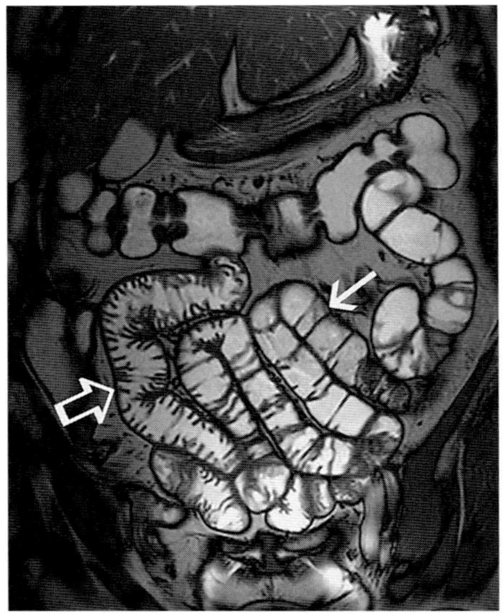

2

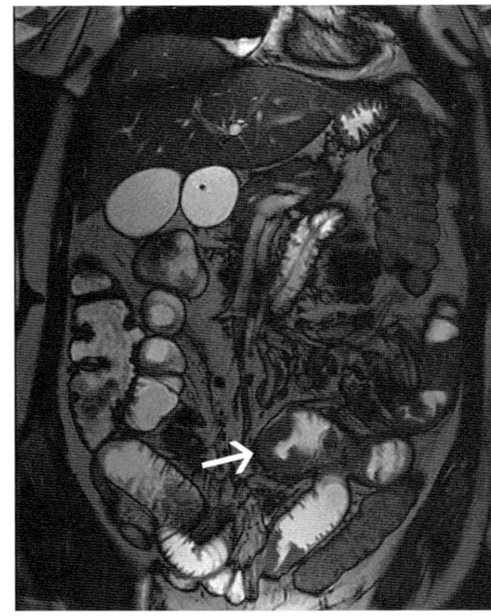

Fig. 1. Coronal MR enteroclysis image shows JFPR in a 45-year-old female with RCD type I. The number of jejunal folds per 5 cm is 2 (arrow), whereas the number of ileal folds per 5 cm is 7 (open arrow).
Fig. 2. Coronal MR enteroclysis image shows EATL (arrow) in a patient with RCD type II.

With the development of fast imaging sequences, small bowel imaging by MR has become possible as well. Advantages include excellent soft tissue contrast and the lack of ionizing radiation. The latter allows for repeated dynamic imaging, so multiple series can be obtained during the same study. This is especially helpful to follow the progression of bowel distention during MR enteroclysis, and allows discrimination between intermittent spasms and stenosis, which often appear the same on static imaging [4]. As in CT, enteroclysis is considered to be more reliable than enterography, although more invasive.

Abdominal US is an easy to perform, noninvasive and readily available imaging modality. However, the lack of bowel preparation often results in intestinal gas or collapse of the bowel wall hindering detailed imaging of the small bowel. However, abdominal US provides better functional evaluation than static small bowel imaging modalities, and especially in case of small bowel obstruction when loops are filled with fluid, the detail with which the intestine can be depicted is impressive [1].

Radiology in Uncomplicated CD

Diagnosis of CD in adults is by serology and duodenal biopsy while the patient is on a gluten-containing diet [5]. The performance of currently available methods for serological diagnosis of CD is very good [6]. For instance, the sensitivity and specificity of IgA anti-endomysial antibodies have been reported to be around 0.84 and 1.00, respectively. For IgA tissue transglutaminase (tTG) antibodies, the sensitivity and specificity have been reported to be around 0.93 and 0.95, respectively [6]. When combined, the diagnostic accuracy of serological tests may approximate 1.0. Despite these performance characteristics, it is generally advised to perform duodenal biopsies, especially in adult patients with gastrointestinal symptoms, before a diagnosis of CD is established [5]. Diagnostic accuracy of duodenal (and bulbar) biopsy specimens for the diagnosis of CD is high, especially when over 4 specimens are obtained [7]. However, one has to be aware that villous atrophy can be caused by more conditions than CD alone, which is why the combination of serology and histology is advocated. In children, the diagnostic accuracy of tTG antibodies is considered that good that in case of tTG raised more than 10× the upper limit of normal, confirmatory duodenal biopsies are no longer required in order to avoid invasive endoscopy [8].

From the above, it can be concluded that modern diagnostic tests for CD are that good that there is no need for radiological methods to investigate the suspected presence of CD in children or adults. However, serological tests for CD, and to a lesser extent duodenal biopsies, are disease-specific tests. In other words, these tests are usually only ordered when a distinct suspicion of CD has arisen. However, the heterogeneous clinical picture of CD remains a challenge to many physicians, and often results in a diagnostic delay of up to 12 years, as well as excessive use of health services [9]. Although there is increasing awareness of CD, this may not be the case for CD present-

Table 2. Radiological findings in CD and its complications

Condition	Intestinal findings	Extraintestinal findings
Untreated CD	Decreased number of jejunal folds Increased number of ileal folds JFPR Jejunal dilatation Wall thickening Intussusception	Presence of nonenlarged mesenteric lymph nodes Presence of enlarged mesenteric lymph nodes Decreased splenic volume Vascular engorgement
RCD type I	As in untreated CD	As in untreated CD
RCD type II	Ulcers Strictures Decreased number of jejunal folds Diffuse bowel wall thickening	Mesenteric fat infiltration Cavitated lymph nodes Severely decreased splenic volume
EATL	Long, smooth small bowel mass Focal small bowel wall thickening	Presence of enlarged mesenteric lymph nodes
Small bowel adenocarcinoma	Circular apple core-like lesion Focal wall thickening Prestenotic dilatation	Presence of enlarged mesenteric lymph nodes

ing with nonspecific, or nongastrointestinal symptoms, which is especially cumbersome now that the classical presenting symptom of CD is less prevalent [10]. For instance, a recent survey among practicing hematologists in the United States revealed that only 8.6% believed that patients with iron deficiency anemia should be screened for CD [11]. In patients with anemia, unintentional weight loss, liver test abnormalities or abdominal pain, it is not unlikely that radiological imaging is performed before CD is considered an option. Radiological imaging has quite often been performed in the diagnostic process of symptoms that were not recognized as being part of the spectrum of CD. This may especially be true in older individuals, where radiological imaging is often used to exclude malignancy. Therefore, it is important that clinicians are aware of the spectrum of radiological findings that may indicate the presence of CD (table 2).

The most striking radiological abnormalities encountered in CD are abnormalities of the intestinal fold pattern (fig. 1). The normal jejunum has over 10 folds per 5 cm, whereas the ileum usually has less than 4 folds per 5 cm [12]. In CD, the number of jejunal folds is often decreased. In severe cases, complete loss of jejunal folds can result in an appearance not unlike that of the colon ('moulage sign') [13]. In contrast, the number of ileal folds is often increased in CD. This probably is the result of ileal adaptation in order to compensate for the loss of absorptive capacity of the jejunum. When the number of ileal folds per 5 cm exceeds the number of jejunal folds per 5 cm, this is called jejunoileal fold pattern reversal (JFPR). This finding, which was first described by Bova in 1985, is considered to be the most specific radiological finding in CD [14]. Lomoschitz et al. [15] identified JFPR on conventional enteroclysis studies in 16/27 patients with CD, compared to 0/123 control patients. Using CT enteroclysis, Soyer et al. [12] found the median number of jejunal and ileal folds in patients with CD was 7 and 8 per 5 cm, respectively, compared to 10 and 4 per 5 cm in controls. The sensitivity and specificity of JFPR in the diagnosis of CD was 0.64 and 1.00, respectively, with an overall accuracy of 0.82. Adequate distention of the small intestine is however mandatory. In a study on abdominal CT after oral administration of 800–1,000 ml Gastrografin, it was not possible to count the number of jejunal folds in 7/52 (13.5%) study subjects [16]. Again, JFPR was only found in patients with CD. Despite the lack of special bowel preparation, Bartusek et al. [17] were able to diagnose a decreased number of jejunal folds in 90%, and an increase in ileal folds in 75% of patients with CD using abdominal US. Abnormalities in fold pattern usually resolve after the introduction of a gluten-free diet [18].

Measurements of small bowel wall thickness usually require cross-sectional imaging and optimal distention of the small intestine in order to prevent false-positive findings caused by collapsed loops. In optimally distended loops, the small bowel wall is usually <3–4 mm thick.

With CT enterography, Tomei et al. [19] found this feature in 21% of patients with CD, the mean thickness being 9 mm (range 5–18). In a study on CT enteroclysis that included 44 patients with CD and 44 control subjects, the sensitivity and specificity of diffuse jejunal wall thickening were 0.66 and 0.98 [12]. Establishing bowel wall thickness with fluoroscopy is less reliable.

Small bowel hypotonia associated with CD may result in jejunal dilatation. In normal subjects, the diameter of the jejunum is usually <4 cm, although this depends on the way it is studied. Using SBFT, McCrae and Sweet [20] showed that in children with CD, the diameter of the jejunum was increased when compared to controls. It could be that the process of enteroclysis diminishes the value of jejunal diameter as a relevant feature. Lomoschitz et al. [15] identified jejunal dilatation in 5/27 patients with CD, and in 9/123 control subjects using conventional enteroclysis. Soyer et al. [12] in a study on CT enteroclysis found the sensitivity and specificity of jejunal dilatation to be 0.16 and 0.95, respectively. In older days, the dilatation of the jejunum as well as the excess fluid in the jejunum resulted in the uneven distribution of barium throughout the jejunum. This finding, called flocculation, has been reported in up to 66% of patients with CD undergoing SBFT, but was much less prevalent with enteroclysis techniques [15, 21]. With modern barium solutions, flocculation is now very rare.

Intussusception is a finding in which one part of the intestine slides into the adjacent part. It is important to realize that intussusceptions in CD are usually transient and may be completely asymptomatic. Intussusception is the most common cause of small bowel obstruction in children aged 3 months to 5 years [22]. Usually, no lead point can be identified. A study from the United States showed that 1.2% of children with CD had experienced a symptomatic intussusception <9 months before the diagnosis of CD. In a large control population, this had occurred in 0.07% of children, within the same time frame [23]. On SBFT, intussusception results in a spring coil-like configuration. On US and cross-sectional imaging, a target sign, reflecting the bowel-in-bowel, is pathognomonic [13]. In adults with CD, intussusception has been reported in up to 20% of patients examined with SBFT [24]. Using abdominal US, Bartusek et al. [17] found transient intussusception in 30% of patients with CD, which reflects the dynamic nature of US.

Extraintestinal findings in CD include changes in blood vessels, lymph nodes and splenic atrophy. All these findings can only be reliably depicted in cross-sectional imaging and to a lesser extent with abdominal US.

Changes in blood flow in CD result in several findings. Abdominal US studies have shown that basal mesenteric blood flow is increased in patients with CD, and that the caliber of the superior mesenteric artery is increased [25]. On cross-sectional imaging, increased blood flow results in a specific image often referred to as vascular engorgement, which is defined as an increase in size and number of proximal and mesenteric vessels, as well as an increase in the number of distal mesenteric vessels adjacent to the small bowel loops [12]. This finding has a reported sensitivity and specificity of 0.64 and 0.91, respectively [12]. This increased blood flow can also be observed in the bowel wall itself. Masselli et al. [26] found that in CD dynamic contrast-enhanced MR imaging showed increased enhancement of the duodenal wall after administration of intravenous contrast. Additionally, this enhancement was very fast, as was the washout of contrast, which probably indicates increased capillary permeability associated with chronic inflammation. As is clear, such measurements require repeated imaging, which is one of the main benefits of MR imaging, compared to CT.

The presence of nonenlarged lymph nodes frequently occurs in the general population, although it is more frequently encountered in patients with CD. Using abdominal US, Bartusek et al. [17] found mesenteric lymph nodes in 95% of patients with CD. Enlarged mesenteric lymph nodes, defined as measuring >1 cm in their short-axis length, were found in 18% of patients with CD [12]. Care is needed in evaluating the aspect of enlarged lymph nodes: enlarged lymph nodes with central hypoattenuation (CD) or a hypoechoic core (abdominal US) are highly suggestive of cavitating lymph node syndrome, especially when associated with splenic atrophy. This very rare syndrome may indicate the presence of lymphoma. Although mortality rates of up to 50% have been reported, spontaneous recovery has been reported as well [13]. Hyposplenism is associated with CD, although the exact mechanism is unclear. On imaging studies, splenic atrophy is often encountered. With CT, Soyer et al. [12] found the median splenic volume of controls was 254 cm^3 compared to 157 cm^3 in patients with untreated CD. Using receiver operating characteristics curve analysis, splenic atrophy was defined as the presence of a splenic volume <145 cm^3. Sensitivity and specificity of this finding were 0.47 and 0.98, respectively.

One has to be aware that many signs associated with CD can also be observed in other conditions resulting in malabsorption. The reported sensitivities and specificities of signs may be inflated by the much larger prevalence of CD than other conditions, like auto-immune enteropathy and Whipple's disease. In many more rare or emerging small-intestinal conditions, no studies on radiological findings have been performed. Therefore, radiological findings that may indicate CD need serological and histological confirmation before a diagnosis of CD can be established.

Radiology in Complicated CD

The role of radiology in patients with complicated CD is much more important than it is in patients with uncomplicated CD. In patients with nonresponsive CD, symptoms may be caused by RCD, or small-intestinal malignancies like small bowel adenocarcinoma or enteropathy-associated T-cell lymphoma (EATL). In these patients, abnormalities are often not within reach of conventional gastroscopes, and especially in the presence of symptoms that may indicate small bowel obstruction, video capsule endoscopy is contraindicated [27, 28]. Therefore, small bowel radiology can be a helpful tool to investigate these patients (fig. 2). However, little is known on radiological findings in patients with complicated CD, and unfortunately, most recent studies were all performed in one expert center, limiting their generalizability.

Ulcerative jejunitis may appear on double-contrast enteroclysis studies as thickened segments with ulcerative lesions and stenosis [13]. On cross-sectional imaging, the bowel wall thickening is the most striking abnormality. Discrimination from lymphoma is often not possible. However, there are no studies that have investigated the diagnostic accuracy of these findings.

Mallant et al. [29] reported on CT enterography performed in patients with CD because of persisting abdominal symptoms and/or suspicion of EATL. The final diagnosis was uncomplicated CD in 14, RCD type I in 10, RCD type II in 15 and EATL in 7. For analysis, patients with uncomplicated CD or RCD type II were put in group A, and patients with RCD II and EATL in group B. There were no statistical differences regarding fold patterns. However, because of lack of intraluminal contrast or lack of distention of small bowel loops, the number of jejunal folds could not be counted in 43% of all patients. Jejunal dilation or increased wall thickness did not differ significantly between both groups. Intussusception was found in 1 patient in group A, and in 5 patients in group B, although this difference failed to reach statistical significance. The presence of mesenteric lymph nodes was similar in both groups, but the presence of enlarged lymph nodes was only found in 5 patients in group B. Splenic volume <122 cm^3 was observed in 27% of patients in group A, and 73% of patients in group B, a difference that was statistically significant.

Researchers from the same group also studied MR enteroclysis in patients with nonresponsive CD [30]. Patients with de-novo EATL were not included in this study. Radiological parameters were evaluated in a test group consisting of 28 patients (uncomplicated CD, n = 10; RCD type I, n = 8; RCD type II, n = 10). No differences between patients with uncomplicated CD or RCD type I could be observed. Multivariate analysis identified three parameters associated with the presence of RCD type II: the presence of <10 jejunal folds per 5 cm, diffuse thickening of the small bowel wall, and infiltration of the mesenteric fat. The median splenic volume in patients with RCD type II was 117 cm^3 compared to 212 cm^3 in patients without RCD II. Using the optimal cutoff value of <160 cm^3, splenic atrophy was present in 33% of patients without RCD type II, and 70% of patients with RCD type II, although this difference was not statistically significant in multivariate analysis. The three identified features associated with RCD II were tested in a validation group consisting of 40 patients, 15 of whom had RCD type II. For the presence of <10 jejunal folds per 5 cm, sensitivity and specificity were 0.93 and 0.88, respectively. For mesenteric fat infiltration, this was 0.87 and 0.80, and for diffuse bowel wall thickening, this was 0.47 and 0.84. A positive MR score was defined as 2 or more of these three features present, and showed sensitivity and specificity of 0.87 and 0.96, respectively, for the diagnosis of RCD type II. This MR score was also associated with mortality: 5-year survival was 95% in patients with a negative MR score, and 56% in patients with a positive MR score. In 8 patients, a small bowel malignancy was present, which was detected by MR enteroclysis in 7, resulting in a specificity and sensitivity of 0.88 and 0.97, respectively, for the diagnosis of small bowel malignancy in patients with CD.

The Amsterdam group also compared findings of CT enterography and ^{18}F-FDG-PET performed in 8 patients with EATL and 30 patients with RCD type II [31]. ^{18}F-FDG-PET could reveal sites histologically proven to be EATL in all 8 patients, whereas CT showed normal findings in 1 patient with EATL. ^{18}F-FDG-PET detected unsuspected extraintestinal sites affected by EATL in 2 patients. CT showed abnormalities such as a thickened small bowel wall or lymphadenopathy in 14 patients with RCD lacking evidence of EATL at follow-up. ^{18}F-FDG-PET findings were positive in 3 and equivocal in another 3 patients with RCD. ^{18}F-FDG-PET was more sensitive and specific than CT (100 vs. 87% and 90 vs. 53%, respectively).

Lohan et al. [32] found that lymphomas in patients with CD were more often solitary, over 10 cm in length and appearing smoother than lymphomas in patients who did not have CD.

Small bowel adenocarcinomas in CD are often, but not solely, located in the proximal jejunum. On SBFT and in conventional enteroclysis studies, they appear as apple core lesions. On cross-sectional imaging, they usually show as solitary, mass-forming lesions, with a predominant intraluminal growth pattern [33, 34].

Besides the studies mentioned, there is limited additional information on the reliability of small bowel imaging for detecting cancer in patients with CD. However, there is emerging evidence that in the detection of small bowel neoplasms in other patient groups, cross-sectional enteroclysis studies are the preferred method, and may even perform better than video capsule endoscopy [2, 33, 35]. Enterography studies often do not result in adequate distention of the jejunum, which is essential in the diagnosis of intraluminal abnormalities.

Conclusions

Small bowel radiology may reveal striking abnormalities in patients with uncomplicated CD. However, in light of the excellent performance characteristics of CD serology and small bowel histology, its role in the diagnosis is limited. However, radiological findings may be the first clues that point physicians to the diagnosis of CD.

The role of radiology in complicated CD seems to be more important, especially when patients present with symptoms that may indicate RCD type II or small bowel malignancy. However, more studies from more centers are needed, which should include a comparison with capsule endoscopy and flexible enteroscopy. Future research should also investigate combined modalities such as PET-CT and PET-MR imaging.

Disclosure Statement

All authors declare that they have no competing interests.

References

1 Van Weyenberg SJ, Van Waesberghe JH, Ell C, Pohl J: Enteroscopy and its relationship to radiological small bowel imaging. Gastrointest Endosc Clin N Am 2009;19:389–407.
2 Masselli G, Gualdi G: MR imaging of the small bowel. Radiology 2012;264:333–348.
3 Maglinte DD, Kohli MD, Romano S, Lappas JC: Air (CO2) double-contrast barium enteroclysis. Radiology 2009;252:633–641.
4 Masselli G, Gualdi G: CT and MR enterography in evaluating small bowel diseases: when to use which modality? Abdom Imag 2013;38: 249–259.
5 Ludvigsson JF, Bai JC, Biagi F, Card TR, Ciacci C, Ciclitira PJ, et al: Diagnosis and management of adult coeliac disease: guidelines from the British Society of Gastroenterology. Gut 2014;63:1210–1228.
6 Schyum AC, Rumessen JJ: Serological testing for celiac disease in adults. United European Gastroenterol J 2013;1:319–325.
7 Rubio-Tapia A, Hill ID, Kelly CP, Calderwood AH, Murray JA, American College of G: ACG clinical guidelines: diagnosis and management of celiac disease. Am J Gastroenterol 2013;108:656–676; quiz 77.
8 Murch S, Jenkins H, Auth M, Bremner R, Butt A, France S, et al: Joint BSPGHAN and Coeliac UK guidelines for the diagnosis and management of coeliac disease in children. Arch Dis Childhood 2013;98:806–811.
9 Fuchs V, Kurppa K, Huhtala H, Collin P, Maki M, Kaukinen K: Factors associated with long diagnostic delay in celiac disease. Scand J Gastroenterol 2014:1–7.
10 Rampertab SD, Pooran N, Brar P, Singh P, Green PH: Trends in the presentation of celiac disease. Am J Med 2006;119:355 e9–e14.
11 Smukalla S, Lebwohl B, Mears JG, Leslie LA, Green PH: How often do hematologists consider celiac disease in iron-deficiency anemia? Results of a national survey. Clin Adv Hematol Oncol 2014;12:100–105.
12 Soyer P, Boudiaf M, Dray X, Fargeaudou Y, Vahedi K, Aout M, et al: CT enteroclysis features of uncomplicated celiac disease: retrospective analysis of 44 patients. Radiology 2009;253:416–424.
13 Buckley O, Brien JO, Ward E, Doody O, Govender P, Torreggiani WC: The imaging of coeliac disease and its complications. Eur J Radiol 2008;65:483–490.
14 Bova JG, Friedman AC, Weser E, Hopens TA, Wytock DH: Adaptation of the ileum in nontropical sprue: reversal of the jejunoileal fold pattern. Am J Roentgenol 1985;144:299–302.
15 Lomoschitz F, Schima W, Schober E, Turetschek K, Kaider A, Vogelsang H: Enteroclysis in adult celiac disease: diagnostic value of specific radiographic features. Eur Radiol 2003;13:890–896.
16 Tomei E, Marini M, Messineo D, Di Giovambattista F, Greco M, Passariello R, et al: Computed tomography of the small bowel in adult celiac disease: the jejunoileal fold pattern reversal. Eur Radiol 2000;10:119–122.
17 Bartusek D, Valek V, Husty J, Uteseny J: Small bowel ultrasound in patients with celiac disease. Retrospective study. Eur J Radiol 2007; 63:302–306.
18 van den Bosch HC, Tjon a Tham RT, Gooszen AW, Fauquenot-Nollen JM, Lamers CB: Celiac disease: small-bowel enteroclysis findings in adult patients treated with a gluten-free diet. Radiology 1996;201:803–808.
19 Tomei E, Diacinti D, Marini M, Mastropasqua M, Di Tola M, Sabbatella L, et al: Abdominal CT findings may suggest coeliac disease. Dig Liver Dis 2005;37:402–406.
20 McCrae WM, Sweet EM: Radiology in diagnosis of coeliac disease. BMJ 1964;2:163–164.
21 Herlinger H, Maglinte DD: Jejunal fold separation in adult celiac disease: relevance of enteroclysis. Radiology 1986;158:605–611.
22 Lehnert T, Sorge I, Till H, Rolle U: Intussusception in children – clinical presentation, diagnosis and management. Int J Colorect Dis 2009;24:1187–1192.
23 Reilly NR, Aguilar KM, Green PH: Should intussusception in children prompt screening for celiac disease? J Pediatr Gastroenterol Nutr 2013;56:56–59.

24 Cohen MD, Lintott DJ: Transient small bowel intussusception in adult coeliac disease. Clin Radiol 1978;29:529–534.

25 Rettenbacher T, Hollerweger A, Macheiner P, Huber S, Gritzmann N: Adult celiac disease: US signs. Radiology 1999;211:389–394.

26 Masselli G, Picarelli A, Di Tola M, Libanori V, Donato G, Polettini E, et al: Celiac disease: evaluation with dynamic contrast-enhanced MR imaging. Radiology 2010;256:783–790.

27 Van Weyenberg SJ, Smits F, Jacobs MA, Van Turenhout ST, Mulder CJ: Video capsule endoscopy in patients with nonresponsive celiac disease. J Clin Gastroenterol 2013;47:393–399.

28 Van Weyenberg SJ, Van Turenhout ST, Bouma G, Van Waesberghe JH, Van der Peet DL, Mulder CJ, et al: Double-balloon endoscopy as the primary method for small-bowel video capsule endoscope retrieval. Gastrointest Endosc 2010;71:535–541.

29 Mallant M, Hadithi M, Al-Toma AB, Kater M, Jacobs M, Manoliu R, et al: Abdominal computed tomography in refractory coeliac disease and enteropathy associated T-cell lymphoma. World J Gastroenterol 2007;13:1696–1700.

30 Van Weyenberg SJ, Meijerink MR, Jacobs MA, van Kuijk C, Mulder CJ, van Waesberghe JH: MR enteroclysis in refractory celiac disease: proposal and validation of a severity scoring system. Radiology 2011;259:151–161.

31 Hadithi M, Mallant M, Oudejans J, van Waesberghe JH, Mulder CJ, Comans EF: 18F-FDG PET versus CT for the detection of enteropathy-associated T-cell lymphoma in refractory celiac disease. J Nucl Med 2006;47:1622–1627.

32 Lohan DG, Alhajeri AN, Cronin CG, Roche CJ, Murphy JM: MR enterography of small-bowel lymphoma: potential for suggestion of histologic subtype and the presence of underlying celiac disease. Am J Roentgenol 2008;190:287–293.

33 Van Weyenberg SJ, Meijerink MR, Jacobs MA, Van der Peet DL, Van Kuijk C, Mulder CJ, et al: MR enteroclysis in the diagnosis of small-bowel neoplasms. Radiology 2010;254:765–773.

34 Masselli G, Gualdi G: Evaluation of small bowel tumors: MR enteroclysis. Abdom Imaging 2010;35:23–30.

35 Van Weyenberg SJ, Bouman K, Jacobs MA, Halloran BP, Van der Peet DL, Mulder CJ, et al: Comparison of MR enteroclysis with video capsule endoscopy in the investigation of small-intestinal disease. Abdom Imaging 2013;38:42–51.

Dig Dis 2015;33:260–263
DOI: 10.1159/000371476

Wheat Amylase Trypsin Inhibitors as Nutritional Activators of Innate Immunity

Detlef Schuppan   Victor Zevallos

Institute for Translational Immunology and Research Center for Immunotherapy, University Medical Center, Johannes Gutenberg University, Mainz, Germany

Key Words

Amylase trypsin inhibitors · Autoimmunity · Celiac disease · Dendritic cell · Gluten · Innate immunity · Macrophage · Monocyte · T cell · Toll-like receptor 4 · Wheat

Abstract

While the central role of an adaptive, T cell-mediated immune response to certain gluten peptides in celiac disease is well established, the innate immune response to wheat proteins remains less well defined. We identified wheat amylase trypsin inhibitors (ATIs), but not gluten, as major stimulators of innate immune cells (dendritic cells > macrophages > monocytes), while intestinal epithelial cells were nonresponsive. ATIs bind to and activate the CD14-MD2 toll-like receptor 4 (TLR4) complex. This activation occurs both in vitro and in vivo after oral ingestion of purified ATIs or gluten, which is usually enriched in ATIs. Wheat ATIs represent a family of up to 17 proteins with molecular weights of around 15 kDa and a variable primary but conserved secondary structure characterized by 5 intrachain disulfide bonds and alpha helices. They mostly form di- and tetramers that appear to equally activate TLR4. Relevant biological activity is confined to ATIs in gluten-containing cereals, while gluten-free cereals display no or minimal activities. ATIs represent up to 4% of total wheat protein and are highly resistant to intestinal proteases. In line with their dose-dependent function as co-stimulatory molecules in adaptive immunity of celiac disease, they appear to play a role in promoting other immune-mediated diseases within and outside the GI tract. Thus, ATIs may be prime candidates of severe forms of non-celiac gluten (wheat) sensitivity.

Introduction

A condition termed non-celiac gluten sensitivity (NCGS) which can be defined as intolerance to wheat in the absence of celiac disease and wheat allergy was described more than 3 decades ago [1]. Between 2010 and 2014, three consensus conferences convened to confirm the existence of this entity and to refine the diagnostic criteria of NCGS, which are largely based on a clear connection of symptoms to the consumption of wheat and the exclusion of celiac disease and wheat allergy. In addition, a significant contribution of irritable bowel syndrome (IBS) or intolerance to sugars and polysaccharides (FODMAPs: fermentable oligo, di-, monosaccharides and polyols) should be ruled out. While wheat allergy, IBS or FODMAP intolerance may contribute to NCGS, there is consensus that they cannot explain the syndrome of NCGS which frequently manifests with extraintestinal symptoms, including fatigue, 'foggy mind', headache, joint or

KARGER 125

E-Mail karger@karger.com
www.karger.com/ddi

0257–2753/15/0332–0260$39.50/0

Detlef Schuppan, MD, PhD
Institute of Translational Immunology, Small Intestinal and Celiac Disease Center
University Medical Center, Johannes Gutenberg University
Langenbeckstrasse 1, DE–55131 Mainz (Germany)
E-Mail detlef.schuppan@unimedizin-mainz.de

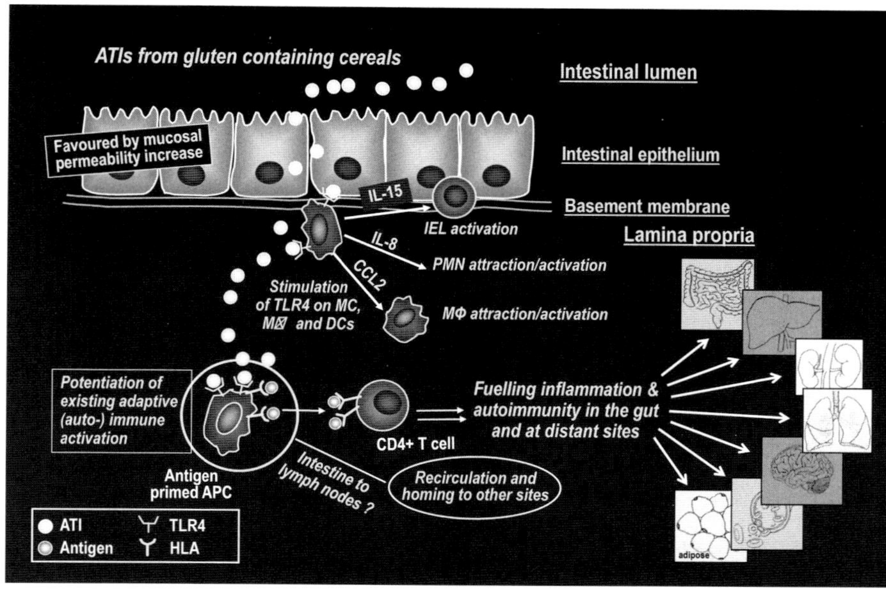

Fig. 1. Nutritional ATIs as innate triggers of intestinal and extraintestinal immune activation. ATIs are resistant to intestinal proteolysis and are sensed by mucosal innate immune cells where they stimulate the release of proinflammatory chemokines and cytokines via activation of TLR4. ATIs potentiate antigen presentation on antigen-presenting cells (APCs), especially dendritic cells, and thus serve as adjuvants for an ongoing adaptive T-cell response, as occurs in chronic inflammatory and especially autoimmune diseases. It is likely that the contact between ATI-activated APCs and specific T cells occurs at extraintestinal sites, such as mesenteric lymph nodes. DC = Dendritic cell; IEL = intraepithelial lymphocyte; HLA = human lymphocyte antigen; MC = monocyte; MΦ = macrophage; PMN = polymorphonuclear leukocyte.

Color version available online

muscle pain, or worsening of a given chronic neurological, psychiatric, or (auto-)immune disease [2–5]. Most experts believe that NCGS is caused by an innate immune response to wheat proteins (as opposed to the adaptive, T cell-mediated response to gluten in celiac disease, or to gluten and non-gluten proteins in wheat allergy) [6–8]. While certain gluten peptides that are different from those that activate T cells in celiac disease elicited innate immune responses in epithelial cells and macrophages, and in intestinal biopsy cultures of celiac patients in vitro, evidence for their role as effective immune activators in vivo is lacking [9–12]. Moreover, the receptor was not identified, except for a study that implicated the chemokine receptor CXCR3 on intestinal epithelial cell cultures and another report suggesting the toll-like receptor pathway [11, 12]. Finally, patients with suspected NCGS and intestinal complaints do not show characteristic inflammatory changes of the small-intestinal mucosa, though likely minimal inflammatory pathology [13], and to date there is no serum biomarker to diagnose the condition. Notably, a substantial proportion of patients with IBS may indeed have NCGS. Thus, a recent study using confocal laser endomicroscopy found an immediate response (epithelial breaks and leakage) to a mucosal wheat challenge through the endoscope in 13/22 patients with food-related IBS in whom celiac disease and common food allergies were excluded [14]. All positively identified patients reported a dramatic, long-term (12 months) improvement when following the exclusion diet. Still, while NCGS was the likely cause, some of these responses may also have been due to an undetected, IgE negative form of wheat allergy.

In search for specific gluten peptides that would activate innate immunity, we failed to confirm published gliadin sequences, such as alpha gliadin peptide p31–49, as activators in intestinal cell cultures. However, a pepsin-trypsin gliadin digest that mimicks (partial) digestion of gliadin as occurs during upper intestinal passage strongly activated myeloid cells in vitro (dendritic cells > macrophages > monocytes). This activity was clearly associated with proteins or peptides of the digest, but absent in purified gliadin or gluten fractions, or synthetic glisadon peptides. Finally, activity could be recovered in a non-gluten fraction that was present in standard gliadin and that was identified as the family of amylase trypsin inhibitors (ATIs) [15]. ATIs represents ~2–4% of total wheat protein (as compared to ~80–90% for gluten) [16].

ATIs engage the toll-like receptor 4 (TLR4)-MD2-CD14 complex and lead to upregulation of maturation markers and release of proinflammatory cytokines in myeloid cells of celiac patients but also of nondiseased controls, as is expected for innate immune triggers. Importantly, mice deficient in TLR4 or TLR4 signaling are protected from the intestinal and systemic immune responses upon oral challenge with ATIs [15].

ATIs are present in many plants, where they inhibit enzymes of common parasites such as mealworms and mealybugs in wheat. They may also regulate metabolic processes occurring during seed development [17]. In vivo feeding experiments in mice showed that ATIs increased intestinal and systemic release of cytokines and chemokines like IL-8, TNFα and CCL-2 within 2–12 h, and ex vivo celiac biopsy studies demonstrated an adjuvant effect of added ATIs for the gluten specific T-cell response [15]. Therefore, ATIs appear to be the sought-for triggers of innate immunity in CD and NCGS. Importantly, ATIs are present and even enriched in commercial gluten and resist proteolytic digestion, e.g. by the gastric/enteric proteases pepsin and trypsin, maintaining their biological activity of TLR4 activation throughout their intestinal passage after oral ingestion. This protease resistance is due to their compact secondary structure which is characterized by 5 intra-chain disulfide bonds [18]. The modern wheat genome encodes 17 different ATI species of ~120- to 150-amino acid length that vary in amino acid sequence but have similar secondary structures [19]. TLR4-activating activity is dependent on the secondary structure and is lost after reduction of disulfide bonds [15]. Wheat ATIs form mainly noncovalent homodimers and tetramers with the dimeric and tetrameric variants 0.19 and CM3 representing the major ATI species in modern wheat. We could demonstrate that dimeric 0.19 and tetrameric CM3, as isolated from wheat or expressed as recombinant proteins in eukaryotic cells, display comparable TLR4-activating activity [15].

Plants other than wheat, rye, barley, and their early ancestors also contain inhibitors of amylase and trypsin-like activities, but show only minimal or absent TLR4-activating activity. Therefore, a gluten-free diet is also essentially ATI free. Modern hexaploid wheat contains higher ATI activity than some ancient variants like diploid (einkorn) and tetraploid (emmer) wheat, or older hexaploid variants like kamut or spelt [own unpubl. results].

An adult person usually consumes between 150 and 250 g of wheat flour per day and will therefore be exposed to 0.5–1 g of ATIs. As predicted by the mechanism of action that indicates a mild to moderate activation of innate immunity in the gut, the majority of (healthy) people ingesting ATI-containing grains should not develop symptoms. Morphological effects of ATIs in the gut are discrete and more reflective of dendritic cell or macrophage activation than characterized by an increase in inflammatory cell numbers, which is well in line with histology previously described in patients with NCGS.

However, this may change in subjects with preexisting inflammation. Thus, our unpublished data indicate that in mouse models of autoimmunity like inflammatory bowel disease, systemic lupus erythematodes, autoimmune encephalitis, or inhalative allergy the feeding of ATIs at doses comparable to human daily consumption exacerbates disease manifestation and induces a stronger antigen-specific adaptive immune response compared to their disease controls fed a defined ATI- or gluten-free diet. Here, ATIs serve as co-stimulants (adjuvants) of an already ongoing immune reaction which is not limited to the gut, but apparently extends to nearby or more remote lymph nodes or lymphatic organs where T-cell priming to specific antigen occurs (fig. 1). This effect is dose dependent, and a reduction of daily ATI ingestion by 90–95% may be sufficient to abolish their co-stimulatory effect on chronic T cell-mediated inflammation. This contrasts with celiac disease (or nutritional wheat allergy) where a strictly gluten-free diet has to be maintained. These activities of wheat ATIs may also partly explain the increasing prevalence of allergies and autoimmune diseases in developing countries where nutrition was originally based on gluten-free staples and where consumption of wheat has increased dramatically in the last years or decades. Finally, these findings should sharpen the definition of NCGS as a syndrome in which extraintestinal symptoms and disease would predominate, and which could affect a larger number of patients with chronic disease who are not aware of this nutritional connection. Clinical studies to show if this translates to human chronic inflammatory diseases are in progress.

Disclosure Statement

The authors have no commercial interest to disclose.

References

1 Ellis A, Linaker BD: Non-coeliac gluten sensitivity? Lancet 1978;1:1358–1359.
2 Ludvigsson JF, Leffler DA, Bai JC, et al: The Oslo definitions for coeliac disease and related terms. Gut 2013;62:43–52.
3 Catassi C, Bai JC, Bonaz B, et al: Non-celiac gluten sensitivity: the new frontier of gluten related disorders. Nutrients 2013;5:3839–3853.
4 Carroccio A, Mansueto P, Iacono G, Soresi M, D'Alcamo A, Cavataio F, Brusca I, Florena AM, Ambrosiano G, Seidita A, Pirrone G, Rini GB: Non-celiac wheat sensitivity diagnosed by double-blind placebo-controlled challenge: exploring a new clinical entity. Am J Gastroenterol 2012;107:1898–1906.
5 Volta U, Bardella MT, Calabrò A, Troncone R, Corazza GR; Study Group for Non-Celiac Gluten Sensitivity: An Italian prospective multicenter survey on patients suspected of having non-celiac gluten sensitivity. BMC Med 2014;23:85.

6 Schuppan D, Junker Y, Barisani D: Celiac disease: from pathogenesis to novel therapies. Gastroenterology 2009;137:1912–1933.
7 Sollid LM, Jabri B: Triggers and drivers of autoimmunity: lessons from coeliac disease. Nat Rev Immunol 2013;13:294–302.
8 Tatham AS, Shewry PR: Allergens to wheat and related cereals. Clin Exp Allergy 2008;38: 1712–1726.
9 Jelinkova L, Tuckova L, Cinova J, Flegelova Z, Tlaskalova-Hogenova H: Gliadin stimulates human monocytes to production of IL-8 and TNF-alpha through a mechanism involving NF-kappaB. FEBS Lett 2004;571:81–85.
10 Nikulina M, Habich C, Flohe SB, Scott FW, Kolb H: Wheat gluten causes dendritic cell maturation and chemokine secretion. J Immunol 2004;173:1925–1933.
11 Lammers KM, Lu R, Brownley J, Lu B, Gerard C, Thomas K, Rallabhandi P, Shea-Donohue T, Tamiz A, Alkan S, Netzel-Arnett S, Antalis T, Vogel SN, Fasano A: Gliadin induces an increase in intestinal permeability and zonulin release by binding to the chemokine receptor CXCR3. Gastroenterology 2008;135:194–204.
12 Thomas KE, Sapone A, Fasano A, Vogel SN: Gliadin stimulation of murine macrophage inflammatory gene expression and intestinal permeability are MyD88-dependent: role of the innate immune response in celiac disease. J Immunol 2006;176:2512–2521.5.
13 Sapone A, Lammers KM, Mazzarella G, Mikhailenko I, Cartenì M, Casolaro V, Fasano A: Differential mucosal IL-17 expression in two gliadin-induced disorders: gluten sensitivity and the autoimmune enteropathy celiac disease. Int Arch Allergy Immunol 2010;152: 75–80.
14 Fritscher-Ravens A, Schuppan D, Ellrichmann M, Schoch S, Röcken C, Brasch J, Bethge J, Böttner M, Klose J, Milla PJ: Confocal endomicroscopy shows food-associated changes in the intestinal mucosa of patients with irritable bowel syndrome. Gastroenterology 2014;147:1012–1020.
15 Junker Y, Zeissig S, Kim SJ, Barisani D, Wieser H, Leffler DA, Zevallos V, Libermann TA, Dillon S, Freitag TL, Kelly CP, Schuppan D: Wheat amylase trypsin inhibitors drive intestinal inflammation via activation of toll-like receptor 4. J Exp Med 2012;209:2395–2408.
16 Dupont FM, Vensel WH, Tanaka CK, Hurkman WJ, Altenbach SB: Deciphering the complexities of the wheat flour proteome using quantitative two-dimensional electrophoresis, three proteases and tandem mass spectrometry. Proteome Sci 2011;9:10.
17 Finnie C, Melchior S, Roepstorff P, Svensson B: Proteome analysis of grain filling and seed maturation in barley. Plant Physiol 2002;129: 1308–1319.
18 Oda Y, Matsunaga T, Fukuyama K, Miyazaki T, Morimoto T: Tertiary and quaternary structures of 0.19 α-amylase inhibitor from wheat kernel determined by X-ray analysis at 2.06 Å resolution. Biochemistry 1997;36: 13503–13511.
19 Altenbach SB, Vensel WH, Dupont FM: The spectrum of low molecular weight alpha-amylase/protease inhibitor genes expressed in the US bread wheat cultivar Butte 86. BMC Res Notes 2011;4:242.

Dig Dis 2015;33:264–268
DOI: 10.1159/000369509

Gluten-Related Disorders: Gluten Ataxia

Marios Hadjivassiliou[a] David D. Sanders[b] Daniel P. Aeschlimann[c]

[a]Academic Department of Neurosciences, and [b]Department of Gastroenterology, Royal Hallamshire Hospital, Sheffield, and [c]Matrix Biology & Tissue Repair Research Unit, School of Dentistry, College of Biomedical and Life Sciences, Cardiff University, Cardiff, UK

Key Words

Gluten ataxia · Cerebellar ataxia · Myoclonic ataxia · TG6 antibodies

Abstract

The term gluten-related disorders (GRD) refers to a spectrum of diverse clinical manifestations triggered by the ingestion of gluten in genetically susceptible individuals. They include both intestinal and extraintestinal manifestations. Gluten ataxia (GA) is one of the commonest neurological manifestations of GRD. It was originally defined as otherwise idiopathic sporadic ataxia in the presence of circulating antigliadin antibodies of IgA and/or IgG type. Newer more specific serological markers have been identified but are not as yet readily available. GA has a prevalence of 15% amongst all ataxias and 40% of all idiopathic sporadic ataxias. It usually presents with gait and lower limb ataxia. It is of insidious onset with a mean age at onset of 53 years. Up to 40% of patients have evidence of enteropathy on duodenal biopsy. Gastrointestinal symptoms are seldom prominent and are not a reliable indicator for the presence of enteropathy. Furthermore, the presence of enteropathy does not influence the response to a gluten-free diet. Most patients will stabilise or improve with strict adherence to gluten-free diet depending on the duration of the ataxia prior to the treatment. Up to 60% of patients with GA have evidence of cerebellar atrophy on MR imaging, but all patients have spectroscopic abnormalities primarily affecting the vermis. Recent evidence suggests that patients with newly diagnosed coeliac disease presenting to the gastroenterologists have abnormal MR spectroscopy at presentation associated with clinical evidence of subtle cerebellar dysfunction. The advantage of early diagnosis and treatment (mean age 42 years in patients presenting with gastrointestinal symptoms vs. 53 years in patients presenting with ataxia) may protect the first group from the development and/or progression of neurological dysfunction.

Introduction

Gluten-related disorders (GRD) represent a spectrum of diverse manifestations sharing a common trigger, the ingestion of gluten [1]. The most widely recognised and best characterised disease within this spectrum is coeliac disease (CD) also known as gluten-sensitive enteropathy.

Classic presentations of CD such as abdominal bloating, weight loss, diarrhoea, anaemia and malabsorption are no longer the norm and patients can present with minimal or no gastrointestinal symptoms but with diverse extraintestinal manifestations affecting other organs such as the skin and the nervous system. Dermatitis herpetiformis (DH) is the typical gluten-related dermatopathy, often associated with enteropathy and responsive to a gluten-free diet [2]. In an analogous way, neurological manifestations can be the presenting feature of GRD with cerebellar ataxia being by far the commonest neurological manifestation. Other neurological manifestations include sensorimotor axonal peripheral neuropathy, sensory ganglionopathy, gluten encephalopathy (headache with white matter abnormalities on MR imag-

KARGER 125

E-Mail karger@karger.com
www.karger.com/ddi

0257–2753/15/0332–0264$39.50/0

Marios Hadjivassiliou
Academic Department of Neurosciences, Royal Hallamshire Hospital
Glossop Road
Sheffield S10 2JF (UK)
E-Mail m.hadjivassiliou@sheffield.ac.uk

ing), epilepsy with and without occipital calcifications, myopathy, myelopathy and rarely chorea. This review will concentrate on gluten ataxia (GA).

Epidemiology

GA was originally defined as otherwise idiopathic sporadic ataxia with positive serological markers for gluten sensitivity [3]. The original definition was based on the serological tests available at the time (antigliadin antibodies, AGA). In a series of 1,000 patients with progressive ataxia evaluated over a period of 18 years in a specialist ataxia clinic, Sheffield, UK, there were 168 patients (17%) who had serological evidence (AGA) of sensitivity to gluten. Amongst patients with sporadic ataxia the prevalence was 168/805 (21%), and amongst patients with idiopathic sporadic ataxia 168/388 (43%). Using the same AGA assay, the prevalence of positive AGA in genetically confirmed ataxias (disease control group) was 14/109 (13%) and in healthy volunteers 149/1,200 (12%). A number of studies looking at the prevalence of AGA in ataxias have been published [4–12]. The variations in prevalence may relate to geographical differences in the prevalence of CD, referral bias, variability in the AGA assays used, patient selection (e.g. some studies included as idiopathic sporadic ataxia, patients with cerebellar variant of multi-system atrophy), small number of patients studied and no controls. The potential role of geographical variation was highlighted in a recent observation that the prevalence of TG6 antibodies (possibly a more specific marker of GA) amongst UK patients newly diagnosed with CD who presented to gastroenterologists was 38%, whereas the prevalence of TG6 antibodies in an equivalent Finnish cohort was only 14% [13]. The common theme in most of these studies is the consistently high prevalence of AGA antibodies in sporadic ataxias when compared to healthy controls. GA is the commonest potentially treatable cerebellar ataxia.

Clinical and Laboratory Features

GA usually presents with pure cerebellar ataxia or rarely ataxia in combination with myoclonus, palatal tremor, opsoclonus-myoclonus [14–16]. GA is usually of insidious onset with a mean age at onset of 53 years. Rarely, the ataxia can be rapidly progressive mimicking paraneoplastic cerebellar degeneration. Gaze-evoked nystagmus and other ocular signs of cerebellar dysfunction are seen in up to 80% of cases. All patients have gait ataxia, almost all have lower limb ataxia and some also have upper limb ataxia. Less than 10% of patients with GA will have any gastrointestinal symptoms, yet 40% will have evidence of enteropathy (triad of villous atrophy, crypt hyperplasia and increased intraepithelial lymphocytes) on duodenal biopsy. Anti-TG2 IgA antibodies are present in up to 40% of patients, usually in those with an enteropathy. Lower levels of TG2 antibodies are found in those patients with GA and no enteropathy. A more specific serological marker, TG6 antibodies, has recently been found to be present in 73% of patients with ataxia and positive AGA [13]. Of interest was also the finding of TG6 antibodies in 32% of patients with idiopathic sporadic ataxia and negative other serological markers for GRD. This may suggest that the prevalence of GA may even be higher than previously thought. Gluten-free diet results in reduction of TG6 antibodies in the same way as with TG2 antibodies [13].

Up to 60% of patients with GA have evidence of cerebellar atrophy on MR imaging. Investigation of the metabolic status of the cerebellum in 15 patients with GA and 10 controls using proton MR spectroscopy demonstrated significant differences in mean N-acetyl aspartate/creatine ratios between patients with GA and healthy controls, suggesting that cerebellar neuronal physiology in these patients is abnormal even before the development of atrophy (fig. 1) [17]. There is emerging evidence that MR spectroscopy is often abnormal in patients with newly diagnosed CD and that such abnormalities improve with the introduction of a gluten-free diet [18]. The improvement on MR spectroscopy manifests after a year on the diet but continues for at least 2 years.

Myoclonic ataxia, as mentioned above, is another less common ataxic manifestation of GRD that merits brief consideration. A recent publication of a series of 9 patients with this phenotype described asymmetrical irregular myoclonus involving one or more limbs and sometimes the face [14]. The myoclonus was often stimulus sensitive and became widespread over time. Five of these patients had a history of at least one secondarily generalised seizure. Electrophysiology showed evidence of cortical myoclonus. Despite the fact that all patients adhered to a strict gluten-free diet, all had ongoing inflammation of the bowel suggestive of refractory CD. Two patients died of enteropathy-associated lymphoma. Even with immunosuppression (usually in the form of mycophenolate), these patients remained disabled, primarily due to the troublesome myoclonus which proved to be resistant to all medication used. When encountering such phenotype, it is essential to monitor closely with repeat biopsies and a low threshold for using immunosuppression.

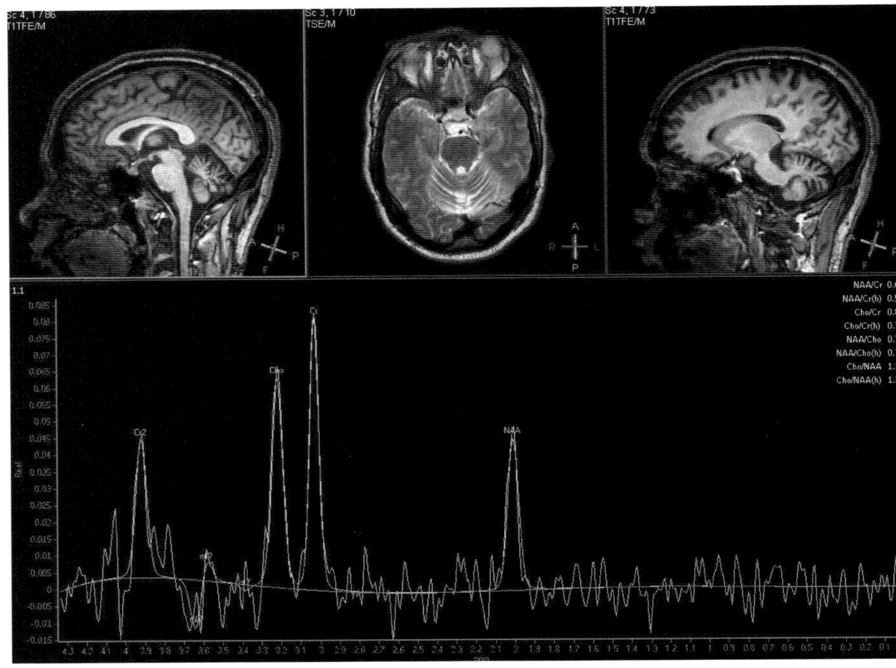

Fig. 1. MR spectroscopy of the cerebellum of a patient with GA showing the typical involvement of the cerebellar vermis (causing gait ataxia) with significant reduction of the NAA/Cr ratio at 0.66. Normal ratio should be over 1.

Color version available online

Treatment

The response to treatment with a gluten-free diet depends on the duration of the ataxia prior to the diagnosis. Loss of Purkinje cells in the cerebellum, the end result of prolonged gluten exposure in patients with GA, is irreversible, and prompt treatment is more likely to result in improvement rather than just stabilisation of the ataxia. Whilst the benefits of a gluten-free diet in the treatment of patients with CD and DH have long been established, there are very few studies, mainly case reports, of the effect of gluten-free diet on the neurological manifestations of gluten sensitivity. Most of these reports primarily concern patients with established CD who then develop neurological symptoms [19–22]. These studies suggest variable but overall favourable responsiveness to a gluten-free diet. A small, uncontrolled study looked at the use of intravenous immunoglobulins in the treatment of 4 patients with GA without enteropathy [23]. All patients improved. In all of these reports, strict adherence to the gluten-free diet was assumed, and no serological evidence of elimination of the gluten sensitivity-related antibodies was provided. Only one systematic study of the effect of gluten-free diet on a cohort of patients presenting with ataxia, with or without an enteropathy, has been published [24]. This study also reported serological evidence of elimination of the AGA as a confirmation of strict adherence to the diet. Forty-three patients with GA were enrolled. Twenty-six adhered strictly to the gluten-free diet, had serological evidence of elimination of antibodies and comprised the treatment group. Fourteen patients refused the diet and comprised the control group. Patient and control groups were matched at baseline for all variables (age, duration of ataxia, etc.). There was no significant difference in the baseline performance for each ataxia test between the two groups. There was significant improvement in performance in test scores and in the subjective global clinical impression scale in the treatment group when compared to the control group. The improvement was apparent even after excluding patients with an enteropathy. The study concluded that strict gluten-free diet is an effective treatment for GA.

Pathophysiology

There is evidence to suggest that the cerebellar insult in GA is immune-mediated. Vitamin deficiencies (e.g. B_{12}, folic acid, vitamin E, copper) are rarely implicated and, given that the majority of patients do not have enteropathy, they do not have such deficiencies that could explain the neurological deficit. Post-mortem examination from patients with GA show patchy loss of Purkinje cells throughout the cerebellar cortex [3, 25, 26]. The cerebellar white matter showed astrocytic gliosis, vacuolation of the neutrophil and a diffuse infiltrate mainly of T lymphocytes. In addition, there was perivascular cuffing with inflammatory cells, mainly T lymphocytes, with smaller numbers of B lymphocytes and macrophages.

Experimental evidence suggests that there is antibody cross-reactivity between antigenic epitopes on Purkinje and other cerebellar cells (granular layer) and gluten peptides. For example, AGA have been shown to react with human and rat cerebellar Purkinje cells in vitro [27]. However, sera from patients with GA appear to contain additional antibodies targeting Purkinje cell epitopes. This is shown by the failure to eliminate such reactivity with Purkinje cells when using sera from patients with GA after removal of AGA using crude gliadin.

There is increasing evidence of the involvement of transglutaminases in the pathogenesis of GA [28]. Transglutaminase 2, the autoantigen in CD is one of a family of enzymes that covalently crosslink or modify proteins by formation of an isopeptide bond between a peptide-bound glutamine residue and a primary amine, either within the same or a neighbouring polypeptide chain. In some instances, TG2 may react with H_2O in preference over an amine leading to the deamidation of glutamine residues. The significance of this latter activity has been established in connection with CD. Gliadin proteins, the immunological trigger of gluten sensitivity are glutamine-rich donor substrates amenable to deamidation [29]. TG2 may contribute to disease development by deamidating gluten peptides and thereby increasing their reactivity with HLA-DQ2/DQ8 (found in almost 100% of patients with CD), which potentiates the T cell response. The absence of intestinal T cell responses to gluten in the majority of individuals carrying HLA-DQ2/DQ8 and the preferential T cell responses to deamidated gluten fragments in patients with CD indicates that there is tolerance to unmodified gluten peptides. Activation of TG2 and deamidation of gluten peptides appears to be central to disease development.

Why should these patients develop autoantibodies to TG2 remains unclear. The formation of complexes of gluten and TG2 may permit gluten-reactive T cells to provide the necessary help to TG2-specific B cells. This would also explain why serum antibodies to TG disappear when patients adopt a gluten-free diet. However, it has also been suggested that molecular mimicry, i.e. shared epitopes between deamidated gliadin and TG2, or exposure of masked epitopes upon reaction of the enzyme with antigenic gliadin peptides could lead to antibody production [30].

Like TG2 in CD, TG3, an epidermal transglutaminase, has been shown to be the autoantigen in DH [31]. DH is a gluten-sensitive dermatopathy that presents with an itchy vesicular rash and is one example of extraintestinal manifestations of gluten sensitivity. Whilst the majority of patients with DH have evidence of enteropathy on duodenal biopsy, these patients rarely experience or complain of gastrointestinal symptoms. This form of gluten sensitivity may be determined by autoimmunity directed primarily towards TG3 rather than TG2, suggesting that the explanation for the heterogeneity in disease manifestation may lie in the specificity of the immune response.

In an analogous way TG6, a brain-expressed transglutaminase, has been shown to be a target antigen in patients with GA [13, 32]. Thus, patients with GA have evidence of circulating anti-TG6 antibodies. Such antibodies are gluten dependent and are eliminated by gluten-free diet. TG6 antibodies produced using phage display methods have been shown to react with both Purkinje cells and cells within the granular layer. Work on brain PM tissue of GA patients demonstrates the accumulation of IgA deposits in the cerebellum and brain stem, most prominently within the muscular layer surrounding vessels but also in brain tissue proper [33]. There was evidence of co-distribution of TG6 with these IgA deposits in the cerebellum and medulla. The perivascular areas where an endomysium-associated IgA deposition occurs were intensely positive for TG6, and to a lesser extent brain tissue itself was also stained, while staining was absent in the parietal lobe. In contrast, TG6 could not be detected in vascular structures of normal cerebellum.

Such intense perivascular changes may imply a perivascular inflammation that may compromise blood brain barrier and allow the entry of gluten-related antibodies into the central nervous system. Evidence that such antibodies may potentially be pathogenic comes from mice experiments [28]. Intraventricular injection of phage display-produced antibodies against TG2 and TG6 was capable of inducing ataxia in mice within 3 h of injection. A similar observation was made using serum from patients with GA.

Conclusions

GA is the commonest potentially treatable form of cerebellar ataxia. It is also the commonest neurological manifestation of sensitivity to gluten. It is imperative that clinicians are aware of this manifestation to be able to diagnose it and treat it early. Strict gluten-free diet may improve and/or stabilise the ataxia. Whilst a lot of insight as to the pathophysiology of GA can be gained from a number of scientific studies, there are still a number of unanswered questions, namely the reason behind the target of the autoimmune reaction (TG2 vs. TG3 vs. TG6 or any combination) and ultimately the trigger for the development of symptomatic disease in genetically susceptible individuals.

Disclosure Statement

The authors declare that no financial or other conflict of interest exists in relation to the content of the article.

References

1 Sapone A, Bai JC, Ciacci C, Dolinsek J, Green PHR, Hadjivassiliou M, Kaukinen K, Rostami K, Sanders DS, Schumann M, Ullrich R, Villalta D, Volta U, Catassi C, Fasano A: Spectrum of gluten-related disorders: consensus on nomenclature and classification. BMC Med 2012;10:13.

2 Marks J, Shuster S, Watson AJ: Small bowel changes in dermatitis herpetiformis. Lancet 1966;ii:1280–1282.

3 Hadjivassiliou M, Grünewald RA, Chattopadhyay AK, Davies-Jones GAB, Gibson A, Jarratt JA, Kandler RH, Lobo A, Powell T, Smith CML: Clinical, radiological, neurophysiological and neuropathological characteristics of gluten ataxia. Lancet 1998;352: 1582–1585.

4 Hadjivassiliou M, Gibson A, Davies-Jones GAB, Lobo A, Stephenson TJ, Milford-Ward A: Does cryptic gluten sensitivity play a part in neurological illness? Lancet 1996;347:369–371.

5 Pellecchia MT, Scala R, Filla A, De Michele G, Ciacci C, Barone P: Idiopathic cerebellar ataxia associated with celiac disease: lack of distinctive neurological features. J Neurol Neurosurg Psychiatry 1999;66:32–35.

6 Luostarinen LK, Collin PO, Paraaho MJ, Maki MJ, Pirttila TA: Coeliac disease in patients with cerebellar ataxia of unknown origin. Ann Med 2001;33:445–449.

7 Bürk K, Bösch S, Müller CA, Melms A, Zuhlke C, Stern M, Bessenthal L, Skalej M, Ruck P, Ferber S, Klockgether T, Dichgans J: Sporadic cerebellar ataxia associated with gluten sensitivity. Brain 2001;124:1013–1019.

8 Bushara KO, Goebel SU, Shill H, Goldfarb LG, Hallett M: Gluten sensitivity in sporadic and hereditary ataxia. Ann Neurol 2001;49: 540–543.

9 Abele M, Bürk K, Schöls L, Schwartz S, Bessenthal I, Dichgans J, Zuhlke C, Riess O, Klockgether T: The aetiology of sporadic adult-onset ataxia. Brain 2002;125:961–968.

10 Hadjivassiliou M, Grünewald RA, Sharrack B, Sanders DS, Lobo A, Wood N, Williamson C, Woodroofe N, Davies-Jones GAB: Gluten ataxia in perspective: epidemiology, genetic susceptibility and clinical characteristics. Brain 2003;126:685–691.

11 Ihara M, Makino F, Sawada H, Mezaki T, Mizutani K, Nakase H: Gluten sensitivity in Japanese patients with adult-onset cerebellar ataxia. Intern Med 2006;45:135–140.

12 Anheim M, Degos B, Echaniz-Laguna A, Fleury M, Grucker M, Tranchant C: Ataxia associated with gluten sensitivity, myth or reality? Rev Neurol 2006;162:214–221.

13 Hadjivassiliou M, Aeschlimann P, Sanders DS, Maki M, Kaukinen K, Grunewlad RA, Bandmann O, Woodroofe N, Haddock G, Aeschlimann DP: Transglutaminase 6 antibodies in the diagnosis of gluten ataxia. Neurology 2013;80:1–6.

14 Sarrigiannis PG, Hoggard N, Aeschlimann DP, Sanders DS, Grunewald RA, Unwin ZC, Hadjivassiliou M: Myoclonus ataxia and refractory coeliac disease. Cerebellum Ataxias 2014;1:11.

15 Kheder A, Currie S, Romanowski C, Hadjivassiliou M: Progressive ataxia with palatal tremor due to gluten sensitivity. Mov Disord 2012;27:62–63.

16 Deconinck N, Scaillon M, Segers V, Groswasser JJ, Dan B: Opsoclonus-myoclonus associated with celiac disease. Pediatr Neurol 2006; 34:312–314.

17 Wilkinson ID, Hadjivassiliou M, Dickson JM, Wallis L, Grunewald RA, Coley SC, Widjaja E, Griffiths PD: Cerebellar abnormalities on proton MR spectroscopy in gluten ataxia. J Neurol Neurosurg Psychiatry 2005;76:1011–1013.

18 Currie S, Hoggard N, Sanders DS, Wilkinson I, Griffiths PD, Hadjivassiliou M: Coeliac disease and neurological dysfunction: a case-control study. Lancet 2014;383:S39.

19 Beversdorf D, Moses P, Reeves A, Dunn J: A man with weight loss, ataxia, and confusion for 3 months. Lancet 1996;347:448.

20 Hahn JS, Sum JM, Bass D, Crowley RC, Horoupian DS: Celiac disease presenting as gait disturbance and ataxia in infancy. J Child Neurol 1998;13:351–353.

21 Pellecchia MT, Scala R, Perretti A: Cerebellar ataxia associated with subclinical celiac disease responding to gluten-free diet. Neurology 1999;53:1606–1607.

22 Sander HW, Magda P, Chin RL, Wu A, Brannagan TH, Green PH: Cerebellar ataxia and celiac disease. Lancet 2003;362:1548.

23 Bürk K, Melms A, Schulz JB, Dichgans J: Effectiveness of intravenous immunoglobulin therapy in cerebellar ataxia associated with gluten sensitivity. Ann Neurol 2001;50:827–828.

24 Hadjivassiliou M, Davies-Jones GAB, Sanders DS, Grünewald RAG: Dietary treatment of gluten ataxia. J Neurol Neurosurg Psychiatry 2003;74:1221–1224.

25 Cooke WT, Smith WT: Neurological disorders associated with adult coeliac disease. Brain 1966;89:683–722.

26 Hadjivassiliou M, Sanders DS, Grunewald RA, Woodroofe N, Boscolo S, Aeschlimann DP: Gluten sensitivity: from gut to brain. Lancet Neurol 2010;3:318–330.

27 Hadjivassiliou M, Boscolo S, Davies Jones GA, Grunewald RA, Not T, Sanders DS, Simpson J, Tongiorgi E, Williamson C, Woodroofe N: The humoral response in the pathogenesis of gluten ataxia. Neurology 2002;58:1221–1226.

28 Boscolo S, Lorenzon A, Sblattero D, Florian F, Stebel M, Marzari R, Not T, Aeschlimann D, Venture A, Hadjivassiliou M, Tongiorgi E: Anti-transglutaminase antibodies cause ataxia in mice. PLoS One 2008;3:e1580.

29 Molberg O, McAdam SN, Sollid LM: Role of tissue transglutaminase in celiac disease. J Paediatr Gastroenterol Nutr 2000;30:232–240.

30 Korponay-Szabo IR, Vecsei Z, kiraly R, Danlbom I, Chirdo F, Nemes E, Fesus L, Maki M: Deamidated gliadin peptides form epitopes that transglutaminase antibodies recognize. J Paediatr Gastroenterol Nutr 2008;46:253–261.

31 Sardy M, Karpati S, Merkl B, Paulsson M, Smyth N: Epidermal transglutaminase (TGase 3) is the autoantigen of dermatitis herpetiformis. J Exp Med 2002;195:747–757.

32 Hadjivassiliou M, Aeschlimann P, Strigun A, Sanders DS, Woodroofe N, Aeschlimann DP: Autoantibodies in gluten ataxia recognize a novel neuronal transglutaminase. Ann Neurol 2008;64:332–343.

33 Hadjivassiliou M, Maki M, Sanders DS, Williamson CA, Grunewald RA, Woodroofe N, Korponay-Szabo I: Autoantibody targeting of brain and intestinal transglutaminase in gluten ataxia. Neurology 2006;66:373–377.

Dig Dis 2015;33:269–276
DOI: 10.1159/000371401

Other Dietary Confounders: FODMAPS et al.

Peter R. Gibson[a] Jane G. Muir[a] Evan D. Newnham[b]

[a]Department of Gastroenterology, Alfred Hospital and Monash University, and [b]Department of Gastroenterology and Hepatology, Eastern Health and Monash University, Melbourne, Vic., Australia

Key Words
Amylase-trypsin inhibitors · Depression · Exorphins · FODMAPs · Fructans · Gastrointestinal symptoms · Irritable bowel syndrome · Lectins · Wheat germ agglutinin

Abstract
Background: While it is well documented and widely appreciated that ingestion of wheat (and less so rye and barley) is associated with gastrointestinal symptoms such as bloating or abdominal pain, the component of wheat to which such an effect is attributed is less well established. ***Key Messages:*** Wheat is a complex of proteins (80% gluten, 20% metabolic proteins), carbohydrates (starch, non-starch polysaccharides, fructans), lipids and other components. The majority of attention has focused on gluten as the culprit in triggering symptoms, but re-challenge studies have nearly all used wheat flour-related products (such as bread) as the stimulus. When carbohydrate-deplete gluten was used as the challenge agent, gluten-specific feelings of depression and not gut symptoms were observed in those who fulfilled strict criteria of 'non-coeliac gluten sensitivity', thereby underlining the complexity of cereals and of undertaking research in this area. Candidate components other than gluten include poorly absorbed oligosaccharides (mainly fructans), non-gluten wheat proteins such as amylase-trypsin inhibitors or wheat germ agglutinin, and exorphins released during the digestion of gluten. Specific biological and/or clinical effects associated with gluten-free diets or wheat ingestion need to be carefully dissected before attribution to gluten can be claimed. ***Conclusions:*** Currently, coeliac disease is the only common condition that has been unequivocally linked to gluten. Inaccurate attribution will be associated with suboptimal therapeutic advice and at least partly underlies the current gluten-free epidemic gripping the Western world.

Introduction

It is well documented and widely appreciated that ingestion of wheat (and less so rye and barley) is associated with gastrointestinal symptoms such as bloating or abdominal pain. The evidence for the association principally involves exclusion diet methodology with reproducible induction of symptoms on re-challenge with wheat and ongoing improvement of symptoms when wheat is avoided. In Australia, about 10% of the non-coeliac adult population avoid wheat or are strictly gluten-free, 80% doing so in response to symptoms, especially bloating, abdominal pain and fatigue [1]. Furthermore, those avoiding wheat are rational people and not psychologically disturbed. Unfortunately, the major focus of atten-

KARGER 125

© 2015 S. Karger AG, Basel
0257–2753/15/0332–0269$39.50/0

E-Mail karger@karger.com
www.karger.com/ddi

Prof. Peter R. Gibson
Department of Gastroenterology
Alfred Hospital
99 Commercial Road, Melbourne, VIC 3004 (Australia)
E-Mail peter.gibson@monash.edu

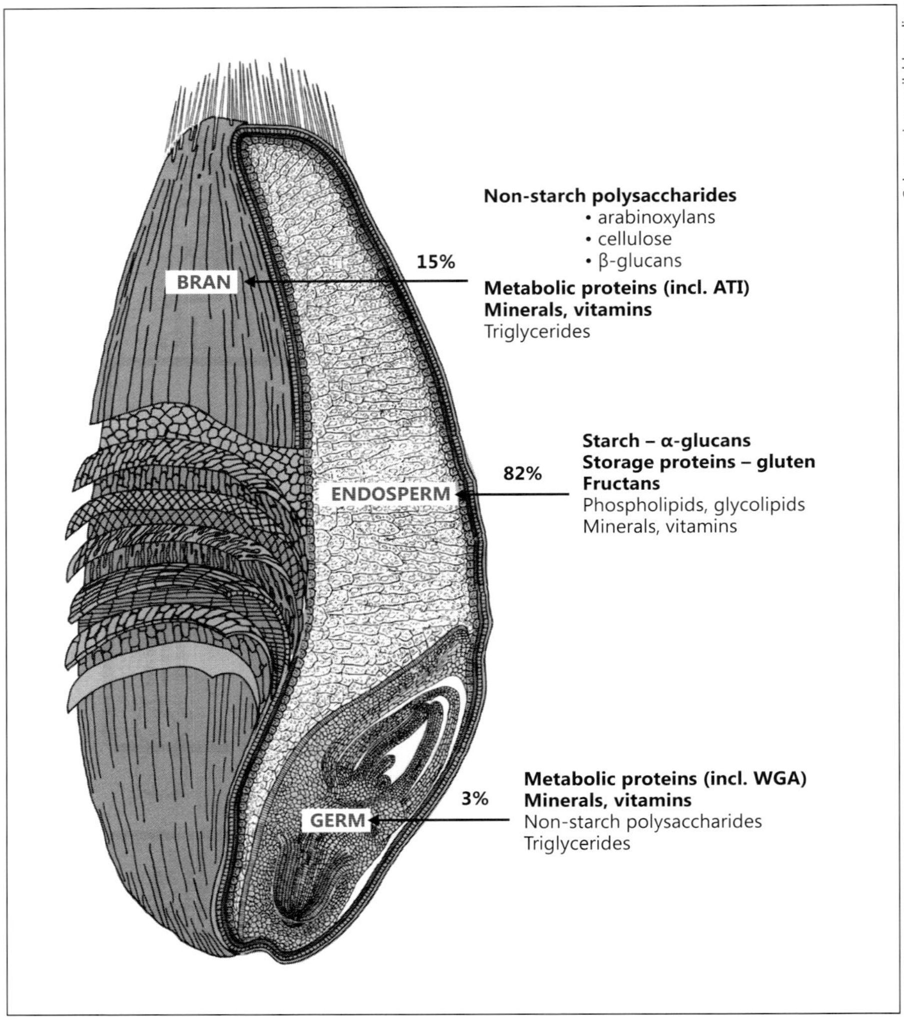

Color version available online

Fig. 1. A wheat kernel and its regional composition.

tion has been on whether gluten causes problems outside coeliac disease, so-called non-coeliac gluten sensitivity (NCGS). The real controversy is what component(s) of wheat is/are the culprits in inducing these effects. On the one hand, popular media have decided that gluten is the cause, and websites, books and a commercial industry have been built around this belief, with liberal use of scientific observations out of context as 'proof'. The evidence base for such a conclusion is very poor in all but coeliac disease, where gluten's role is now incontrovertible including knowledge of the inciting antigenic sequences [2, 3]. An open-minded approach to the role or not of gluten in inducing physiological or other effects is necessary. The use of the term non-coeliac wheat sensitivity has been proposed to divert attention away from gluten specifically [4].

Evidence Base for Gluten Causing Non-Coeliac Effects

Gluten has been implicated in multiple effects that mainly involve the gut (such as irritable bowel syndrome), the skin (such as dermatitis herpetiformis) and the brain (such as ataxia, depression and autism). The principal evidence that gluten causes those effects has comprised the reported response to a gluten-free diet and re-challenge with wheat [5–7]. Gluten-specific immunological effects, notably the production of circulating antibodies to gluten components, have also had significance attached to them despite their poor sensitivity and specificity in coeliac disease [8, 9]. Only coeliac disease, dermatitis herpetiformis and ataxia syndromes have a reasonable to high level of evidence in their immunological response and pathophysiology. An example of the difficulties in defining the offending agents is the recent demonstration that carbohydrate-depleted gluten induced current feelings of depression in a randomised controlled re-challenge study [10]; the challenged agent used was 70% gluten, and it cannot be concluded that gluten caused the effect. Thus, it is essential to address the complexity of wheat both by examining its other components and by addressing how gluten might induce problems by mechanisms other than specific immune responses (as in coeliac disease).

The other confusing and controversial area is the target population in which potential effects of wheat/gluten are examined. Some groups have confined their work to those without evidence of abnormal immune responses or injury to the gut [11, 12] characterised by inflammation and mucosal structural changes, while others have examined mixed groups with a proportion having evidence of mucosal injury or abnormalities [5, 9, 13]. The problem with having evidence of immune activation to gluten is that it is not easy to exclude coeliac disease or coeliac-specific immune events such as specific T-cell sensitivity to 'toxic' gluten peptides [14]. It has become evident over recent years that coeliac disease represents a spectrum from severe intestinal injury to minimal injury and that the evidence that fulfils the diagnostic criteria for coeliac disease may evolve over time for reasons that are poorly understood. Furthermore, the effects of wheat/gluten are clearly heterogeneous with several pathogenic pathways involving or independent of inflammation likely. This is best illustrated by the range of events from wheat allergy syndromes [15] to coeliac disease [16] to wheat sensitivity with eosinophilic gut infiltration [9] to gluten-induced feeling of depression where no markers of inflammation or gluten-related immune phenomena exist [10].

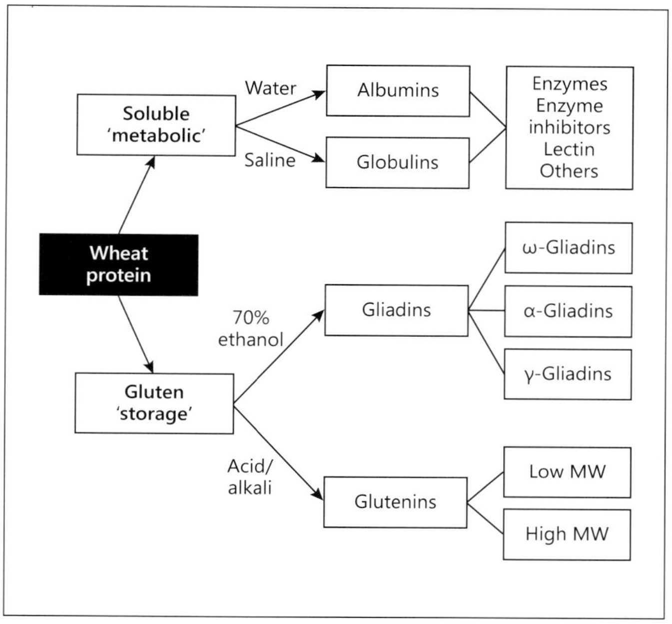

Fig. 2. Classification of proteins derived from wheat including the solubility characteristics used to separate the fractions. MW = Molecular weight.

Components of Wheat

Wheat kernels are complex structures comprising outer layers (bran), the germ and the starchy endosperm (fig. 1). These make up approximately 2–3, 13–17 and 80–85% of the dry weight, respectively [17]. Wheat grain contains multiple components that include proteins (gluten and non-gluten), carbohydrates (long- and short-chain, digestible and indigestible), lipids and lignin, ash, vitamins and anti-nutrients such as phytates. Digestion of gluten in the human upper gut also releases bioactive peptides. Details of these components, their locations and functions within the kernel, and known or potential effects on health and biological processes in the human consuming wheat are shown in table 1.

Proteins

The main storage protein of wheat, rye and barley is referred to as 'gluten', which comprises about 80% of wheat protein. The protein content of these cereals is a complex of a large number of different but related proteins that include storage proteins comprising: glutenins of both high and low molecular weight; prolamins, being gliadin in wheat, secalin in rye and hordein in barley [20], and albumin and globulins that are principally metabolic proteins involved with enzymatic or enzyme-inhibiting functions important for providing nutrients and energy during germination and for protecting against pests and disease. Two of interest with the latter function are α-amylase/trypsin inhibitors (ATI), a family of small-molecular-weight proteins that protect the plants from parasites and other pests [21, 22], and small glycoproteins relatively resistant to enzymatic or heat-derived degradation that avidly bind to sugars and hence act as lectins [23]. Grains have selectively been bred to have higher concentrations of both groups as they confer survival advantages.

Table 1. Chemical composition of wheat and peptides exposed to the gastrointestinal tract and functional correlates [17 – 21]

	Fractions	Proportion	Where	Functions	Disease associations/biological effects
Proteins	Glutenins Gliadins	72–75% of protein	Starchy endosperm	Storage in mealy endosperm Technologically active (formation of dough)	Food allergy Coeliac disease, baker's asthma, atopic dermatitis, food allergy, WDEIA
	Albumins Globulins	25–28% of protein	Seed coats, aleurone cells, germ	Enzymes, enzyme inhibitors – metabolic and protective	Baker's asthma, food allergy, WDEIA
				– ATI	Activates innate immune system
				– WGA	Pro-inflammatory, increase epithelial permeability
	Peptides following digestion	–	Released in the gut	–	Opioid activity (exorphins)
Carbo-hydrates	Starch (α-glucans) – amylose – amylopectins	 20–30% 70–80%	Starchy endosperm	Storage – nutrition	Important nutritional source
	Non-starch polysaccharides – arabinoxylans (insoluble) – cellulose (insoluble) – β-glucans (soluble)	wheat bran: 70% 24% 6%	Cell walls outer → inner layers bran → endosperm	Structural roles	Laxation, prevention of colorectal cancer, lower cholesterol, improved metabolic syndrome
	Fructans	–	Mealy endosperm	Storage; confer resistance to cold and drought stress	Prebiotic effects (favourable) Trigger gastrointestinal symptoms (unfavourable)
Lignin	Complex polymer of aromatic alcohols (monolignols)	–	Cell walls	Mechanical strength, water conduction	–
Lipids	Triglycerides Phospholipids, glycolipids	0.5–3% of whole kernel	Germ, aleurone layer endosperm	Structural, nutrition	–
Other	Ash (minerals), vitamins, polyphenols, phytates, other	–	Concentrated in outer layers	Nutritional; phytates – storage of phosphorus	Phytates reduce bioavailability of zinc, magnesium, iron and calcium

WDEIA = Wheat-dependent exercise-induced anaphylaxis.

All of these protein groups have been implicated in disease genesis. The toxic peptide sequences in coeliac disease are now well defined and exist in the γ-gliadin fraction of the gluten complex (fig. 2) [3]. Distinct wheat allergy syndromes have been described – wheat-dependent exercise-induced anaphylaxis in which all protein types have been implicated, baker's asthma in which inhaled gliadin and ATI have been implicated, and atopic dermatitis in which gliadin and low-molecular-weight glutenins have been blamed (table 1) [15].

More recently, non-IgE-mediated hypersensitivity to wheat proteins has been described in detail by Carroccio et al. [9]. Two general types appear to occur; 75% had sensitivity on double-blind placebo-controlled food challenge to wheat and other foods, especially milk proteins, while 25% reacted only to wheat. The specific proteins involved have not been studied, but antibodies to whole gliadin are present in 65% of such patients. The scenario described is one of chronic gut symptoms consistent with IBS, often with an atopic history, and inflammatory changes on small bowel biopsy that include increased density of intra-epithelial lymphocytes (in 90%) and eosinophilic infiltrates in addition to intraepithelial eosinophils in colonic biopsies in 75%. Somewhat surprisingly, this group comprised nearly one third of patients referred with IBS. The patients can also be identified with reasonable sensitivity (80%) by testing in vitro using the basophil activation test [24]. Importantly, gratifying improvement in symptoms at least in the short term occurs in nearly all of the patients with subsequent exclusion of wheat and other foods identified on challenge testing. Study in other centres is required as these patients are not currently being widely recognised.

ATI are of additional interest. They are able to activate the TLR4-MD2-CD14 complex and thus elicit innate immune effects [22]. All data in vivo derive from animal studies in which biologically significant activation was observed after oral and systemic challenge. Whether ATI can cause similar effects in humans ingesting dietary wheat remains to be determined, and their role in coeliac disease or non-coeliac wheat sensitivity remains speculative.

Of the lectins, wheat germ agglutinin (WGA) has received most attention, as recently reviewed [25]. It binds to N-glycolylneuraminic acid found in cell membranes (including those in epithelia of the gut), permitting it to be internalised. Studies in vitro have shown WGA to have a range of effects on polymorphs, monocytes and macrophages that are potentially pro-inflammatory and can increase paracellular permeability in cell lines. Studies in vivo have been limited to experimental animals, but increase in intestinal permeability and pro-inflammatory effects have been reported. Thus, it can potentially play a pro-inflammatory role alone or act in an adjunctive way with gluten in coeliac disease. In humans, some degree of penetration across the mucosal barrier may occur as circulating antibodies to WGA have been reported in healthy subjects and patients with coeliac disease [26, 27]. There are moderate to large amounts present in wheat germ, whole grains and some processed grains, and these are unlikely to be significantly degraded in the gastrointestinal tract. Only minute concentrations of the lectin are needed for its actions in epithelial models in vitro [28]. Thus, it would appear that WGA is a likely candidate to exert effects on epithelia and inflammatory cells in the human intestine, and this would be exaggerated if epithelial permeability was compromised. However, whether WGA plays a pathogenic role in humans is unknown.

Bioactive Peptides from Gluten Digests

Bioactive peptides, particularly those with opioid agonist actions (exorphins), released from proteins during digestion in the gastrointestinal tract have been described for gluten and other dietary proteins such as casein and rubisco (from spinach) [29]. Five distinct exorphin peptides (A4, A5, B4, B5 and E) from trypsin digests were originally described more than 30 years ago, mostly but not all from the gliadin fraction [30, 31]. An additional exorphin, gliadinomorphin-7, has also been described [32]. Exorphins are also released from pancreatic elastase digests [33]. They are probably absorbed since they have been measured in peripheral blood, at least in infants [34] and in patients with untreated coeliac disease [35].

Detailed study of the effects in vivo of exorphins has been limited, and few studies have been performed in humans. For the casein-derived exorphin β-casomorphin-7 effects on the gastrointestinal effects are likely since sufficient concentrations are released in the intestinal lumen during casein digestion [36]. Intestinal transit is reduced in animals fed milk containing A1 β-casein [37] and evidence of changes to gut function has recently been reported in healthy volunteers [38]. Whether systemically delivered exorphins exert biologically significant opioid actions remains contentious, but is the basis of exorphin hypothesis for autism and schizophrenia. Two observations in humans might potentially be exorphin-mediated – gluten-mediated increase in current feelings of depression in patients who believe they have NCGS [10] and reduction of diarrhoea in patients with diarrhoea-predominant IBS on a gluten-free diet [39]. However, the role of exorphins in these is purely speculative, and other explanations are possible. Sensitive accessible assays for exorphins are few and have yet to be applied to these settings to determine systemic exposure.

Carbohydrates

It is the indigestible carbohydrate component of wheat, barley and rye that has incited interest in having health-modulating roles. Non-starch polysaccharides and other indigestible long-chain carbohydrates play key roles in laxation and possibly also in prevention of colorectal cancer [40]. Wheat bran is widely used as a ready source of fibre that promotes faecal bulk and more rapid transit through the colon in healthy subjects. Only recently have the importance of indigestible oligosaccharides, notably fructans and to a lesser extent galacto-oligosaccharides, in colonic health and induction of gut symptoms been highlighted. Fructans are an important natural food prebiotic and increasing their intake can have major effects on the structure and presumably function of the gut microbiota [41]. On the detrimental side, fructans are a major member of the FODMAPs (fermentable oligo-, di- and monosaccharides and polyols); these can induce functional gut symptoms and reducing their intake is associated with considerable reduction of gut symptoms in about 70% of patients with IBS [42]. Evidence suggests they induce symptoms by distending the intestine with gas, via their rapid bacterial fermentation, and water, via their osmotic effects [43].

The contribution of oligosaccharides to gut symptoms in patients with apparent NCGS has been strongly suggested by the observation that gut symptoms of patients who previously gained benefit from a gluten-free diet, but had no evidence of coeliac disease or duodenal inflammation, were further improved by additionally reducing FODMAP intake from vegetables, fruits and beverages

[12]. Many people who believe they are gluten-sensitive do have persisting symptoms of not inconsiderable severity despite adhering to a gluten-free diet [44]. The hypothesis is that the perceived improvement of symptoms is due to the avoidance of fructan-containing cereals, but that their ongoing symptoms are due to FODMAPs present in non-cereal-based vegetables and fruits.

Of importance, FODMAPS and gluten coexist in grains – gluten-free cereals have very low levels and gluten-containing cereals have high levels of FODMAP oligosaccharides [45, 46]. This coexistence, also shared by rye and barley, has led to confusion regarding food challenges, which have generally involved the ingestion of wheat-based bread, to detect 'gluten sensitivity'. Indeed, two consecutive randomised controlled cross-over rechallenge studies in patients with NCGS and no inflammation in their duodenal biopsies failed to reveal specific induction of symptoms with FODMAP-devoid gluten, indicating that, at least in the 37 patients studied, gluten was not the cause of their gut symptoms [12].

In wheat, fructans are a reserve source of energy used when environmental conditions are unfavourable. In that way, they protect wheat in time of drought. Not surprisingly, modern wheat that has been bred for its hardiness under multiple conditions has higher content of fructans than ancient wheats such as spelt [45]. Traditional sourdough bread-making methods involve a long fermentation time with a live sourdough culture. Short-chain carbohydrates are used by the sourdough culture that includes yeasts and lactic acid bacteria thereby reducing level of sugars and presumably fructans in the bread [47]. Both of these factors have led to the idea that the increased content of fructans in bread is a factor contributing to the increasing prevalence of wheat sensitivity.

Other Wheat Components

Little is known of the functional significance to humans of consuming the lipids in wheat, which comprise 2–4% of the whole grain. Wheat also contains minerals (ash), vitamins and other chemicals that include polyphenols and phytates. Phytates are regarded as 'anti-nutrients' because they bind zinc, magnesium, iron and calcium, and reduce the bioavailability of these minerals.

The Way Forward

There are several lessons for future research into clinical syndromes or symptoms that appear to relate to the ingestion of wheat.

(1) It is essential to take into account the multiple components of wheat when interpreting findings associated with its ingestion, so that attribution of an effect to a specific part (e.g. to gluten) is not incorrectly made. This might involve using specific parts of the wheat (e.g. carbohydrate-depleted gluten) when challenging a subject [11, 12]. The amount of wheat used is another less direct method of making an educated guess as to the culprit; for example, the amount of wheat contained within capsules used in some challenge protocols is too small to anticipate carbohydrate-mediated effects to be observed [9]. Likewise, the presence of inflammatory lesions due to its ingestion is less likely to be carbohydrate associated.

(2) The definition of the target population is essential. Much controversy about NCGS has revolved around different study populations who have responded to a gluten-free diet. For example, some are defined histologically and immunologically [11, 12], some defined by symptom response to blinded placebo-controlled challenges with wheat [9], some with a variety of symptom clusters from intestinal to extra-intestinal alone or in combination, and some with a variety of histological and immunological features in which some might indeed have coeliac disease [13].

(3) The need for biomarkers is paramount since the use of patient-reported outcomes (i.e. symptom induction) during re-challenges with wheat/gluten or placebo may be fraught with nocebo responses, although not all groups have experienced this. Circulating anti-whole-gliadin antibodies have been proposed, but their frequency in the non-wheat-sensitive population is too high for it to be discriminatory [9] and may be related to increased exposure to gliadin secondary to increased epithelial permeability from the intestinal lesion itself. The report of the high positive predictive value of the basophil activation test for those with wheat hypersensitivity is promising in this way [20].

(4) Longer-term, prospective data on clinical outcomes following dietary interventions are essential to define the true value of that dietary intervention. To date, the literature is devoid of such information.

(5) The current definitions and terminology used create confusion. The consensus definition of gluten sensitivity recently reached [48, 49] is difficult to carry through since there is no available challenge that is purely gluten and the gluten-free diet leads to a concomitant reduction of all wheat components in addition to gluten. There is no problem with the term if strong evidence

implicates gluten in the symptom genesis, but, as outlined above, this has been a general weakness of many studies as uncovered by the cross-over study of Biesiekierski et al. [12]. The proposal that the term NCGS is replaced with 'non-coeliac wheat sensitivity' is helpful in taking attention away from gluten as the culprit [9], but would apply to perhaps 10% of the population since wheat induces symptoms presumably via the ingestion of fructans in the majority of patients with IBS. Furthermore, it would in many cases inappropriately excuse a similar role for other cereals such as rye and barley.

Only with carefully designed studies addressing many of these issues will clarity emerge from the current confusion that is present in both the clinical and general community. Currently, coeliac disease is the only common condition that has been unequivocally linked to gluten. Inaccurate attribution will be associated with suboptimal therapeutic advice and at least partly underlies the current gluten-free epidemic gripping the Western world.

Disclosure Statement

No perceived conflicts of interest.

References

1 Golley S, Corsini N, Topping D, Morell M, Mohr P: Motivations for avoiding wheat consumption in Australia: results from a population survey. Public Health Nutr 2014;1–10.

2 Anderson RP, Degano P, Godkin AJ, Jewell DP, Hill AV: In vivo antigen challenge in celiac disease identifies a single transglutaminase-modified peptide as the dominant A-gliadin T-cell epitope. Nat Med 2000;6:337–342.

3 Tye-Din JA, Stewart JA, Dromey JA, Beissbarth T, van Heel DA, Tatham A, Henderson K, Mannering SI, Gianfrani C, Jewell DP, Hill AV, McCluskey J, Rossjohn J, Anderson RP: Comprehensive, quantitative mapping of T cell epitopes in gluten in celiac disease. Sci Transl Med 2010;2:41ra51.

4 Carroccio A, Rini G, Mansueto P: Non-celiac wheat sensitivity is a more appropriate label than non-celiac gluten sensitivity. Gastroenterology 2014;146:320–321.

5 Volta U, Bardella MT, Calabrò A, Troncone R, Corazza GR; Study Group for Non-Celiac Gluten Sensitivity: An Italian prospective multicenter survey on patients suspected of having non-celiac gluten sensitivity. BMC Med 2014;12:85.

6 Lu W, Gwee KA, Siah KT, Kang JY, Lee R, Ngan CC: Prevalence of anti-deamidated gliadin peptide antibodies in Asian patients with irritable bowel syndrome. J Neurogastroenterol Motil 2014;20:236–241.

7 Kabbani TA, Vanga RR, Leffler DA, Villafuerte-Galvez J, Pallav K, Hansen J, Mukherjee R, Dennis M, Kelly CP: Celiac disease or non-celiac gluten sensitivity? An approach to clinical differential diagnosis. Am J Gastroenterol 2014;109:741–746.

8 Volta U, Tovoli F, Cicola R, Parisi C, Fabbri A, Piscaglia M, Fiorini E, Caio G: Serological tests in gluten sensitivity (nonceliac gluten intolerance). J Clin Gastroenterol 2012;46:680–685.

9 Carroccio A, Mansueto P, D'Alcamo A, Iacono G: Non-celiac wheat sensitivity as an allergic condition: personal experience and narrative review. Am J Gastroenterol 2013;108:1845–1852.

10 Peters SL, Biesiekierski JR, Yelland GW, Muir JG, Gibson PR: Randomised clinical trial: gluten may cause depression in subjects with non-coeliac gluten sensitivity – an exploratory clinical study. Aliment Pharmacol Ther 2014;39:1104–1112.

11 Biesiekierski JR, Newnham ED, Irving PM, Barrett JS, Haines M, Doecke JD, Shepherd SJ, Muir JG, Gibson PR: Gluten causes gastrointestinal symptoms in subjects without celiac disease: a double-blind randomized placebo-controlled trial. Am J Gastroenterol 2011;106:508–514.

12 Biesiekierski JR, Peters SL, Newnham ED, Rosella O, Muir JG, Gibson PR: No effects of gluten in patients with self-reported non-celiac gluten sensitivity after dietary reduction of fermentable, poorly absorbed, short-chain carbohydrates. Gastroenterology 2013;145:320–328.

13 Wahnschaffe U, Schulzke JD, Zeitz M, Ullrich R: Predictors of clinical response to gluten-free diet in patients diagnosed with diarrhea-predominant irritable bowel syndrome. Clin Gastroenterol Hepatol 2007;5:844–850.

14 Ontiveros N, Tye-Din JA, Hardy MY, Anderson RP: Ex-vivo whole blood secretion of interferon (IFN)-γ and IFN-γ-inducible protein-10 measured by enzyme-linked immunosorbent assay are as sensitive as IFN-γ enzyme-linked immunospot for the detection of gluten-reactive T cells in human leucocyte antigen (HLA)-DQ2 · 5(+)-associated coeliac disease. Clin Exp Immunol 2014;175:305–315.

15 Uvackova L, Skultety L, Bekesova S, McClain S, Hajduch M: The MS(E)-proteomic analysis of gliadins and glutenins in wheat grain identifies and quantifies proteins associated with celiac disease and baker's asthma. J Proteomics 2013;93:65–73.

16 Kaukinen K, Lindfors K, Mäki M: Advances in the treatment of coeliac disease: an immunopathogenic perspective. Nat Rev Gastroenterol Hepatol 2014;11:36–44.

17 Šramkováa Z, Gregovráb E, Šturdíka E: Chemical composition and nutritional quality of wheat grain. Acta Chimica Slovaca 2009;2:115–138.

18 Koehler P, Wieser H: Chemistry of cereal grains; in Boetti M, Ganzle M (eds): Handbook on Sourdough Biotechnology. Springer, New York, 2013, pp 11–45.

19 Stevenson L, Phillips F, O'Sullivan K, Walton J: Wheat bran: its composition and benefits to health, a European perspective. Int J Food Sci Nutr 2012;63:1001–1013.

20 Wieser H: Chemistry of gluten proteins. Food Microbiol 2007;24:115–119.

21 Altenbach SB, Vensel WH, Dupont FM: The spectrum of low molecular weight alpha-amylase/protease inhibitor genes expressed in the US bread wheat cultivar Butte 86. BMC Res Notes 2011;4:242.

22 Junker Y, Zeissig S, Kim SJ, Barisani D, Wieser H, Leffler DA, Zevallos V, Libermann TA, Dillon S, Freitag TL, Kelly CP, Schuppan D: Wheat amylase trypsin inhibitors drive intestinal inflammation via activation of toll-like receptor 4. J Exp Med 2012;209:2395–2408.

23 Pusztai A, Ewen SW, Grant G, Brown DS, Stewart JC, Peumans WJ, Van Damme EJ, Bardocz S: Antinutritive effects of wheat-germ agglutinin and other N-acetylglucosamine-specific lectins. Br J Nutr 1993;70:313–321.

24 Carroccio A, Brusca I, Mansueto P, Pirrone G, Barrale M, Di Prima L, Ambrosiano G, Iacono G, Lospalluti ML, La Chiusa SM, Di Fede G: A cytologic assay for diagnosis of food hypersensitivity in patients with irritable bowel syndrome. Clin Gastroenterol Hepatol 2010;8:254–260.

25 de Punder K, Pruimboom L: The dietary intake of wheat and other cereal grains and their role in inflammation. Nutrients 2013;5:771–787.

26 Tchernychev B, Wilchek M: Natural human antibodies to dietary lectins. FEBS Lett 1996; 397:139–142.

27 Sollid LM, Kolberg J, Scott H, Ek J, Fausa O, Brandtzaeg P: Antibodies to wheat germ agglutinin in coeliac disease. Clin Exp Immunol 1986;63:95–100.

28 Dalla Pellegrina C, Perbellini O, Scupoli MT, Tomelleri C, Zanetti C, Zoccatelli G, Fusi M, Peruffo A, Rizzi C, Chignola R: Effects of wheat germ agglutinin on human gastrointestinal epithelium: insights from an experimental model of immune/epithelial cell interaction. Toxicol Appl Pharmacol 2009;237:146–153.

29 Teschemacher H: Opioid receptor ligands derived from food proteins. Curr Pharm Design 2003;9:1331–1344.

30 Zioudrou C, Streaty RA, Klee WA: Opioid peptides derived from food proteins. The exorphins. J Biol Chem 1979;254:2446–2449.

31 Huebner FR, Lieberman KW, Rubino RP, Wall JS: Demonstration of high opioid-like activity in isolated peptides from wheat gluten hydrolysates. Peptides 1984;5:1139–1147.

32 Trivedi MS, Shah JS, Al-Mughairy S, Hodgson NW, Simms B, Trooskens GA, Van Criekinge W, Deth RC: Food-derived opioid peptides inhibit cysteine uptake with redox and epigenetic consequences. J Nutr Biochem 2014;25:1011–1018.

33 Fukudome S, Jinsmaa Y, Matsukawa T, Sasaki R, Yoshikawa M: Release of opioid peptides, gluten exorphins by the action of pancreatic elastase. FEBS Lett 1997;412:475–479.

34 Kost NV, Sokolov OY, Kurasova OB, Dmitriev AD, Tarakanova JN, Gabaeva MV, Zolotarev YA, Dadayan AK, Grachev SA, Korneeva EV, Mikheeva IG, Zozulya AA: Beta-casomorphins-7 in infants on different type of feeding and different levels of psychomotor development. Peptides 2009;30:1854–1860.

35 Pennington CL, Dufresne CP, Fanciulli G, Wood TD: Detection of gluten exorphin B4 and B5 in human blood by liquid chromatography-mass spectrometry/mass spectrometry. Open Spectroscopy J 2007;1:9–16.

36 Boutrou R, Gaudichon C, Dupont D, Jardin J, Airinei G, Marsset-Baglieri A, Benamouzig R, Tomé D, Leonil J: Sequential release of milk protein-derived bioactive peptides in the jejunum in healthy humans. Am J Clin Nutr 2013; 97:1314–1323.

37 Barnett MP, McNabb WC, Roy NC, Woodford KB, Clarke AJ: Dietary A1 β-casein affects gastrointestinal transit time, dipeptidyl peptidase-4 activity, and inflammatory status relative to A2 β-casein in Wistar rats. Int J Food Sci Nutr 2014;65:720–727.

38 Ho S, Woodford K, Kukuljan S, Pal S: Comparative effects of A1 versus A2 beta-casein on gastrointestinal measures: a blinded randomised cross-over pilot study. Eur J Clin Nutr 2014;68:994–1000.

39 Vazquez-Roque MI, Camilleri M, Smyrk T, Murray JA, Marietta E, O'Neill J, Carlson P, Lamsam J, Janzow D, Eckert D, Burton D, Zinsmeister AR: A controlled trial of gluten-free diet in patients with irritable bowel syndrome-diarrhea: effects on bowel frequency and intestinal function. Gastroenterology 2013;144:903–911.

40 Muir JG, Gibson PR: Manipulating dietary carbohydrates to treat irritable bowel syndrome; in Simren M (ed): Clinical Insights. London, Future Medicine, pp 81–103.

41 Halmos EP, Christophersen CT, Bird AR, Shepherd SJ, Gibson PR, Muir JG: Diets that differ in their FODMAP content alter the colonic luminal microenvironment. Gut 2015; 64:93–100.

42 Halmos EP, Power VA, Shepherd SJ, Gibson PR, Muir JG: A diet low in FODMAPs reduces symptoms of irritable bowel syndrome. Gastroenterology 2014;146:67–75.

43 Tuck CJ, Muir JG, Barrett JS, Gibson PR: Fermentable oligosaccharides, disaccharides, monosaccharides and polyols: role in irritable bowel syndrome. Expert Rev Gastroenterol Hepatol 2014;8:819–834.

44 Biesiekierski JR, Newnham ED, Shepherd SJ, Muir JG, Gibson PR: Characterization of adults with a self-diagnosis of nonceliac gluten sensitivity. Nutr Clin Pract 2014;29:504–509.

45 Biesiekierski JR, Rosella O, Rose R, Liels K, Barrett JS, Shepherd SJ, Gibson PR, Muir JG: Quantification of fructans, galacto-oligosaccharides and other short-chain carbohydrates in processed grains and cereals. J Hum Nutr Diet 2011;24:154–176.

46 Gibson PR, Muir JG: Not all effects of a gluten-free diet are due to removal of gluten. Gastroenterology 2013;145:693.

47 Vrancken G, Rimaux T, Weckx S, Leroy F, De Vuyst L: Influence of temperature and backslopping time on the microbiota of a type I propagated laboratory wheat sourdough fermentation. Appl Environ Microbiol 2011;77: 2716–2726.

48 Sapone A, Bai JC, Ciacci C, Dolinsek J, Green PH, Hadjivassiliou M, Kaukinen K, Rostami K, Sanders DS, Schumann M, Ullrich R, Villalta D, Volta U, Catassi C, Fasano A: Spectrum of gluten-related disorders: consensus on new nomenclature and classification. BMC Med 2012;10:13.

49 Ludvigsson JF, Leffler DA, Bai JC, Biagi F, Fasano A, Green PH, Hadjivassiliou M, Kaukinen K, Kelly CP, Leonard JN, Lundin KE, Murray JA, Sanders DS, Walker MM, Zingone F, Ciacci C: The Oslo definitions for coeliac disease and related terms. Gut 2013; 62:43–52.

Novel Therapies

Dig Dis 2015;33:277–281
DOI: 10.1159/000369536

Novel Treatments for Celiac Disease: Glutenases and Beyond

Katri Kaukinen[a, b] Katri Lindfors[c]

[a]School of Medicine, University of Tampere, [b]Department of Internal Medicine, Tampere University Hospital, and
[c]Tampere Center for Child Health Research, University of Tampere and Tampere University Hospital, Tampere, Finland

Key Words
Celiac disease · Gluten · Glutenase · Enzyme supplement · Villous atrophy

Abstract
Currently, the only effective treatment for celiac disease is a strict lifelong gluten-free diet. However, gluten-free dieting is restrictive, difficult to maintain and nutritionally less than optimal. The improved knowledge on celiac disease pathogenesis has enabled researchers to suggest alternative strategies to treat the disorder. The drug development poses a challenge as any novel drug for celiac disease should be simultaneously effective and as safe as the gluten-free diet. The rationale behind enzyme supplementation therapy as a future treatment option for celiac patients lies in the fact that gluten is only poorly digested by gastrointestinal proteases. Due to incomplete degradation in the gastrointestinal tract, fairly long gluten peptides enter the small-intestinal lumen and come into contact with the mucosal epithelium, and in celiac disease patients this encounter launches deleterious downstream effects. Enzyme supplement therapy using either bacterial or fungal endopeptidases or proteases from germinating cereals has been proposed to promote complete digestion of prolamins and destroy disease-inducing gluten peptides. A major advantage of these glutenases is that they work in the lumen of the small intestine and do not themselves take part in the immunological cascade of events in the lamina propria, thus being unlikely to cause harmful side effects to the host. Studies to test this rationale, e.g. with *Aspergillus niger* prolyl endoprotease and a combination enzyme product ALV003, are already ongoing. The development of a novel medication for celiac disease is still in its early days, and thus the conventional dietary treatment will hold its place for the time being.

Introduction

In celiac disease, the benefit of treatment with a strict gluten-free diet is obvious. The diet improves the damaged small-bowel mucosal villous architecture and decreases the number of intraepithelial lymphocytes, alleviates gastrointestinal symptoms, and it may reduce the risk of long-term complications such as malignancies and osteoporosis [1]. Gluten-free diet excluding all food products containing wheat, rye and barley is currently the only treatment option for celiac disease. The high cost, and often poor availability of gluten-free foods makes it difficult to maintain [2]. Furthermore, removal of gluten from baked products renders them less palatable than comparable items in the normal diet. Due to the particularly restricted nature of the gluten-free diet, changing eating habits for life can be an enormous challenge for many celiac disease patients [3] and the compliance with the diet easily remains inadequate [4]. It has been found that in clinical practice even 20–80% of the celiac disease patients

KARGER 125
E-Mail karger@karger.com
www.karger.com/ddi

0257–2753/15/0332–0277$39.50/0

Prof. Katri Kaukinen, MD, PhD
School of Medicine
University of Tampere
FI–33014 Tampere (Finland)
E-Mail katri.kaukinen@uta.fi

adhere only partially to the gluten-free diet [4]. Despite a good adherence to the diet, a subgroup of patients may remain symptomatic and still have small-intestinal damage and inflammation [5]. In such cases, ongoing inadvertent gluten indigestion is frequently found [6]. Products on the market may contain trace amounts of contaminating gluten, and in real life a diet completely devoid of gluten is difficult if not even impossible to maintain [7]. Furthermore, even if appropriately maintained, a gluten-free diet is not nutritionally optimal, and it may predispose to an undesirable intake of fat and carbohydrates and lead to poor vitamin status and detrimental weight gain [8]. Due to these obvious problems with gluten-free dieting, celiac disease patients express an unmet need for alternative therapies to treat their condition [9–10]. However, the development of any new drug is a very slow and expensive process. In the context of celiac disease, one must remember that the new drug should be as effective and safe as a gluten-free diet. This article reviews recent knowledge about gluten-based therapies including enzymatic alteration of wheat and oral enzyme supplementation by glutenases as novel treatment options for celiac disease.

Rationale behind Enzyme Supplementation Therapy

Gluten, the major structural storage protein of wheat, rye and barley, has unique viscoelastic properties that are essential for dough formations and gives bread its distinctive texture and taste. Due to this, gluten-containing products are widely consumed, and currently the daily gluten intake in Western world is high, often ranging between 15 and 20 g per day [11]. The rationale behind enzyme supplementation therapy as a future treatment option for celiac disease patients lies in the fact that food-derived gluten consists of considerable amounts of proline and glutamine amino acids, and therefore gluten is only poorly digested in human gastrointestinal tract by gastric, pancreatic and intestinal brush border proteases even in individuals without celiac disease [12]. Incomplete degradation leads to fairly long gluten peptides entering the small-intestinal lumen, and they first come into contact with the small-intestinal mucosal epithelium. In celiac disease patients, this encounter launches downstream various innate and adaptive immune responses which eventually lead to the development of small bowel mucosal damage and symptomatic clinical condition [13].

There are approaches by which gluten could be detoxified during food processing even before it is digested. Bacteria and fungi have an advanced ability to process food proteins by means of a variety of specific proteases, and e.g. the lactobacilli of sourdough, possess such enzymes. Specific combinations of lactobacilli and fungal proteases may result in complete hydrolyzation of gluten in wheat flour [14]. In recent small clinical studies, there are implications that goods baked using sourdough fermentation are not harmful for celiac patients [15, 16]. However, so far only few short-term challenge studies have been carried out, and therefore firm conclusions cannot be drawn. Furthermore, enzymatic pretreatment of wheat flour and removal of the celiac-harmful components might result in a loss of characteristics that make gluten-containing products preferable for food processing. Still, these studies provide valuable data on enzymatic detoxification of gluten, and such information can be exploited in drug development.

Per oral enzyme supplementation therapy is currently the most studied approach for alternative celiac disease treatment [17]. It is based on digesting food-derived gluten peptides further into small nontoxic peptides by glutenases before they enter the intestinal epithelium. Glutenases are endopeptidases that are designed to target and destroy proline and glutamine residues in gluten peptides and thereby decrease the immunogenicity of gluten and prevent the downstream activation of celiac disease type pathogenic cascade [18–20]. Microbial prolyl endopeptidases (PEPs) from species including *Aspergillus niger*, *Flavobacteruim meningosepticum*, *Sphingomonas capsulata* and *Myxococcus xanthus* as well as germinating cereal enzymes (e.g. EP-B2 from barley) possess the capacity to hydrolyze gluten peptides in various in vitro and in vivo conditions (table 1). These enzymes are also able to exert their proteolytic function in the pH range present in the gastrointestinal tract, and they are at least moderately resistant to the prevailing harsh environment [20]. As shown in table 1, detoxification capacity of these enzymes has been supported by extensive in vitro, in vivo (in rats and macaques) and ex vivo (using biopsy-derived T cells and small bowel biopsies in organ culture systems) studies [21–28]. As PEP and EP-B2 are complementary as regards their sequence specificities, investigators have thought that a combination of these enzymes would be a dramatically superior therapeutic approach for the treatment of celiac disease [19]. Based on this, a combination enzyme product ALV003, consisting of 1:1 mixture of barley EP-B2 and *Sphingomonas capsulata* PEP has been formulated [23]. Following the line of thinking of the combination enzyme therapy, also an entire range of germinating cereal enzymes have been tested for their capability to degrade gluten [26, 27]. The major advance in

Table 1. Preclinical studies on detoxifying gluten with glutenases

First author	Glutenase	Study design	Main findings
Matysiak-Budnik [21]	Bacterial PEP	In vitro degradation of gliadin peptides 56–88 (33-mer) and 31–49 HPLC, mass spectrometry Ex vivo: using chamber with CD duodenal biopsies	Gliadin was degraded partly by PEP High PEP concentrations were required to achieve full detoxification of peptides and to prevent intestinal transport of active fragments
Gass [22]	EP-B2 from barley	Rats, meals containing 1 g of gluten HPCL, mass spectrometry	Pretreatment of gluten with EP-B2: the gastric concentration of the highly immunogenic 33-mer gliadin peptide was reduced
Gass [23]	Bacterial PEP EP-B2 from barley	Whole-wheat bread gluten In vitro and in vivo (rat) experimental systems developed to simulate human gastric digestion: HPLC, enzyme-linked immunoabsorbent assay, patient-derived T-cell proliferation assays	PEP and EP-B2 have synergetic potential to detoxify gluten; the efficacy of this 2-enzyme glutenase was verified in a rat model of gastric gluten digestion
Bethune [24]	EP-B2 from barley	Gluten-sensitive macaque Orally dosed labeled 33-mer gluten peptide ± EP-B2 Intestinal permeability, serum gliadin and transglutaminase antibodies	Administration of EP-B2 prevented clinical relapse in response to a dietary gluten challenge; unexpectedly celiac antibody titers increased
Mitea [25]	Fungal AN-PEP	Human gastrointestinal tract model Slice of wheat bread and fast-food meal Gliadin peptides and glutenins were assessed by monoclonal antibody-based competition assays, Western blot analysis and proliferation T-cell assays	AN-PEP accelerated the degradation of gluten in the stomach compartment to such an extent that hardly any gluten reached the duodenum compartment
Stenman [26, 27]	Proteases from germinating wheat and rye	Pepsin and trypsin digested gliadin pretreated with germinating wheat/rye proteases HPLC and mass spectrometry, polyacrylamide gel, Caco-2 epithelial cells, celiac patient-derived T cells, human small-intestinal mucosal organ culture biopsies	Germinating cereal enzymes reduce the toxicity of gliadin in vitro and ex vivo
Toft-Hansen [28]	25 proteases	Gluten-specific CD4+ T-cell clone and 7 gluten-reactive T-cell lines	AN-PEP was particularly efficient at diminishing proliferation of gluten-reactive T cells

HPCL = High-performance liquid chromatography.

such an approach is that the protease preparation contains all the enzymes that are evolutionarily selected for total cleavage of storage proteins in germinating kernels. First proof-of-concept studies in these enzyme cocktails have shown that this approach might be successful and subject to further development and optimization.

Clinical Studies with Glutenases

The first clinical intervention study with glutenases in celiac disease was published in 2005 (table 2). In that randomized, double-blind, crossover study, 20 asymptomatic treated celiac disease patients were challenged with 5 g of gluten for 14 days and were subsequently crossed over to consume gluten pretreated with *F. meningosepticum*-derived PEP for an additional 14 days [29]. The study found that pretreatment of gluten with PEP alleviated the development of fat or carbohydrate malabsorption in most celiac patients who otherwise developed these abnormalities after the 14-day gluten challenge [29].

In a recent Dutch double-blind randomized study, 14 treated celiac disease adults were challenged daily with 7 g of gluten for 2 weeks either with *A. niger*-derived PEP (AN-PEP) or placebo [31]. Unfortunately, the short-term gluten challenge was not able to induce small bowel mucosal damage (primary end point), and thus it was impossible to evaluate the effects of AN-PEP on detoxification of gluten in celiac disease [31]. However, there was some evidence that AN-PEP was able to prevent local gluten-induced small bowel mucosal autoantibody responses in celiac disease patients (table 2).

The glutenase ALV003 has been shown to be safe, well tolerated, and during the clinical studies no serious adverse events or allergic reactions have been observed [33]. Moreover, it has been found to be highly effective in degrading gluten primarily in the stomach before it reached the duodenal compartment. Based on these encouraging results, this drug candidate has entered phase 2 clinical trials (table 2). In a study of 20 adults with biopsy-proven celiac disease who were randomly assigned to gluten (16 g daily for 3 days) pretreated with ALV003 or placebo,

Table 2. Clinical studies on detoxifying gluten with glutenases in CD patients

First author	Glutenase	Study design	Main findings
Pyle [29]	Bacterial PEP	20 treated CD adults Double-blind randomized, crossover study 5 g gluten 14 days with PEP pretreatment/placebo Fecal fat, D-xylose urine excretion	Pretreatment of gluten with PEP prevented from the development of fat or carbohydrate malabsorption in the majority of CD patients who developed malabsorption after a 2-week gluten challenge
Tye-Din [30]	ALV003[1]	20 treated CD adults Randomized study: a large gluten meal (16 g daily) for 3 days pretreated with ALV003 or placebo Peripheral blood T-cell IFN-γ ELISpot responses to gliadin and an immunogenic 33-mer, symptoms	6 out of 10 had significant ELISPOT responses in placebo group; 0 out of 10 in ALV003 group Symptoms typically associated with gluten ingestion occurred in both groups
Tack [31]	Fungal AN-PEP	14 treated CD adults Double-blind randomized study 7 g gluten per day for 2 weeks with AN-PEP or placebo Duodenal biopsies (Marsh grade, IgA TG2 deposits, immunophenotyping of T cells) complaints, quality of life, serum antibodies	Primary end point was not met due to lack of clinical deterioration upon placebo, impeding an effect of AN-PEP IgA-TG2 deposit staining increased after gluten compared to baseline in 4 out of 7 patients on placebo; in the 7 patients receiving AN-PEP, 1 patient showed increased and 1 showed decreased IgA-TG2 deposits
Lähdeaho [32]	ALV003[1]	34 treated CD adults Double-blind randomized study 2 g gluten per day for 6 weeks with ALV003 or placebo Duodenal biopsies (villus height to crypt depth and densities of intraepithelial lymphocytes, IgA TG2 deposits), complaints, quality of life, serum antibodies	Biopsies from subjects in the placebo group showed evidence of mucosal injury after gluten challenge; no significant mucosal deterioration was observed in biopsies from the ALV003 group There were no statistically significant differences in symptoms between groups

TG2 = Transglutaminase 2. [1] Consists of two proteases: bacterial PEP and EP-B2 from barley.

enzymatic pretreatment was able to decrease peripheral blood gluten-specific immune response, even if no significant improvement was seen in clinical responses (the occurrence nausea, bloating, abdominal pain, lethargy, vomiting and diarrhea) with ALV003 [30].

In the next phase 2 study, the primary objective was to determine whether ALV003 was able to attenuate gluten-induced small-intestinal mucosal damage in celiac disease (table 2). Interestingly, glutenase ALV003 was able to diminish gluten-induced small-intestinal mucosal injury in patients with treated celiac disease in the context of an everyday gluten-free diet containing up to 2 g of gluten per day for 6 weeks [32]. Phase 2b studies are currently in progress (Alvine Pharmaceuticals, San Carlos, Calif., USA; ClinicalTrials.gov identifier: NCT01917630).

Future Aspects

An alternative treatment for celiac disease is called for. In addition to enzyme supplementation therapy, suggested therapeutic approaches include modulation of intestinal permeability, prevention of gluten presentation to T cells by blocking the binding of gluten epitopes to HLA-DQ2 molecules, use of transglutaminase 2 inhibitors, downregulation of immune response by antibodies against proinflammatory cytokines, and promotion of tolerance by other immunomodulatory strategies [17]. Some of the novel treatment options have already entered clinical trials, but before any of the candidates can enter phase 3 trials, researchers must develop novel reliable noninvasive surrogate markers for intestinal injury and disease activity. Currently, no novel drugs or new treatments are available on the market. The first medication to become available will most likely be marketed as a supplement to a gluten-free diet, although patients would prefer the medication to replace the burdensome diet. As the development of a novel medication for celiac disease is still in its early days, the conventional dietary treatment will hold its place for the time being.

Acknowledgements

The Celiac Disease Study Group and this work were supported by grants from the Competitive State Research Financing of the Expert Responsibility Area of Tampere University Hospital, the Academy of Finland, and the Sigrid Juselius Foundation.

Disclosure Statement

The authors report no conflict of interest.

References

1 Ludvigsson JF, Bai JC, Biagi F, Card TR, Ciacci C, Ciclitira PJ, Green PH, Hadjivassiliou M, Holdoway A, van Heel DA, Kaukinen K, Leffler DA, Leonard JN, Lundin KE, McGough N, Davidson M, Murray JA, Swift GL, Walker MM, Zingone F, Sanders DS: BSG Coeliac Disease Guidelines Development Group: Diagnosis and management of adult coeliac disease: guidelines from the British Society of Gastroenterology. Gut 2014;63:1210–1228.

2 Lee AR, Ng DL, Zivin J, Green PH: Economic burden of a gluten-free diet. J Hum Nutr Diet 2007;20:423–430.

3 Shah S, Akbari M, Vanga R, Kelly CP, Hansen J, Theethira T, Tariq S, Dennis M, Leffler DA: Patient perception of treatment burden is high in celiac disease compared with other common conditions. Am J Gastroenterol DOI: 10.1038/ajg.2014.29.

4 Hall NJ, Rubin G, Charnock A: Systematic review: adherence to a gluten-free diet in adult patients with coeliac disease. Aliment Pharmacol Ther 2009;30:315–330.

5 Ilus T, Lähdeaho MT, Salmi T, Haimila K, Partanen J, Saavalainen P, Huhtala H, Mäki M, Collin P, Kaukinen K: Persistent duodenal intraepithelial lymphocytosis despite a long-term strict gluten-free diet in celiac disease. Am J Gastroenterol 2012;107:1563–1569.

6 Leffler DA, Dennis M, Hyett B, Kelly E, Schuppan D, Kelly CP: Etiologies and predictors of diagnosis in nonresponsive celiac disease. Clin Gastroenterol Hepatol 2007;5:445–450.

7 Collin P, Thorell L, Kaukinen K, Mäki M: The safe threshold for gluten contamination in gluten-free products. Can trace amounts be accepted in the treatment of coeliac disease? Aliment Pharmacol Ther 2004;19:1277–1283.

8 Wild D, Robins GG, Burley VJ, Howdle PD: Evidence of high sugar intake, and low fibre and mineral intake, in the gluten-free diet. Aliment Pharmacol Ther 2010;32:573–581.

9 Aziz I, Evans KE, Papageorgiou V, Sanders DS: Are patients with coeliac disease seeking alternative therapies to a gluten-free diet? J Gastrointest Liver Dis 2011;20:27–31.

10 Ukkola A, Mäki M, Kurppa K, Collin P, Huhtala H, Kekkonen L, Kaukinen K: Patients' experiences and perceptions of living with coeliac disease – implications for optimizing care. J Gastrointest Liver Dis 2012;21:17–22.

11 van Overbeek FM, Uil-Dieterman IG, Mol IW, Köhler-Brands L, Heymans HS, Mulder CJ: The daily gluten intake in relatives of patients with coeliac disease compared with that of the general Dutch population. Eur J Gastroenterol Hepatol 1997;9:1097–1099.

12 Shan L, Molberg Ø, Parrot I, Hausch F, Filiz F, Gray GM, Sollid LM, Khosla C: Structural basis for gluten intolerance in celiac sprue. Science 2002;297:2275–2279.

13 Abadie V, Sollid LM, Barreiro LB, Jabri B: Integration of genetic and immunological insights into a model of celiac disease pathogenesis. Annu Rev Immunol 2011;29:493–525.

14 De Angelis M, Cassone A, Rizzello CG, Gagliardi F, Minervini F, Calasso M, Di Cagno R, Francavilla R, Gobbetti M: Mechanism of degradation of immunogenic gluten epitopes from *Triticum turgidum* L. var. *durum* by sourdough lactobacilli and fungal proteases. Appl Environ Microbiol 2010;76:508–518.

15 Di Cagno R, Barbato M, Di Camillo C, Rizzello CG, De Angelis M, Giuliani G, De Vincenzi M, Gobbetti M, Cucchiara S: Gluten-free sourdough wheat baked goods appear safe for young celiac patients: a pilot study. J Pediatr Gastroenterol Nutr 2010;51:777–783.

16 Greco L, Gobbetti M, Auricchio R, Di Mase R, Landolfo F, Paparo F, Di Cagno R, De Angelis M, Rizzello CG, Cassone A, Terrone G, Timpone L, D'Aniello M, Maglio M, Troncone R, Auricchio S: Safety for patients with celiac disease of baked goods made of wheat flour hydrolyzed during food processing. Clin Gastroenterol Hepatol 2011;9:24–29.

17 Kaukinen K, Lindfors K, Mäki M: Advances in the treatment of coeliac disease: an immunopathogenic perspective. Nat Rev Gastroenterol Hepatol 2014;11:36–44.

18 Bethune MT, Strop P, Tang Y, Sollid LM, Khosla C: Heterologous expression, purification, refolding, and structural-functional characterization of EP-B2, a self-activating barley cysteine endoprotease. Chem Biol 2006;13:637–647.

19 Siegel M, Bethune MT, Gass J, Ehren J, Xia J, Johannsen A, Stuge TB, Gray GM, Lee PP, Khosla C: Rational design of combination enzyme therapy for celiac sprue. Chem Biol 2006;13:649–658.

20 Stepniak D, Spaenij-Dekking L, Mitea C, Moester M, de Ru A, Baak-Pablo R, van Veelen P, Edens L, Koning F: Highly efficient gluten degradation with a newly identified prolyl endoprotease: implications for celiac disease. Am J Physiol Gastrointest Liver Physiol 2006;291:G621–G629.

21 Matysiak-Budnik T, Candahl C, Collier C, Dugave C, Namane A, Vidal-Martinez, Cerf-Bensussan N, Heyman M: Limited efficiency of prolyl-endopeptidase in the detoxification of gliadin peptides in celiac disease. Gastroenterology 2005;129:786–796.

22 Gass J, Vora H, Bethune MT, Gray GM, Khosla CJ: Effect of barley endoprotease EP-B2 on gluten digestion in the intact rat. Pharmacol Exp Ther 2006;318:1178–1186.

23 Gass J, Bethune MT, Siegel M, Spencer A, Khosla C: Combination enzyme therapy for gastric digestion of dietary gluten in patients with celiac sprue. Gastroenterology 2007;133:472–480.

24 Bethune MT, Ribka E, Khosla C, Sestak K: Transepithelial transport and enzymatic detoxification of gluten in gluten-sensitive rhesus macaques. PLoS One 2008;3:e1857.

25 Mitea C, Havenaar R, Drijfhout JW, Edens L, Dekking L, Koning F: Efficient degradation of gluten by a prolyl endoprotease in a gastrointestinal model: implications for coeliac disease. Gut 2008;57:25–32.

26 Stenman SM, Venäläinen JI, Lindfors K, Auriola S, Mauriala T, Kaukovirta-Norja A, Jantunen A, Laurila K, Qiao SW, Sollid LM, Männisto PT, Kaukinen K, Mäki M: Enzymatic detoxification of gluten by germinating wheat proteases: implications for new treatment of celiac disease. Ann Med 2009;41:390–400.

27 Stenman SM, Lindfors K, Venäläinen JI, Hautala A, Männistö PT, Garcia-Horsman JA, Kaukovirta-Norja A, Auriola S, Mauriala T, Mäki M, Kaukinen K: Degradation of coeliac disease-inducing rye secalin by germinating cereal enzymes: diminishing toxic effects in intestinal epithelial cells. Clin Exp Immunol 2010;161:242–249.

28 Toft-Hansen H, Rasmussen KS, Staal A, Roggen EL, Sollid LM, Lillevang ST, Barington T, Husby S: Treatment of both native and deamidated gluten peptides with an endo-peptidase from *Aspergillus niger* prevents stimulation of gut-derived gluten-reactive T cells from either children or adults with celiac disease. Clin Immunol 2014;153:323–331.

29 Pyle GG, Paaso B, Anderson BE, Allen DD, Marti T, Li Q, Siegel M, Khosla C, Gray GM: Effect of pretreatment of food gluten with prolyl endopeptidase on gluten-induced malabsorption in celiac sprue. Clin Gastroenterol Hepatol 2005;3:687–694.

30 Tye-Din JA, Anderson RP, Ffrench RA, Brown GJ, Hodsman P, Siegel M, Botwick W, Shreeniwas R: The effects of ALV003 pre-digestion of gluten on immune response and symptoms in celiac disease in vivo. Clin Immunol 2010;134:289–295.

31 Tack GJ, van de Water JM, Bruins MJ, Kooy-Winkelaar EM, van Bergen J, Bonnet P, Vreugdenhil AC, Korponay-Szabo I, Edens L, von Blomberg BM, Schreurs MW, Mulder CJ, Koning F: Consumption of gluten with gluten-degrading enzyme by celiac patients: a pilot-study. World J Gastroenterol 2013;19:5837–5847.

32 Lähdeaho ML, Kaukinen K, Laurila K, Vuotikka P, Koivurova OP, Kärjä-Lahdensuu T, Marcantonio A, Adelman DC, Mäki M: Glutenase ALV003 attenuates gluten-induced mucosal injury in patients with celiac disease. Gastroenterology 2014;146:1649–1658.

33 Siegel M, Garber ME, Spencer AG, Botwick W, Kumar P, Williams RN, Kozuka K, Shreeniwas R, Pratha V, Adelman DC: Safety, tolerability, and activity of ALV003: results from two phase 1 single, escalating-dose clinical trials. Dig Dis Sci 2012;57:440–450.

Dig Dis 2015;33:282–289
DOI: 10.1159/000369511

Vaccination and Other Antigen-Specific Immunomodulatory Strategies in Celiac Disease

Mauro Rossi

Institute of Food Sciences, CNR, Avellino, Italy

Key Words

Celiac disease · Epitope masking · Gliadin · Immunomodulation · Regulatory T cells

Abstract

Background: Celiac disease (CD) results from an alteration in the oral tolerance to dietary gluten. The response to gluten is normally tightly regulated and involves the secretion of TGF-β and IL-10 from different subtypes of regulatory T cells (Tregs). Interestingly, in addition to proinflammatory cytokines, the inflamed CD mucosa also contains high levels of T cell-derived IL-10 compared with treated CD patients or normal donors. Furthermore, most studies describe an increase in the number of Foxp3+ Tregs in the small intestinal mucosa in CD patients compared to controls. This paradoxical condition suggests that regulatory mechanisms might operate to counterbalance the abnormal gliadin-triggered immune activation in untreated mucosa. Indeed, addition of exogenous IL-10 to mucosal cultures from treated CD patients can suppress gliadin-induced T cell activation. Considering the central role of adaptive immunity in CD, the development of strategies to stimulate these mechanisms is a primary goal of efforts to restore gluten tolerance. ***Key Messages:*** Different immunomodulatory strategies have been explored. NexVax2, a desensitizing vaccine that uses three dominant gluten peptides administered subcutaneously to induce a tolerogenic response in CD patients, is under development. Alternatively, the potential of substituted, cyclic or dimeric peptide analogues as blockers to prevent HLA from binding to the immunodominant gliadin epitopes has been demonstrated in vitro. In line with these results, we recently found that modified (transamidated) gliadins influenced the immune response in intestinal biopsy samples from CD patients with overt disease by drastically reducing the production of IFN-γ. Notably, in a mouse model, transamidated gliadins reverted the phenotype of the gliadin-inducible immune response from an inflammatory phenotype to an anti-inflammatory phenotype. ***Conclusions:*** Various approaches are currently under investigation to recover gluten tolerance based on the use of both modified and native antigen molecules. More specific studies are now required to test the efficacy of such strategies for preventing CD.

Introduction

Celiac disease (CD) is the most common food-sensitive enteropathy in humans. This condition is caused by the lack of immune tolerance (oral tolerance) to wheat gluten and the prolamin fractions of rye and barley.

KARGER 125

E-Mail karger@karger.com
www.karger.com/ddi

0257–2753/15/0332–0282$39.50/0

Dr. Mauro Rossi
Istituto di Scienze dell'Alimentazione
CNR, via Roma 64
IT–83100 Avellino (Italy)
E-Mail mrossi@isa.cnr.it

The underlying pathogenic process of CD can be reverted, and in most CD patients on a gluten-free diet (GFD), the clinical symptoms disappear together with normalization of the levels of autoimmune antibodies in the serum and the recovery of the mucosal architecture. Genetic factors play a central role in CD. Virtually all CD patients express MHC class II HLA-DQ2 or HLA-DQ8 molecules [1, 2], which accounts for the main pathogenic mechanism leading to CD. An adaptive immune response to gluten-derived peptides driven by activated CD4+ T cells takes place in the lamina propria (LP) of the small intestinal mucosa [3]. Furthermore, in vitro studies indicate that gluten also has other biological effects and directly influences innate immunity in CD.

Because the protein responsible for CD is known, CD appears to be a suitable model for establishing a therapeutic immunomodulatory protocol that selectively targets T cells to reestablish tolerance. Moreover, an approach for inducing tolerance to this antigen in susceptible individuals could provide an alternative to the only treatment for CD that is currently available, which is the dietary exclusion of grains containing gluten (i.e. wheat, rye, barley, triticale, couscous, spelt, and kamut) [4]. However, significant changes are needed to begin and maintain a GFD, and they can have a major impact on daily life. In addition, gluten cross-contamination, high costs, the restricted availability of gluten-free food alternatives, low palatability and cultural practices make a GFD difficult to sustain. Therefore, there is an increasing interest in the development of new strategies for CD patients [5]. Some of these strategies include the production of engineered grains, the degradation of immunodominant gliadin peptides by microbial peptidases and decreasing the permeability of the intestine to gluten by blocking of the zonulin receptor [6]. Other approaches include immunomodulatory strategies, which are the subject of this review. Although some of these strategies are already in phase 1 or 2 clinical trials, others are extremely challenging and will require further work to achieve the ambitious goal of CD prevention.

The Complex Picture of T-Cell Adaptive Immunity in CD

More than 99% of people with CD express the MHC class II molecules HLA-DQ2.5, HLA-DQ8 and HLA-DQ2.2, with HLA-DQ2.5 being the major genetic risk factor present in 90% of patients [7]. This association indicates the central role of the adaptive arm of mucosal immunity in the pathogenesis of CD. In particular, CD4+ T cell activation in the LP triggered by specific gluten peptides bound to DQ2 and DQ8 heterodimers on the surface of APCs is typically found in CD [8].

The mucosal intestinal lesions are believed to be mainly induced by the production of IFN-γ by gluten-specific Th1 T cells [3]. However, in addition to gluten-specific CD4+ LP T cells, CD8+ intraepithelial lymphocytes (IELs) also contribute to this massive Th1 response [9]. Furthermore, a pathogenic role for proinflammatory IL-17A, which is mainly secreted by gluten-specific Th17 T cells, has been hypothesized in CD, but the experimental evidence remains contradictory [10].

It is now evident that the detrimental cross talk between the LP and IELs governs the events that lead to the mucosal damage. Specifically, activated monocyte-derived CD11c+ dendritic cells (DCs) are preferentially involved in the stimulation of gluten-reactive CD4+ T cells in LP [11], thus generating the proinflammatory milieu that might also be responsible for the increased number of CD8+ IELs in active CD [12]. On the other hand, in vitro evidence indicates that gluten has an innate stimulatory effect: non-HLA-restricted gliadin peptides can directly stimulate epithelial cells, macrophages, and DCs to secrete IL-15, which in turn may recruit and activate cytotoxic IELs, leading to enhanced epithelial apoptosis and, consequently, villus atrophy [13]. Furthermore, recent data indicate that another wheat component, the amylase trypsin inhibitors, is also involved in the activation of innate immunity via engagement of Toll-like receptor 4 [14].

The interplay between epithelial and LP compartments in CD also involves IL-21, which is produced by LP CD4+ T cells that might amplify and stabilize the induced Th1 cell phenotype [15]. Finally, IL-15 might also act in concert with retinoic acid, a derivative of vitamin A produced by a subset of intestinal DCs and enterocytes. Together, IL-15 and retinoic acid inhibit the differentiation of regulatory T cells (Tregs) and, accordingly, stimulate inflammatory Th1 CD4+ T cells [16].

The toxicity of gluten in CD is also a consequence of its biochemical properties. Specifically, both components of gluten, the gliadins and the glutenins, are characterized by a high content of glutamine and proline residues. To date, most of the identified T-cell gliadin and glutenin epitopes have been identified after deamidation catalyzed by tissue transglutaminase (tTG), which resulted in specific glutamine residues being converted to glutamic acid [17]. The molecular basis of deamidation dependence can differ, depending on which HLA molecule is involved:

Table 1. Subtypes of CD4+ Tregs and their gluten specificity

Types of CD4+ Tregs	Presence in CD	Gluten specificity
Tr1 (IL-10 dependent, Foxp3–)	+	+
iCD25+Foxp3+	+	+
nCD25+Foxp3+	+	–
Th3 (TGF-β dependent, Foxp3–LAP+)	n.d.	n.d.

n.d. = Not determined.

DQ8-restricted gluten peptides can require deamidation at the P1 and/or P9 positions [18, 19]; DQ2-restricted gluten determinants are frequently dependent on deamidation of a single glutamine at P4 or P6 for optimal T cell reactivity [20, 21]. In both cases, in vitro studies have clearly shown that the negative charges introduced by this deamidation process greatly increase the binding affinity of gluten peptides to DQ2 [20, 22, 23] and DQ8 [24] molecules. The presence of proline protects gliadins and glutenins against digestive proteolysis and directs the tTG-mediated deamidation of glutamines [25]. Interestingly, some DQ2-restricted gliadin peptides are part of a single immunoactive 33-mer gliadin peptide that has been found to be resistant to digestion by gastric and pancreatic enzymes [26]. An updated list of gluten motifs recognized by the intestinal T cells of CD patients encompasses 15 DQ2.5- and 5 DQ8-restricted epitopes, respectively (http://www.isscd.net/EpitopeNomenclature.htm). Therefore, a relatively large number of gluten epitopes have been implicated in the development of CD.

The Occurrence of T-Cell Regulatory Pathways in CD

In recent years, a more complex picture of the ongoing interplay between cytokines in the mucosa of CD patients has emerged, supported by findings of high levels of inhibitory cytokines (IL-10 and TGF-β) produced by intestinal T cells from patients with active CD [27, 28]. Furthermore, other studies have unexpectedly shown that the number of regulatory Foxp3+ T cells (Tregs) is increased in the LP of patients with active CD [29, 30], and this phenomenon could be induced in situ by gliadin [31] (table 1). These findings argue against the hypothesis that a defect in the recruitment or in the de novo generation of intestinal Tregs is involved in the pathogenesis of CD. The presence of this apparently paradoxical milieu of both proinflammatory and suppressive cytokines also suggests that regulatory mechanisms might operate to counterbalance the abnormal immune activation in active CD.

Interestingly, both in vitro proliferation and IFN-γ secretion by effector CD4+ T cells in the LP were not inhibited by autologous or even control peripheral Tregs in active CD, whereas the suppressive effect of autologous Tregs in treated patients with normal histology and in controls was comparable, suggesting that the defect was not primary but secondary to the inflammatory process [32]. In agreement with these findings, LP Tregs isolated from active CD patients have been found to be functional [31]. Notably, exogenous IL-15 impaired the suppressive activity of Tregs [31] and, in active CD, IL-15 was found to be involved in the downregulation of TGF-β signaling despite strong TGF-β expression in the LP [33]. The ability of TGF-β to maintain the suppressor function of and support Foxp3 expression in Tregs [34] might explain how IL-15 impairs the suppressive activity of Tregs in CD. Furthermore, IL-15 positively regulates IL-21 production in the mucosa of CD patients [35]. In addition to its other activities, IL-21 markedly enhances the proliferation of effector CD4+ T cells and counteracts the suppressive effects of Tregs on these cells without directly affecting the survival of the Tregs [36]. Therefore, therapies that aim to neutralize IL-15 might not only decrease bystander T cell activation but also recover the suppressor function of Tregs. New therapeutic strategies might also be based on immune modulation by IL-10 in view of the findings that exogenous IL-10 suppresses the gliadin-driven IFN-γ response in vitro in intestinal biopsies from treated CD patients [37]. This result also indicates that the high levels of IL-10 normally found in active CD represent a compensatory anti-inflammatory pathway that is not sufficient to suppress the overwhelming Th1-mediated response.

Induction of Gluten Tolerance by Antigen Manipulation

The strong genetic association between specific HLA-DQ alleles and CD is further sustained by the notion that the efficiency of the presentation of the gluten peptides to CD4+ T cells influences the risk of disease development. HLA-DQ2.5 homozygous individuals have a 5-fold higher risk of developing CD than HLA-DQ2.5 heterozygous individuals [38]. The gene-dose effect correlates with findings demonstrating that the number of HLA-DQ2.5

molecules on the surface of the APCs determines the magnitude of the CD4+ T cell response. HLA-DQ2.5 homozygous individuals induce a very strong proliferative T cell response and IFN-γ production in comparison with heterozygous individuals [39]. Taken together, epidemiological and pathogenic data underscore gluten-specific CD4+ T cells as the main immunological target for strategies aiming at restore oral tolerance to gluten in CD.

One promising modulatory methodology is represented by blocking the peptide-binding site of DQ2/8. A systematic approach to the discovery of antagonist peptides was initially conducted by Anderson et al. [40] using the deamidated α/β-gliadin peptide (p57-73 QE65), which harbors two overlapping dominant DQ2-restricted gliadin T cell epitopes (DQ2-α-I and -II) in CD. T cells specific for p57-73 QE65 were present in the blood after an in vivo gluten challenge in CD patients and were analyzed by ELISPOT assay. The authors found that substitutions that conferred antagonistic properties were particularly abundant in three positions and were predicted to have the following roles: anchors for HLA-DQ2 (65E); a TCR contact (64P); a TCR contact for DQ2-α-I, and an anchor between HLA-DQ2 and DQ-α-II (67P). The most potent combined substitutions resulted in 64P→W with 65E→I/T and 64P→W with 67P→I, which produced peptides that were pure antagonists of p57-73 QE65-induced IFN-γ secretion. Notably, the altered versions of the p57-73 QE65 peptide had antagonist activity but lacked IFN-γ stimulatory activity and retained most of the IL-10 stimulatory activity of the parent molecule, making these peptides useful for therapeutic methodologies.

A similar strategy using cyclic and dimeric peptide analogues that can act as MHC blockers has been explored [41]. Internally bridged cyclic peptides, but not disulphide-bridged peptides, containing the DQ2-αI gliadin epitope were found to be effective inhibitors of gliadin peptide-specific T cell proliferation in vitro. Similarly, dimeric peptides were produced with a 20-mer gluten peptide deduced from the immunodominant 33-mer peptide still containing the structural determinants that are important for DQ2 binding [42]. Analogous to the findings with cyclic peptides, dimers with amide crosslinkers, but not with cysteine-maleimide linkers, did not have a stimulatory effect and were able to efficiently inhibit antigen presentation in a dose-dependent manner. To date, these peptides represent the first prototypical examples of pharmacologically relevant DQ2 blockers for the treatment of CD.

By following the same strategy of interfering with peptide antigen presentation, other studies have focused on producing small single-chain MHC mimetics, designated as recombinant TCR ligands (RTLs), that would retain the signaling characteristics of the MHC class II heterodimer [43]. The potential of these molecules has been explored for use in patients suffering from multiple sclerosis [44]. A recombinant HLA-DQ2.5 RTL was produced, and the inhibitory potential of this RTL bearing a covalently tethered α-II gliadin peptide (RTL802) was tested on peptide-specific intestinal T clones. RTL802 blocked proliferation of the α-II peptide-specific clone TCC364.1.0.14 but not of clones recognizing other gliadin peptides. TCC364.1.0.14 produced a wide range of cytokines following gliadin stimulation, including IL-2, IL-5, IL-6, IL-10, IL-17, IFN-γ and TNF-α. Interestingly, RTL802 inhibited all of the secreted cytokines significantly, with the most dramatic reduction observed for IL-2, IL-5 and TNF-α. This finding was in agreement with previous studies showing that RTL therapy induces Ag-specific cytokine changes in T cell lines and clones isolated from both humans and rodents.

Nevertheless, treatment should also consider the vast heterogeneity of gluten epitopes and gluten-reactive T cells involved in CD. To address this issue, we applied an innovative enzyme methodology and tested the possibility of introducing functional modifications in whole gliadin. The effects were analyzed in different biological systems. First, we showed that enzymatic transamidation of whole gliadin was effective at inhibiting IFN-γ secretion by intestinal TCLs from CD patients [45]. In silico analysis of a prototypic dominant gliadin peptide, p56-68, suggested that this occurs because binding of the cognate transamidated gliadin peptide to the DQ2 molecule is strongly reduced, even if it is not completely abolished [45]. Furthermore, in DQ8 transgenic mice, the enzymatic modification of whole gliadin was associated with an alteration of the gliadin-inducible IL-10/IFN-γ ratio, indicative of reversal of the phenotype from inflammatory to anti-inflammatory [46]. Therefore, we speculated that the transamidation of dominant peptides might favor HLA binding of low-affinity, subdominant or cryptic, gliadin determinants with dramatic consequences for the immune outcome. This hypothesis appears to be in line with another study showing that masking B-cell epitopes by coupling carbohydrates to the protein surface made the protein hypoallergenic but still able to elicit elevated IgG titers following intradermal immunization [47]. Importantly, if primed by immunization, T cell populations specific for subdominant/cryptic epitopes were not diluted out by the preferential outgrowth of T cells directed to the dominant epitopes [48]. It is also known that im-

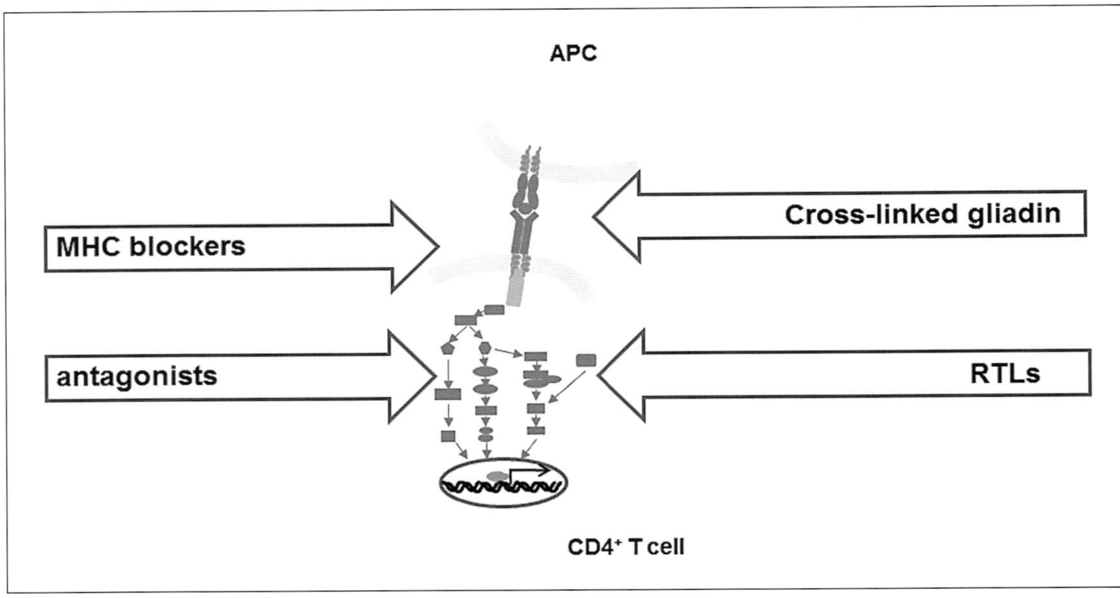

Fig. 1. Schematic view of the mechanisms involved in the re-induction of tolerance by antigen manipulation. They all include T cell-intrinsic pathways: signaling alteration with partial T cell activation (antagonists and RTLs), competition for TCR engagement (MHC blockers) or epitope shift (cross-linked gliadin).

munodominance hierarchies limit the diversity of the elicited T-cell responses. Accordingly, the selective delivery of subdominant/cryptic gliadin epitopes can rescue expansion of less favored CD4+ T cells. This might result in a more balanced T cell repertoire that is stably maintained with positive consequences for the restoration of gluten tolerance. In figure 1, the possible mechanisms involved in the re-induction of tolerance by antigen manipulation are summarized.

Induction of Gluten Tolerance by Vaccination

CD can be seen as a condition in which a breakdown occurs in the immunoregulatory mechanisms that normally guarantee unresponsiveness to dietary proteins (fig. 2). Unfortunately, the classical oral tolerance protocol of native antigen feeding is not applicable in CD because the local administration of gliadin peptides carries the risk of exacerbating the disease. One possibility that has been recently explored as an alternative to the use of modified gliadin is the oral delivery of gliadin by genetically modified *Lactococcus lactis* (LL), a noncolonizing, nonpathogenic bacterium [49]. Oral administration of LL engineered to secrete a deamidated DQ8 gliadin epitope induced suppression of the LP and systemic DQ8-restricted T-cell responses in NOD ABo DQ8 transgenic mice together with downregulation of IL-12 secretion and systemic production of IL-10 and TGF-β. Furthermore, the reported cytokine pattern was also associated with the induction of Foxp3+ Tregs in the LP. Therefore, the data confirmed that the induction of tolerance by LL is related to the intrinsic ability of this strain to alter DC function, which in the presence of simultaneous exposure to a DC-presented Ag might result in the generation of Ag-specific Tregs.

Other studies have addressed this issue by exploiting the tolerogenic ability of other mucosae, such as the nasal mucosa. The existence of a connection between the nasal and gut mucosal systems has been documented [50, 51]. Thus, we performed preliminary tests using this strategy and found a significant suppression of the systemic proliferative response in DQ8 transgenic mice receiving high nasally administered doses of recombinant α-gliadin and mice that were immunized with native gliadin [52]. Therefore, our data indicated that the DQ8-restricted epitopes contained in wheat gliadin were downregulated by the administration of a single recombinant molecule through the nasal route. Interestingly, this treatment was specifically associated with decreased transcript levels of IFN-γ, whereas IL-10 was not influenced, suggesting the lack of a substantial role of Tregs. This result is in accor-

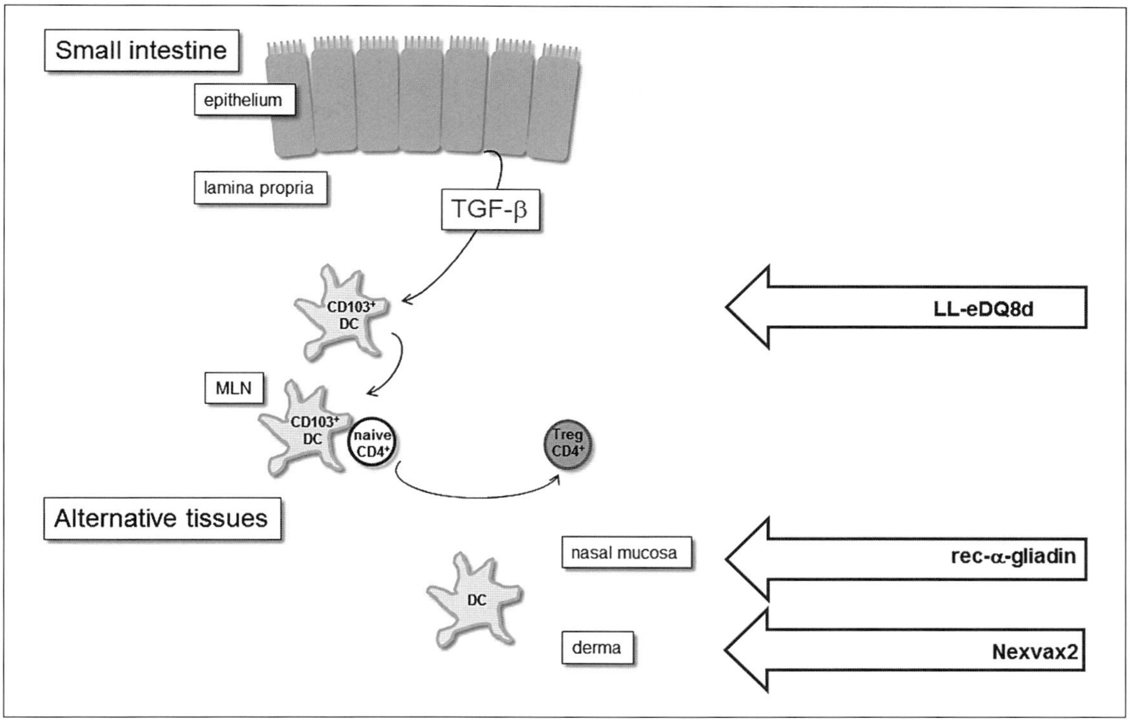

Fig. 2. Schematic view of the exogenous pathway involved in peripheral tolerance. This mechanism is exploited by the different prophylactic approaches under investigation for CD.

dance with data reported in the literature indicating that the administration of high doses of Ag essentially promotes anergy or deletion of effector T cells [53].

However, whether these strategies can efficiently downregulate the inflammatory intestinal response in CD remains to be demonstrated. Although numerous in vivo studies have been performed, only a limited number of experimental approaches have been tested in clinical trials and, in particular, only one clinical trial has been conducted with a gliadin-based immunotherapy. This study, which included a safety assessment and evaluation of an inducible immune response by intradermal injections of Nexvax2 in treated CD patients, has recently been completed (ClinicalTrials.gov Identifier: NCT00879749). The trial design originated from a comprehensive project in which customized libraries were thoroughly screened with PBMCs from 226 HLA-DQ2+ adult CD patients isolated after gluten challenge [54]. These libraries included more than 16,000 peptides containing unique 12-amino acid sequences from all toxic prolamin fractions of wheat, barley, and rye. Specifically, the IFN-γ ELISpot responses revealed that the immunotoxicity of gluten is specifically related to three highly immunogenic peptides containing the DQ2-α-I/II, DQ2-ω-I/II, and DQ2-Hor-I epitopes. These peptides represent the constituents of Nexvax2. Similar to nasal tolerization, the rationale behind the choice of intradermal administration is the requirement for antigen presentation by tolerogenic DCs that can promote gliadin-specific Tregs that express gut homing receptors, thus restoring intestinal tolerance in CD patients. Finally, it is worth noting that the findings demonstrate a strict hierarchy of stimulatory gliadin peptides. This insight may lead to the development of novel immunomodulatory strategies, particularly those involving the design of additional functional antagonists.

Conclusions

Evidence suggests that intestinal Tregs are induced by gluten in CD; however, the function of these Tregs is limited by cytokines such as IL-15 and IL-21, which are produced under inflammatory conditions. Accordingly, antigen-specific HLA-restricted strategies aimed at reverting the Th1 phenotype might reconstitute the suppressor function of Tregs. A number of different approaches are currently under investigation to address this issue. The use of both modified and native antigen molecules is currently being explored. Despite the ongoing in vivo studies and a first clinical trial, the effectiveness of these molecules for preventing CD remains to be established.

Disclosure Statement

The author has no conflicts of interest to declare.

References

1 Bevan S, Popat S, Braegger CP, Busch A, O'Donoghue D, Falth-Magnusson K, Ferguson A, Godkin A, Hogberg L, Holmes G, Hosie KB, Howdle PD, Jenkins H, Jewell D, Johnston S, Kennedy NP, Kerr G, Kumar P, Logan RF, Love AH, Marsh M, Mulder CJ, Sjoberg K, Stenhammer L, Walker-Smith J, Marossy AM, Houlston RS: Contribution of the MHC region to the familial risk of coeliac disease. J Med Genet 1999;36:687–690.

2 Hogberg L, Falth-Magnusson K, Grodzinsky E, Stenhammar L: Familial prevalence of celiac disease: a twenty-year follow-up study. Scand J Gastroenterol 2003;38:61–65.

3 Nilsen EM, Jahnsen FL, Lundin KE, Johansen FE, Fausa O, Sollid LM, Jahnsen J, Scott H, Brandtzaeg P: Gluten induces an intestinal cytokine response strongly dominated by interferon gamma in patients with celiac disease. Gastroenterology 1998;115:551–563.

4 Fasano A, Catassi C: Current approaches to diagnosis and treatment of celiac disease: an evolving spectrum. Gastroenterology 2001; 120:636–645.

5 Tack GJ, Verbeek WH, Schreurs MW, Mulder CJ: The spectrum of celiac disease: epidemiology, clinical aspects and treatment. Nat Rev Gastroenterol Hepatol 2010;7:204–213.

6 Makharia GK: Current and emerging therapy for celiac disease. Front Med 2014;1:1–7.

7 Jabri B, Chen X, Sollid LM: How T cells taste gluten in celiac disease. Nat Struct Mol Biol 2014;21:429–431.

8 Sollid LM: Coeliac disease: dissecting a complex inflammatory disorder. Nat Rev Immunol 2002;2:647–655.

9 Forsberg G, Hernell O, Melgar S, Israelsson A, Hammarstrom S, Hammarstrom M-L: Paradoxical coexpression of proinflammatory and down-regulatory cytokines in intestinal T cells in childhood celiac disease. Gastroenterology 2002;123:667–678.

10 Fernandez S, Molina IJ, Romero P, et al: Characterization of gliadin-specific Th17 cells from the mucosa of celiac disease patients. Am J Gastroenterol 2011;106:528–538.

11 Ráki M, Tollefsen S, Molberg O, Lundin KEA, Sollid LM, Jahnsen FL: A unique dendritic cell subset accumulates in the celiac lesion and efficiently activates gluten-reactive T cells. Gastroenterology 2006;131:428–438.

12 Tjon JM, van Bergen J, Koning F: CD: how complicated can it get? Immunogenetics 2010;62:641–645.

13 Jabri B, Sollid LM: Tissue-mediated control of immunopathology in coeliac disease. Nat Rev Immunol 2009;9:858–870.

14 Junker Y, Zeissig S, Kim SJ, Barisani D, Wieser H, Leffler DA, Zevallos V, Libermann TA, Dillon S, Freitag TL, Kelly CP, Schuppan D: Wheat amylase trypsin inhibitors drive intestinal inflammation via Toll-like receptor 4. J Exp Med 2012;209:2395–2408.

15 Fina D, Sarra M, Caruso R, Del Vecchio Blanco G, Pallone F, MacDonald TT, Monteleone G: Interleukin-21 contributes to the mucosal T helper cell type1 response in celiac disease. Gut 2008;57:887–892.

16 DePaolo RW, Abadie V, Tang F, Fehlner-Peach H, Hall JA, Wang W, Marietta EV, Kasarda DD, Waldmann TA, Murray JA, Semrad C, Kupfer SS, Belkaid Y, Guandalini S, Jabri B: Coadjuvant effects of retinoic acid and IL-15 induce inflammatory immunity to dietary antigens. Nature 2011;471:220–224.

17 Molberg O, McAdam SN, Korner R, Quarsten H, Kristiansen C, Madsen L, Fugger L, Scott H, Noren O, Roepstorff P, Lundin KE, Sjostrom H, Sollid LM: Tissue transglutaminase selectively modifies gliadin peptides that are recognized by gut-derived T cells in celiac disease. Nat Med 1998;4:713–717.

18 Henderson KN, Tye-Din JA, Reid HH, Chen Z, Borg NA, Beissbarth T, Tatham A, Mannering SI, Purcell AW, Dudek NL, van Heel DA, McCluskey J, Rossjohn J, Anderson RP: A structural and immunological basis for the role of human leukocyte antigen DQ8 in celiac disease. Immunity 2007;27:23–34.

19 Tollefsen S, Arentz-Hansen H, Fleckenstein B, Molberg O, Ráki M, Kwok WW, Jung G, Lundin KE, Sollid LM: HLA-DQ2 and -DQ8 signatures of gluten T cell epitopes in celiac disease. J Clin Invest 2006;116:2226–2236.

20 Arentz-Hansen H, Corner R, Molberg O, Quarsten H, Vader W, Kooy YM, Lundin KE, Koning F, Roepstorff P, Sollid LM, McAdam SN: The intestinal T cell response to alpha-gliadin in adult celiac disease is focused on a single deamidated glutamine targeted by tissue transglutaminase. J Exp Med 2000;191: 603–612.

21 Petersen J, Montserrat V, Mujico JR, Loh KL, Beringer DX, van Lummel M, Thompson A, Mearin ML, Schweizer J, Kooy-Winkelaar Y, van Bergen J, Drijfhout JW, Kan W-T, La Gruta NL, Anderson RP, Reid HH, Koning F, Rossjohn J: T-cell receptor recognition of HLA-DQ2-gliadin complexes associated with celiac disease. Nat Struct Mol Biol 2014;21: 480–490.

22 Sjostrom H, Lundin KE, Molberg O, Corner R, McAdam SN, Anthonsen D, Quarsten H, Noren O, Roepstorff P, Thorsby E, Sollid LM: Identification of a gliadin T-cell epitope in coeliac disease: general importance of gliadin deamidation for intestinal T-cell recognition. Scand J Immunol 1998;48:111–115.

23 Vader W, Kooy Y, Van Veelen P, De Ru A, Harris D, Benckhuijsen W, Pena S, Mearin L, Drijfhout JW, Koning F: The gluten response in children with celiac disease is directed toward multiple gliadin and glutenin peptides. Gastroenterology 2002;122:1729–1737.

24 van de Wal Y, Kooy Y, van Veelen P, Pena S, Mearin L, Papadopoulos G, Koning F: Selective deamidation by tissue transglutaminase strongly enhances gliadin-specific T cell reactivity. J Immunol 1998;161:1585–1588.

25 Hausch F, Shan L, Santiago NA, Gray GM, Khosla C: Intestinal digestive resistance of immunodominant gliadin peptides. Am J Physiol Gastrointest Liver Physiol 2002; 283:G996–G1003.

26 Shan L, Molberg O, Parrot I, Hausch F, Filiz F, Gray GM, Sollid LM, Khosla C: Structural basis for gluten intolerance in celiac sprue. Science 2002;297:2275–2279.

27 Lahat N, Shapiro S, Karban A, Gerstein R, Kinarty A, Lerner A: Cytokine profile in coeliac disease Scand J Immunol 1999;49:441–446.

28 Benahmed M, Meresse B, Arnulf B, Barbe U, Mention JJ, Verkarre V, Allez M, Cellier C, Hermine O, Cerf-Bensussan N: Inhibition of TGF-beta signaling by IL-15: a new role for IL-15 in the loss of immune homeostasis in celiac disease. Gastroenterology 2007;132: 994–1008.

29 Vorobjova T, Uibo O, Heilman K Rägo T, Honkanen J, Vaarala O, Tillmann V, Ojakivi I, Uibo R: Increased FOXP3 expression in small-bowel mucosa of children with coeliac disease and type I diabetes mellitus. Scand J Gastroenterol 2009;44:422–430.

30 Tittanen M, Westerholm-ormio M, Verkasalo M, Savilahti E, Vaarala O: Infiltration of forkhead box P3- expression cells in small intestinal mucosa in coeliac disease but not in type 1 diabetes. Clin Exp Immunol 2008;152: 498–507.

31 Zanzi D, Stefanile R, Santagata S, Iaffaldano L, Iaquinto G, Giardullo N, Lania G, Vigliano I, Vera AR, Ferrara K, Auricchio S, Troncone R, Mazzarella G: IL-15 interferes with suppressive activity of intestinal regulatory T cells expanded in celiac disease. Am J Gastroenterol 2011;106:1308–1317.

32 Hmida NB, Ben Ahmed M, Moussa A, Rejeb MB, Said Y, Kourda N, Meresse B, Abdeladhim M, Louzir H, Cerf-Bensussan N: Impaired control of effector T cells by regulatory T cells: a clue to loss of oral tolerance and autoimmunity in celiac disease? Am J Gastroenterol 2012;107:604–611.

33 Benahmed M, Meresse B, Arnulf B, Barbe U, Mention JJ, Verkarre V, Allez M, Cellier C, Hermine O, Cerf-Bensussan N: Inhibition of TGF-β signaling by IL-15: a new role for IL-15 in the loss of immune homeostasis in celiac disease. Gastroenterology 2007;132:994–1008.

34 Marie JC, Letterio JJ, Gavin M, Rudensky AY: TGF-beta1 maintains suppressor function and Foxp3 expression in CD4+CD25+ regulatory T cells. J Exp Med 2005;201:1061–1067.

35 Sarra M, Cupi ML, Monteleone I, Franzè E, Ronchetti G, Di Sabatino A, Gentileschi P, Franceschilli L, Sileri P, Sica G, Del Vecchio Blanco G, Cretella M, Paoluzi OA, Corazza GR, Pallone F, Monteleone G: IL-15 also positively regulates IL-21 production in celiac disease mucosa. Mucosal Immunol 2013;6: 244–255.

36 Peluso I, Fantini MC, Fina D, Caruso R, Boirivant M, MacDonald TT, Pallone F, Monteleone G: IL-21 counteracts the regulatory T cell-mediated suppression of human CD4+ T lymphocytes. J Immunol 2007;178:732–739.

37 Salvati VM, Mazzarella G, Gianfrani C, Levings MK, Stefanile R, De Giulio B, Iaquinto G, Giardullo N, Auricchio S, Roncarolo MG, Troncone R: Recombinant human interleukin 10 suppresses gliadin dependent T cell activation in ex vivo cultured coeliac intestinal mucosa. Gut 2005;54:46–53.

38 Mearin ML, Biemond I, Pena AS, Polanco I, Vazquez C, Schreuder GT, de Vries RR, van Rood JJ: HLA-DR phenotypes in Spanish coeliac children: their contribution to the understanding of the genetics of the disease. Gut 1983;24:532–537.

39 Vader W, Stepniak D, Kooy Y, Mearin L, Thompson A, van Rood JJ, Spaenij L, Koning F: The HLA-DQ2 gene dose effect in celiac disease is directly related to the magnitude and breadth of gluten-specific T cell responses. Proc Natl Acad Sci USA 2003;100:12390–12395.

40 Anderson RP, van Heel DA, Tye-Din JA, Jewell DP, Hill AVS: Antagonists and non-toxic variants of the dominant wheat gliadin T cell epitope in coeliac disease. Gut 2006;55:485–491.

41 Xia J, Bergseng E, Fleckenstein B, Siegel M, Kim C-Y, Khosla C, Sollid LM: Cyclic and dimeric gluten peptide analogues inhibiting DQ2-mediated antigen presentation in celiac disease. Bioorg Med Chem 2007;15:6565–6573.

42 Xia J, Siegel M, Bergseng E, Sollid LM, Khosla C: Inhibition of HLA-DQ2 mediated antigen presentation by analogues of a high affinity 33-residue peptide from α2-gliadin. J Am Chem Soc 2006;128:1859–1867.

43 Huan J, Meza-Romero R, Mooney JL, Vandenbark AA, Offner H, Burrows GG: Single chain recombinant HLA-DQ2.5/peptide molecules block α2-gliadin-specific pathogenic CD4+ T cell proliferation and attenuate production of inflammatory cytokines: a potential therapy for celiac disease. Mucosal Immunol 2011;4:112–120.

44 Burrows GG, Chou YK, Wang C, Chang JW, Finn TP, Culbertson NE, Kim J, Bourdette DN, Lewinsohn DA, Lewinsohn DM, Ikeda M, Yoshioka T, Allen CN, Offner H, Vandenbark AA: Rudimentary TCR signaling triggers default IL-10 secretion by human Th1 cells. J Immunol 2001;167:4386–4395.

45 Gianfrani C, Siciliano RA, Facchiano AM, Camarca A, Mazzeo MF, Costantini S, Salvati VM, Maurano F, Mazzarella G, Iaquinto G, Bergamo P, Rossi M: Transamidation inhibits the intestinal immune response to gliadin in vitro. Gastroenterology 2007;133:780–789.

46 Lombardi E, Maurano F, Bergamo P, Bozzella G, Luongo D, Mazzarella G, Capobianco F, Rotondi Aufiero V, Iaquinto G, Rossi M: Selective inhibition of gliadin immune reactivity by transamidation of wheat flour with microbial transglutaminase, J Leukoc Biol 2013;93: 479–488.

47 Weinberger EE, Himly M, Myschik J, Hauser M, Altmann F, Isakovic A, Scheiblhofer S, Thalhamer J, Weiss R: Generation of hypoallergenic neoglycoconjugates for dendritic cell targeted vaccination: a novel tool for specific immunotherapy. J Control Release 2013;165: 101–109.

48 Aagaard CS, Hoang TT, Vingsbo-Lundberg C, Dietrich J, Andersen P: Quality and vaccine efficacy of CD4+ T cell responses directed to dominant and subdominant epitopes in ESAT-6 from *Mycobacterium tuberculosis*. J Immunol 2009;183:2659–2668.

49 Huibregtse IL, Marietta EV, Rashtak S, Koning F, Rottiers P, David CS, van Deventer SJ, Murray JA: Induction of antigen-specific tolerance by oral administration of *Lactococcus lactis* delivered immunodominant DQ8-restricted gliadin peptide in sensitized nonobese diabetic Abo Dq8 transgenic mice. J Immunol 2009;183:2390–2396.

50 Kiyono H, Fukuyama S: NALT- versus Peyer's-patch-mediated mucosal immunity. Nat Rev Immunol 2004;4:699–710.

51 Rossi M, Maurano F, Luongo D, Senger S, Siciliano RA, Marotti B, Mazzeo MF, Auricchio S, Troncone R: Immunotherapy with gliadin peptides in mice; in Cerf-Bensussan N, Brousse N, Caillat-Zucman S, Cellier C, Schmitz J (eds): Proceedings of 10th International Symposium on Coeliac Disease, Paris 2–5 June 2002. Montrouge, John Libbey Eurotext, 2003, pp 259–267.

52 Senger S, Luongo D, Maurano F, Mazzeo MF, Siciliano RA, Gianfrani C, David C, Troncone R, Auricchio S, Rossi M: Intranasal administration of a recombinant alpha-gliadin downregulates the immune response to wheat gliadin in DQ8 transgenic mice. Immunol Lett 2003;88:127–134.

53 Wolvers DA, Coenen-de Roo CJ, Mebius RE, van der Cammen MJ, Tirion F, Miltenburg AM, Kraal G: Intranasally induced immunological tolerance is determined by characteristics of the draining lymph nodes: studies with OVA and human cartilage GP-39. J Immunol 1999;162:1994–1998.

54 Tye-Din JA, Stewart JA, Dromey JA, Beissbarth T, van Heel DA, Tatham A, Henderson K, Mannering SI, Gianfrani C, Jewell DP, Hill AV, McCluskey J, Rossjohn J, Anderson RP: Comprehensive, quantitative mapping of T cell epitopes in gluten in celiac disease. Sci Transl Med 2010;2:41–51.

Dig Dis 2015;33:290–292
DOI: 10.1159/000375475

Falk Symposium Series

145. Henne-Bruns D, Buttenschön K, Fuchs M, Lohse AW, eds. Artificial Liver Support. Falk Symposium 145. 2005 ISBN 1-4020-3239-0
146. Blumberg RS, Gangl A, Manns MP, Tilg H, Zeitz M, eds. Gut–Liver Interactions: Basic and Clinical Concepts. Falk Symposium 146. 2005 ISBN 1-4020-4143-8
147. Jewell DP, Colombel JF, Peña AS, Tromm A, Warren BS, eds. Colitis: Diagnosis and Therapeutic Strategies. Falk Symposium 147. 2006 ISBN 1-4020-4315-5
148. Kruis W, Forbes A, Jauch KW, Kreis ME, Wexner SD, eds. Diverticular Disease: Emerging Evidence in a Common Condition. Falk Symposium 148. 2006 ISBN 1-4020-4317-1
149. van Cutsem E, Rustgi AK, Schmiegel W, Zeitz M, eds. Highlights in Gastrointestinal Oncology. Falk Symposium 149. 2006 ISBN 1-4020-5108-5
150. Galle PR, Gerken G, Schmidt WE, Wiedenmann B, eds. Disease Progression and Disease Prevention in Hepatology and Gastroenterology. Falk Symposium 150. 2006 ISBN 1-4020-5109-3
151. Fraser A, Gibson PR, Hibi T, Qian JM, Schölmerich J, eds. Emerging Issues in Inflammatory Bowel Disease. Falk Symposium 151. 2006 ISBN 978-1-4020-5701-4
152. Fockens P, Schulz H-J, Rösch T, Špičák J, eds. Endoscopy 2006 – Update and Live Demonstration. Falk Symposium 152. 2008 ISBN 978-1-4020-9147-6
153. Dignass A, Rachmilewitz D, Stange E-F, Weinstock JV, eds. Immunoregulation in Inflammatory Bowel Diseases – Current Understanding and Innovation. Falk Symposium 153. 2007 ISBN 978-1-4020-5888-2
154. Adler G, Fiocchi C, Lazebnik LB, Vorobiev GI, eds. Inflammatory Bowel Disease – Diagnostic and Therapeutic Strategies. Falk Symposium 154. 2007 ISBN 978-1-4020-6115-8
155. Keppler D, Beuers U, Leuschner U, Stiehl A, Trauner M, Paumgartner G, eds. Bile Acids: Biological Actions and Clinical Relevance. Falk Symposium 155. 2007 ISBN 978-1-4020-6251-3
156. Blum HE, Cox DW, Häussinger D, Jansen PLM, Kullak-Ublick GA, eds. Genetics in Liver Diseases. Falk Symposium 156. 2007 ISBN 978-1-4020-6393-0
157. Diehl AM, Hayashi N, Manns MP, Sauerbruch T, eds. Chronic Hepatitis: Metabolic, Cholestatic, Viral and Autoimmune. Falk Symposium 157. 2007 ISBN 978-1-4020-6522-4
158. Gasche G, Herrerías Gutiérrez JM, Gassull M, Monterio E, eds. Intestinal Inflammation and Colorectal Cancer. Falk Symposium 158. 2007 ISBN 978-1-4020-6825-6

KARGER 125

E-Mail karger@karger.com
www.karger.com/ddi

159. Tözün N, Mantzaris G, Dağlı, Schölmerich J, eds. IBD 2007 – Achievements in Research and Clinical Practice. Falk Symposium 159. 2008 ISBN 978-1-4020-6986-4

160. Ferkolj I, Gangl A, Galle PR, Vucelic B, eds. Pathogenesis and Clinical Practice in Gastroenterology. Falk Symposium 160. 2008 ISBN 978-1-4020-8766-0

161. Carey MC, Gabryelewicz A, Díte P, Keim V, Mössner J, eds. Future Perspectives in Gastroenterology. Falk Symposium 161. 2008 ISBN 978-1-4020-8832-2

162. Bosch J, Lammert F, Burroughs AK, Lebrec D, Sauerbruch T, eds. Liver Cirrhosis: From Pathophysiology to Disease Management. Falk Symposium 162. 2008 ISBN 978-1-4020-8655-7

163. Adler G, Fan DM, Jia JD, LaRusso NF, Owyang C, eds. Chronic Inflammation of Liver and Gut. Falk Symposium 163. 2008 ISBN 978-1-4020-9352-4

164. Tulassay Z, Dítě P, Krejs GJ, Schölmerich J, Schultz HJ, eds. Intestinal Disorders. Falk Symposium 164. 2009 ISBN 978-1-4020-9590-0

165. Keppler D, Beuers U, Stiehl A, Trauner M, eds. Bile Acid Biology and Therapeutic Actions. Falk Symposium 165. 2009 ISBN 978-1-4020-9643-3

165A. Lieberman DA, Malfertheiner P, Riemann JF, Spechler SJ, eds. Strategies of Cancer Prevention in Gastroenterology. Falk Workshop. 2009 ISBN 978-90-481-2628-6

166. Ell C, Ponchon T, Riemann JF, Sakai P, Yamamoto H, eds. GI Endoscopy – Standards and Innovations. Falk Symposium 166. 2009 ISBN 978-90-481-2748-1

167. Day CP, Galle PR, Lohse AW, Thorgeirsson SS, eds. Liver under Constant Attack – From Fat to Viruses. Falk Symposium 167. 2009 ISBN 978-90-481-2758-0

168. Rogler G, Gassul M, Levine A, López San Román A, eds. IBD in Different Age Groups. Falk Symposium 168. 2009 ISBN 978-3-8055-9273-4

169. Buhr HJ, Kharchenko NV, Siegmund B, Zacharash MP, Zeitz M, eds. Inflammation in the Intestinal Tract: Pathogenesis and Treatment. Falk Symposium 169. 2009 ISBN 978-3-8055-9282-6

170. Travis SPL, Spiller RC, Colombel JF, Holzer P, eds. IBD and IBS: Novel Mechanisms and Future Practice. Falk Symposium 170. 2009 ISBN 978-3-8055-9420-2

171. Day CP, Diehl AM, Lehnert H, Manns MP, Negro F, eds. Liver and Metabolic Syndrome. Falk Symposium 171. 2009 ISBN 978-3-8055-9446-2

171A. Gershwin ME, Lohse AW, Manns MP, Vergani D, eds. Immunology and Liver Disease. Falk Workshop. 2009 ISBN 978-3-8055-9446-2

172. Rogler G, Sandborn W, eds. The Keys to IBD 2010: Treatment, Diagnosis and Pathophysiology. Falk Symposium 172. 2010 ISBN 978-3-8055-9588-9

173. Dítě P, Krejs GJ, Malfertheiner P, Tulassay Z, eds. From Chronic Inflammation to Cancer. Falk Symposium 173. 2010 ISBN 978-3-8055-9653-4

174. Chen CW, Cheng J, Ginès P, Ouyang Q, Schölmerich J, eds. Gut and Liver. Falk Symposium 174. 2010 ISBN 978-3-8055-9672-5

175. Häussinger D, Beuers U, Stiehl A, Trauner M, eds. Bile Acids as Metabolic Integrators and Therapeutics. Falk Symposium 175. 2010 ISBN 978-3-8055-9804-0

176. Blum HE, Hunt RH, Schölmerich J, eds. Environment and Lifestyle – Effects on Disorders of the Digestive Tract. Falk Symposium 176. 2010 ISBN 978-3-8055-9809-5

WS Singer MV, Dooley S, McClain CJ, Zakhari S, eds. Liver and Pancreatic Diseases: Consequences of Chronic Alcoholic Consumption. Falk Workshop Freiburg. 2010 ISBN 978-3-8055-9732-6

WS Schlitt HJ, Benseler V, Hellerbrand C, Loss M, Weiss TS, Wiest R, eds. Liver and Immunology. Falk Workshop Regensburg. 2011 ISBN 978-3-8055-9845-3

177. Schulz HJ, Rösch T, Siersema PD, eds. Endoscopy Live Berlin 2011-Intestinal Disease Meeting. Falk Symposium 177. 2011 ISBN 978-3-8055-9874-3

178. Kruis W, Spiller RC, Papagigoriadis S, Engel A, Kreis ME, eds. Diverticular Disease: A Fresh Approach to a Neglected Disease. Falk Symposium 178. 2011 ISBN 978-3-8055-9878-8

179. D'Haens G, Dignass A, Vermeire S, eds. Revisiting IBD Management: Dogmas to Be Challenged. Falk Symposium 179. 2012 ISBN 978-3-318-02187-5

WS Tiegs G, Lohse AW, Thimme R, Trautwein C, eds. Inflammation and Cancer. Falk Workshop. 2012 ISBN 978-3-318-02185-1

WS Miehlke S, Munch A, eds. Microscopic Colitis – Creating Awareness for an Underestimated Disease. Falk Workshop Basel. 2012

181. Tilg H, Blumberg RS, Endres S, Kaser A, Manns MP, eds. Innate Immunity in Gastrointestinal Disorder: Basic and Therapeutic Concepts. Falk Symposium 181. 2012 ISBN 978-3-318-02210-0

182. Friess H, Schmid RM, Fried M, van de Velde CJH, eds. Carcinogenesis, Prevention and Treatment of Colorectal Cancer – State of the Art 2012. Falk Sympsium 182. 2012 ISBN 978-3-318-02213-1

183. Rogler C, Beglinger C, Colombel J-F, Michetti P, eds. Dealing with Our 'In-Vironment': New Aspects in IBD Pathogenesis and Therapy. Falk Symposium 183. 2012 ISBN 978-3-318-02258-2

184. Häussinger D, Beuers U, Trauner M, eds. XXII International Bile Acid Meeting – Hepatic and Extrahepatic Targets of Bile Acid Signaling. Falk Symposium 184. 2012

185. Ell C, Galle PR, Mössner J, Meyenberger C, Spechler SJ, Yamamoto H, eds. Interfaces and Controversies in Gastroenterology. Falk Symposium 185. 2013 ISBN 978-3-318-02384-8

186. Galle PR, Clavien P-A, Gores GJ, Protzer U, Schuchmann M, eds. Challenges of Liver Cirrhosis and Tumors: Prevent It, Treat It, Manage Consequences. Falk Symposium 186. 2013 ISBN 978-3-318-02384-8

187. Panés J, Ghosh S, Gomollón F, Louis E, eds. Overcoming Challenges in IBD Management. Falk Symposium 187. 2013 ISBN 978-3-318-02468-5

188. Stange EF, Dignass A, Fellermann K, Herrlinger K, eds. Inflammatory Bowel Diseases: Microbiota versus the Barrier. Falk Symposium 188. 2013 ISBN 978-3-318-02538-5

189. Straumann A, Schoepfer A, Simon H-U, eds. Eosinophilic Esophagitis: A Novel Chronic Inflammatory Disease of the GI Tract. Falk Symposium 189. 2013

WS Krejs GJ, Eherer AJ, Pointner R, eds. GERD: Gastroesophageal Reflux Disease. Falk Workshop Graz. 2013 ISBN 978-3-318-02594-1

190. Levine A, Forbes A, Probert C, eds. Challenges in the Care of IBD in Patients of All Ages. Falk Symposium 190. 2013 ISBN 978-3-318-02662-7

191. Chapman RW, Adams DH, Beuers U, Day CP, Manns MP, eds. Liver Diseases in 2013: Advances in Pathogenesis and Treatment. Falk Symposium 191. 2013 ISBN 978-3-318-02665-8

192. Dignass A, Allez M, Danese S, Marteau P, eds. IBD 2014: Thinking Out of the Box. Falk Symposium 192. 2014 ISBN 978-3-318-02806-5

Author Index

E-Mail karger@karger.com
www.karger.com/ddi

Subject Index

E-Mail karger@karger.com
www.karger.com/ddi